60-AKW-230

**Health Reference Series**

*Volume Sixteen*

# Gastrointestinal DISEASES AND DISORDERS SOURCEBOOK

*Basic Information about Gastroesophageal Reflux Disease (Heartburn), Ulcers, Diverticulosis, Irritable Bowel Syndrome, Crohn's Disease, Ulcerative Colitis, Diarrhea, Constipation, Lactose Intolerance, Hemorrhoids, Hepatitis, Cirrhosis and Other Digestive Problems, Featuring Statistics, Descriptions of Symptoms, and Current Treatment Methods of Interest for Persons Living with Upper and Lower Gastrointestinal Maladies*

*Edited by*
**Linda M. Ross**

Omnigraphics, Inc.
Penobscot Building / Detroit, MI 48226

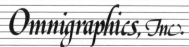

## BIBLIOGRAPHIC NOTE

This volume contains individual publications issued by the National Institutes of Health (NIH), its sister agencies, and subagencies, the Agency for Health Care Policy and Research (AHCPR) along with selected articles from FDA's *FDA Consumer.* Document numbers where applicable and specific source citations are listed on the first page of each publication.

In addition, this volume contains excerpts from copyrighted documents produced by Aspen Publishers, *Southern Medical Journal, The Harvard Health Letter, Patient Care, The Mayo Clinic Health Letter, Contemporary Gastroenterology,* American Liver Foundation, *Practical Gastroenterology,* and *The New York Times*. These are used by permission.

Edited by Linda M. Ross

Peter D. Dresser, Managing Editor, *Health Reference Series*
Karen Bellenir, Series Editor, *Health Reference Series*

RC
806
.G37
1996

Omnigraphics, Inc.

Matthew P. Barbour, *Production Manager*
Laurie Lanzen Harris, *Vice President, Editorial*
Peter E. Ruffner, *Vice President, Administration*
James A. Sellgren, *Vice President, Operations and Finance*
Jane J. Steele, *Vice President, Research*

Frederick G. Ruffner, Jr., *Publisher*

Copyright © 1996, Omnigraphics, Inc.

**Library of Congress Cataloging-in-Publication Data**

Gastrointestinal diseases & disorders sourcebook : basic information about diseases and disorders of the gastrointestinal system . . . / edited by Linda M. Ross.
p. cm. — (Health reference series ; v. 16)
Collection of articles previously published.
Includes bibliographical references and index.
ISBN 0-7808-0078-8 (librarybinding : alk. paper)
1. Gastrointestinal system—Diseases—Popular works. I. Ross, Linda M. (Linda Michelle) II. Series.
[DNLM: 1. Gastrointestinal Diseases—collected works. W1 HE506R v. 16 1996 / WI 140 G2586 1996]
RC806.G37 1996
616.3'3—dc20
DNLM/DLC
for Library of Congress 96-26198
CIP

∞

This book is printed on acid-free paper meeting the ANSI Z39.48 Standard. The infinity symbol that appears above indicates that the paper in this book meets that standard.

Printed in the United States.

34974329

# Contents

## *Part III: Stomach Problems*



## *Part IV: Intestinal and Anorectal Disorders*



## *Part V: Liver, Pancreatic, and Gallbladder Diseases and Disorders*

# Preface

## About This Book

The publications assembled in this book come from a variety of government and private sources and were selected on the basis of their helpfulness to the layperson searching for information on gastrointestinal problems. Some of the diseases and disorders discussed in this volume are rare and lay-oriented material is not available. Where this is the case, articles of a more technical nature are included with the intent that they may be helpful for the patient to discuss with his or her physician.

## How to Use This Book

*Part I: General Information* provides an overview of how the digestive system works and offers suggestions that will help maintain healthy digestion. It also includes statistical information on digestive diseases; debunks commonly held myths about gastrointestinal problems; addresses the harmful effects of smoking, medicines, laxatives, and antacids on the digestive system; and gives an extensive list of resources for the patient and professional.

*Part II: Esophageal Problems* discusses gastroesophageal reflux which includes such conditions as hiatal hernia and heartburn. Coverage in this section includes information on chronic pulmonary aspiration in children.

*Part III: Stomach Problems* focuses on ulcers. Information from the NIH on stomach and duodenal ulcers, peptic ulcer disease, and bleeding ulcers describes each condition and includes the most recent discoveries about the cause of ulcers. Courses of treatment are discussed.

*Part IV: Intestinal and Anorectal Disorders* plague most people at some point in time. This section gives concise information about diverticulosis and diverticulitis, Crohn's disease, ulcerative colitis, Inflammatory Bowel Disease (IBD), Irritable Bowel Syndrome (IBS), diarrhea, constipation, certain malabsorption problems, lactose intolerance, hemorrhoids, and small intestine maladies. Ostomies and transplants are among the treatments discussed.

*Part V: Liver, Pancreatic, and Gallbladder Diseases and Disorders* describes the symptoms and treatments for hepatitis, cirrhosis, primary sclerosing cholangitis, tarcolimus, pancreatitis, and gallstones. Liver function tests, liver transplants, and liver biopsy are discussed as well.

## Acknowledgments

The editor wishes to thank Aspen Publishers, *Southern Medical Journal, The Harvard Health Letter, Patient Care, The Mayo Clinic Health Letter, Contemporary Gastroenterology,* American Liver Foundation, *Practical Gastroenterology,* and *The New York Times* for their permission to include their material in this book. Thanks is due to Margaret Mary Missar for her tireless quest to find the information that made this volume possible. Thanks as well to Karen for her patience, Bruce for his scanning expertise, Jeanne for her negotiation skills, and Sarah for wading through the garbled parts.

## Note from the Editor

This book is part of Omnigraphics' *Health Reference Series.* The series provides basic information about a broad range of medical concerns. It is not intended to serve as a tool for diagnosing illness, in prescribing treatments, or as a substitute for the physician/patient relationship. All persons concerned about medical symptoms or the possibility of disease are encouraged to seek professional care from an appropriate health care provider.

# Part One

# General Information

## Chapter 1

# *Your Digestive System and How It Works*

The digestive system is a series of hollow organs joined in a long, twisting tube from the mouth to the anus (see figure). Inside this tube is a lining called the mucosa. In the mouth, stomach, and small intestine, the mucosa contains tiny glands that produce juices to help digest food.

There are also two solid digestive organs, the liver and the pancreas, which produce juices that reach the intestine through small tubes. In addition, parts of other organ systems (for instance, nerves and blood) play a major role in the digestive system.

## *Why Is Digestion Important?*

When we eat such things as bread, meat, and vegetables, they are not in a form that the body can use as nourishment. Our food and drink must be changed into smaller molecules of nutrients before they can be absorbed into the blood and carried to cells throughout the body. Digestion is the process by which food and drink are broken down into their smallest parts so that the body can use them to build and nourish cells and to provide energy.

## *How Is Food Digested?*

Digestion involves the mixing of food, its movement through the digestive tract, and chemical breakdown of the large molecules of food

NIH Pub. 95-2681.

into smaller molecules. Digestion begins in the mouth, when we chew and swallow, and is completed in the small intestine. The chemical process varies somewhat for different kinds of food.

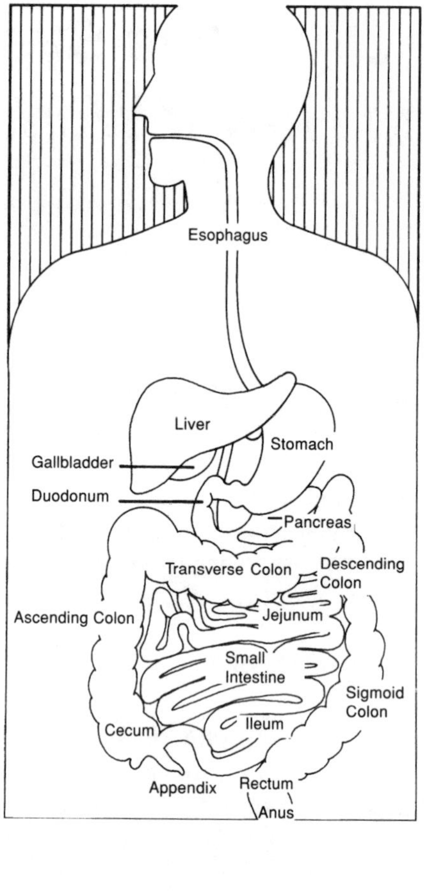


***Figure 1.1.*** *The Digestive System*

## *Movement of Food Through the System*

The large, hollow organs of the digestive system contain muscle that enables their walls to move. The movement of organ walls can propel food and liquid and also can mix the contents within each organ. Typical movement of the esophagus, stomach, and intestine is called peristalsis. The action of peristalsis looks like an ocean wave moving through the muscle. The muscle of the organ produces a narrowing and then propels the narrowed portion slowly down the length of the organ. These waves of narrowing push the food and fluid in front of them through each hollow organ.

The first major muscle movement occurs when food or liquid is swallowed. Although we are able to start swallowing by choice, once the swallow begins, it becomes involuntary and proceeds under the control of the nerves.

The esophagus is the organ into which the swallowed food is pushed. It connects the throat above with the stomach below. At the junction of the esophagus and stomach, there is a ring-like valve closing the passage between the two organs. However, as the food approaches the closed ring, the surrounding muscles relax and allow the food to pass.

The food then enters the stomach, which has three mechanical tasks to do. First, the stomach must store the swallowed food and liquid. This requires the muscle of the upper part of the stomach to relax and accept large volumes of swallowed material. The second job is to mix up the food, liquid, and digestive juice produced by the stomach. The lower part of the stomach mixes these materials by its muscle action. The third task of the stomach is to empty its contents slowly into the small intestine.

Several factors affect emptying of the stomach, including the nature of the food (mainly its fat and protein content) and the degree of muscle action of the emptying stomach and the next organ to receive the stomach contents (the small intestine). As the food is digested in the small intestine and dissolved into the juices from the pancreas, liver, and intestine, the contents of the intestine are mixed and pushed forward to allow further digestion.

Finally, all of the digested nutrients are absorbed through the intestinal walls. The waste products of this process include undigested parts of the food, known as fiber, and older cells that have been shed from the mucosa. These materials are propelled into the colon, where they remain, usually for a day or two, until the feces are expelled by a bowel movement.

### Production of Digestive Juices

Glands of the digestive system are crucial to the process of digestion. They produce both the juices that break down the food and the hormones that help to control the process.

The glands that act first are in the mouth: the salivary glands. Saliva produced by these glands contains an enzyme that begins to digest the starch from food into smaller molecules.

The next set of digestive glands is in the stomach lining. They produce stomach acid and an enzyme that digests protein. One of the unsolved puzzles of the digestive system is why the acid juice of the stomach does not dissolve the tissue of the stomach itself. In most people, the stomach mucosa is able to resist the juice, although food and other tissues of the body cannot.

After the stomach empties the food and its juice into the small intestine, the juices of two other digestive organs mix with the food to continue the process of digestion. One of these organs is the pancreas. It produces a juice that contains a wide array of enzymes to break down the carbohydrates, fat, and protein in our food. Other enzymes that are active in the process come from glands in the wall of the intestine or even a part of that wall.

The liver produces yet another digestive juice: bile. The bile is stored between meals in the gallbladder. At mealtime, it is squeezed out of the gallbladder into the bile ducts to reach the intestine and mix with the fat in our food. The bile acids dissolve the fat into the watery contents of the intestine, much like detergents that dissolve grease from a frying pan. After the fat is dissolved, it is digested by enzymes from the pancreas and the lining of the intestine.

### Absorption and Transport of Nutrients

Digested molecules of food, as well as water and minerals from the diet, are absorbed from the cavity of the upper small intestine. The absorbed materials cross the mucosa into the blood, mainly, and are carried off in the bloodstream to other parts of the body for storage or further chemical change. As noted above, this part of the process varies with different types of nutrients.

*Carbohydrates*—An average American adult eats about half a pound of carbohydrate each day. Some of our most common foods contain mostly carbohydrates. Examples are bread, potatoes, pastries, candy, rice, spaghetti, fruits, and vegetables. Many of these foods contain both starch, which can be digested, and fiber, which the body cannot digest.

The digestible carbohydrates are broken into simpler molecules by enzymes in the saliva, in juice produced by the pancreas, and in the lining of the small intestine. Starch is digested in two steps: First, an enzyme in the saliva and pancreatic juice breaks the starch into molecules called maltose; then an enzyme in the lining of the small intestine (maltase) splits the maltose into glucose molecules that can be absorbed into the blood. Glucose is carried through the bloodstream to the liver, where it is stored or used to provide energy for the work of the body.

Table sugar is another carbohydrate that must be digested to be useful. An enzyme in the lining of the small intestine digests table sugar into glucose and fructose, each of which can be absorbed from the intestinal cavity into the blood. Milk contains yet another type of sugar, lactose, which is changed into absorbable molecules by an enzyme called lactase, also found in the intestinal lining.

*Protein*—Foods such as meat, eggs, and beans consist of giant molecules of protein that must be digested by enzymes before they can be used to build and repair body tissues. An enzyme in the juice of the stomach starts the digestion of swallowed protein. Further digestion of the protein is completed in the small intestine. Here, several enzymes from the pancreatic juice and the lining of the intestine carry out the breakdown of huge protein molecules into small molecules called amino acids. These small molecules can be absorbed from the hollow of the small intestine into the blood and then be carried to all parts of the body to build the walls and other parts of cells.

*Fats*—Fat molecules are a rich source of energy for the body. The first step in digestion of a fat such as butter is to dissolve it into the watery content of the intestinal cavity. The bile acids produced by the liver act as natural detergents to dissolve fat in water and allow the enzymes to break the large fat molecules into smaller molecules, some of which are fatty acids and cholesterol. The bile acids combine with the fatty acids and cholesterol and help these molecules to move into the cells of the mucosa. In these cells the small molecules are formed back into large molecules, most of which pass into vessels (called lymphatic) near the intestine. These small vessels carry the reformed fat to the veins of the chest, and the blood carries the fat to storage depots in different parts of the body.

*Vitamins*—Another vital part of our food that is absorbed from the small intestine is the class of chemicals we call vitamins. There are two different types of vitamins, classified by the fluid in which they can be dissolved: water-soluble vitamins (all the B vitamins and vitamin C) and fat-soluble vitamins (vitamins A, D, and K).

*Water and Salt*—Most of the material absorbed from the cavity of the small intestine is water in which salt is dissolved. The salt and water come from the food and liquid we swallow and the juices secreted by the many digestive glands. In a healthy adult, more than a gallon of water containing over an ounce of salt is absorbed from the intestine every 24 hours.

## How Is the Digestive Process Controlled?

### Hormone Regulators

A fascinating feature of the digestive system is that it contains its own regulators. The major hormones that control the functions of the digestive system are produced and released by cells in the mucosa of the stomach and small intestine. These hormones are released into the blood of the digestive tract, travel back to the heart and through the arteries, and return to the digestive system, where they stimulate digestive juices and cause organ movement.

The hormones that control digestion are gastrin, secretin, and cholecystokinin (CCK):

- Gastrin causes the stomach to produce an acid for dissolving and digesting some foods. It is also necessary for the normal growth of the lining of the stomach, small intestine, and colon.

- Secretin causes the pancreas to send out a digestive juice that is rich in bicarbonate. It stimulates the stomach to produce pepsin, an enzyme that digests protein, and it also stimulates the liver to produce bile.

- CCK causes the pancreas to grow and to produce the enzymes of pancreatic juice, and it causes the gallbladder to empty.

### Nerve Regulators

Two types of nerves help to control the action of the digestive system. Extrinsic (outside) nerves come to the digestive organs from the unconscious part of the brain or from the spinal cord. They release a chemical called acetylcholine and another called adrenaline. Acetylcholine causes the muscle of the digestive organs to squeeze with more force and increase the "push" of food and juice through the digestive tract. Acetylcholine also causes the stomach and pancreas to produce more digestive juice. Adrenaline relaxes the muscle of the stomach and intestine and decreases the flow of blood to these organs.

Even more important, though, are the intrinsic (inside) nerves, which make up a very dense network embedded in the walls of the esophagus, stomach, small intestine, and colon. The intrinsic nerves are triggered to act when the walls of the hollow organs are stretched by food. They release many different substances that speed up or delay the movement of food and the production of juices by the digestive organs.

## Additional Readings

*Facts and Fallacies About Digestive Diseases*. 1991. This fact sheet discusses commonly held beliefs about digestive diseases. Available from the National Digestive Diseases Information Clearinghouse, 2 Information Way, Bethesda, MD 20892-3570. (301) 654-3810.

Larson DE, editor. *Mayo Clinic Family Health Book*. New York: William Morrow and Company, Inc., 1990. General medical guide with section on the digestive system and how it works. Available in libraries and bookstores.

Tapley DF, et al., eds. *The Columbia University College of Physicians and Surgeons Complete Home Medical Guide*, revised edition. New York: Crown Publishers, Inc., 1990. General medical guide with section on the digestive system and how it works. Available in libraries and bookstores.

**National Digestive Diseases Information Clearinghouse**
2 Information Way
Bethesda, MD 20892-3570
(301) 654-3810

The National Digestive Diseases Information Clearinghouse (NDDIC) is a service of the National Institute of Diabetes and Digestive and Kidney Diseases, part of the National Institutes of Health, under the U.S. Public Health Service. The clearinghouse, authorized by Congress in 1980, provides information about digestive diseases and health to people with digestive diseases and their families, health care professionals, and the public. The NDDIC answers inquiries; develops, reviews, and distributes publications; and works closely with professional and patient organizations and government agencies to coordinate resources about digestive diseases.

Publications produced by the clearinghouse are reviewed carefully for scientific accuracy, content, and readability. Publications produced by other sources are also reviewed for scientific accuracy and are used, along with clearinghouse publications, to answer requests.

Chapter 2

# Digestive Diseases Statistics

## All Digestive Diseases[1]

**Prevalence:** 60 to 70 million people affected by all digestive diseases (1985)
**Mortality:** 191,000, including deaths from cancer (1985)
**Hospitalizations:** 10 million (13 percent of all hospitalization) (1985)
**Diagnostic and therapeutic procedures:** 6 million (14 percent of all procedures) (1987)
**Physician office visits:** 50 million (1985)
**Disability:** 1.4 million people (1987)
**Costs:**
$107 billion (1992)
$87 billion direct medical costs
$20 billion indirect costs (e.g., disability and mortality)

## Specific Diseases

### *Abdominal Wall Hernia*

**Incidence:** 800,000 new cases, including 500,000 inguinal hernias (1985)
**Prevalence:** 4.5 million people (1988–90)

---

NIH Pub. 95-3873.

**Hospitalizations:** 640,000 (1980)
**Physician office visits:** 2 to 3 million (1989–90)
**Prescriptions:** 184,000 (1989–90)
**Disability:** 550,000 people (1983–87)

### *Chronic Liver Disease and Cirrhosis*

**Prevalence:** 400,000 people(1976–80)
**Mortality:** 26,050 deaths (1987)
**Hospitalizations:** 300,000 (1987)
**Physician office visits:** 1 million (1985)
**Disability:** 112,000 people (1983–87)

### *Constipation*

**Prevalence:** 4.4 million people (1983–87)
**Mortality:** 29 deaths (1982–85)
**Hospitalizations:** 100,000 (1983–87)
**Physician office visits:** 2 million (1985)
**Prescriptions:** 1 million (1985)
**Disability:** 13,000 people (1983–87)

### *Diverticular Disease*

**Incidence:** 300,000 new cases (1987)
**Prevalence:** 2 million people (1983–87)
**Mortality:** 3,000 deaths (1985)
**Hospitalizations:** 440,000 (1987)
**Physician office visits:** 2 million (1987)
**Disability:** 112,000 people (1983–87)

### *Gallstones*

**Prevalence:** 16 to 22 million people (1976–87)
**Mortality:** 2,975 (1985)
**Hospitalizations:** 800,000 (1987)
**Physician office visits:** 600,000 to 700,000 (1985)
**Prescriptions:** 195,000 (1985)
**Surgical procedures:** 500,000 cholecystectomies (1987)
**Disability:** 48,000 people (1983–87)

## *Gastritis and Nonulcer Dyspepsia (NUD)*

**Incidence:**
Gastritis: 313,000 new cases (1975)
Chronic NUD: 444,000 new cases (1975)
Acute NUD: 8.2 million new cases (1988)

**Prevalence:**
Gastritis: 2.7 million people (1988)
NUD: 5.8 million people (1988)

**Mortality:**
Gastritis: 703 (1980's)
NUD: 49 (1980's)

**Hospitalizations:**
Gastritis: 600 (1980's)
NUD: 65,000 (1980's)

**Physician office visits:**
Gastritis: 3 million (1980's)
NUD: 800,000 (1980's)

**Prescriptions:**
Gastritis: 2 million (1985)
NUD: 649,000 (1985)

**Disability:**
Gastritis: 34,000 people (1983–87)
Chronic NUD: 42,000 people (1983–87)

## *Gastroesophageal Reflux Disease and Related Esophageal Disorders*

**Prevalence:** 3 to 7 percent of U.S. population (1985)
**Mortality:** 1,000 deaths (1984–88)
**Hospitalizations:** 1 million (1985)
**Physician office visits:** 4 to 5 million (1985)

## *Hemorrhoids*

**Incidence:** 1 million new cases
**Prevalence:** 10.4 million people
**Mortality:** 17 deaths
**Hospitalizations:** 316,000
**Physician** office visits: 3.5 million
**Prescriptions:** 1.5 million
**Disability:** 52,000 people

### *Infectious Diarrhea*

**Incidence:** 99 million new cases (1980)
**Mortality:** 3,100 deaths (1985)
**Hospitalizations:** 462,000 to 728,000 (1987)
**Physician office visits:** 8 to 12 million (1985)
**Prescriptions:** 5 to 8 million (1985)

### *Inflammatory Bowel Disease (1987)*

**Incidence:** 2 to 6 new cases per 100,000 people
**Prevalence:** 300,000 to 500,000 people
**Mortality:** Fewer than 1,000 deaths
**Hospitalizations:** 100,000 (64 percent for Crohn's disease)
**Physician office visits:** 700,000
**Disability:** 119,000 people (1983–87)

### *Irritable Bowel Syndrome*

**Prevalence:** 5 million people (1987)
**Hospitalizations:** 34,000 (1987)
**Physician office visits:** 3.5 million (1987)
**Prescriptions:** 2.2 million (1985)
**Disability:** 400,000 people (1983–87)

### *Lactose Intolerance*[2]

**Prevalence:** 30 to 50 million people (1994)

### *Pancreatitis*

**Incidence:** Acute: 17 new cases per 100,000 people (1976-88)
**Mortality:** 2,700 deaths (1985)
**Hospitalizations:**
Acute: 125,000 (1987)
Chronic: 20,000 (1987)
**Physician office visits:**
Acute: 911,000 (1987)
Chronic: 122,000 (1987)

### *Peptic Ulcer*

**Prevalence:** 5 million people (1987)
**Mortality:** 6,500 deaths (1987)
**Hospitalizations:** 630,000 (1987)
**Physician office visits:** 3 to 5 million (1985)
**Prescriptions:** 2 million (1985)
**Disability:** 401,000 people (1983–87)

### *Viral Hepatitis*

**Incidence:**
- **Hepatitis A:** 32,000 new cases (1992)
- **Hepatitis B:** 200,000 to 300,000 new cases (1990)
- **Hepatitis C:** 150,000 new cases (1991)
- **Hepatitis D:** 70,000 new cases (1990

**Prevalence:**
- **Hepatitis A:** 32 to 38 percent of U.S. population that have any history of disease (1991)
- **Hepatitis B:** 4 percent of U.S. population that have any history of disease (1990)
- **Hepatitis C and D:** Not determined

**Mortality:** Fewer than 1,000 deaths (1985)
**Hospitalizations:** 33,000 (1987)
**Physician office visits:** 500,000 (1985)

## Additional Data

**Liver Transplants[3]:** 3,300 transplants performed (1993)
**Number of gastroenterologists in the United States[4]:** 7,493 (1990)

## Sources

[1]Unless noted, the data in this fact sheet are from:

Everhart, JE, editor. *Digestive Diseases in the United States: Epidemiology and Impact*. US Department of Health and Human Services, Public Health Service, National Institutes of Health,

National Institute of Diabetes and Digestive and Kidney Diseases. Washington, DC: US Government Printing Office, 1994; NIH publication no. 94–1447.

The book answers hundreds of questions about the scope and impact of the major infectious, chronic, and malignant digestive diseases. National and special population based data provide information about the prevalence, incidence, medical care, disability, mortality, and research needs regarding specific digestive diseases. The data were compiled primarily from the surveys of the National Center for Health Statistics, supplemented by other Federal agencies and private sources.

The book is available for $15 from the National Digestive Diseases Information Clearinghouse at the address and phone number listed below. Please make checks payable to "NDDIC."

[2]National Institute of Diabetes and Digestive and Kidney Diseases, National Institutes of Health.

[3]United Network for Organ Sharing Scientific Registry

[4]American Medical Association Physician Characteristics and Distribution in the United States. 1992 edition, Chicago, Illinois: American Medical Association, 1992, p.20.

## Glossary

Data for digestive diseases as a group and for specific diseases are provided in various categories. Data do not exist in all categories for some diseases. Following are definitions of the categories as used in this fact sheet:

**Disability:** The number of people in a year whose ability to perform major daily activities such as working, housekeeping, and going to school, is limited and reduced over long periods because of a disease.

**Hospitalizations:** The number of hospitalizations for a disease in a year.

**Incidence:** The number of new cases of a disease in the U.S. population in a year.

**Mortality:** The number of deaths resulting from the disease listed as the underlying or primary cause in a year.

**Physician office visits:** The number of outpatient visits to office-based physicians for a disease in a year.

**Prescriptions:** The number of prescriptions written annually for medications to treat a specific disease.

**Prevalence:** The number of people in the United States affected by a disease or diseases in a year.

**Procedures:** The number of diagnostic and therapeutic procedures performed annually in a hospital setting.

**National Digestive Diseases Information Clearinghouse**
2 Information Way
Bethesda, MD 20892-3570
(301) 654-3810

The National Digestive Diseases Information Clearinghouse (NDDIC) is a service of the National Institute of Diabetes and Digestive and Kidney Diseases, part of the National Institutes of Health, under the U.S. Public Health Service. The clearinghouse, authorized by Congress in 1980, provides information about digestive diseases and health to people with digestive diseases and their families, health care professionals, and the public. The NDDIC answers inquiries; develops, reviews, and distributes publications; and works closely with professional and patient organizations and government agencies to coordinate resources about digestive diseases.

Publications produced by the clearinghouse are reviewed carefully for scientific accuracy, content, and readability. Publications produced by other sources are also reviewed for scientific accuracy and are used, along with clearinghouse publications, to answer requests.

# Chapter 3

# *Digestive Do's and Don'ts*

The digestive system performs the amazing task of changing food into the fuel your body needs to carry on. Most of the time this system stays remarkably free of trouble. With age, however, your body may begin to work less efficiently in some ways and your lifestyle may change. Afterward, digestion may be a problem every now and then.

During the chemical process of digestion, food is broken down into pieces tiny enough to be taken into the blood. The blood, in turn, carries these food elements to cells in all parts of the body where they are changed into energy or used to form new structures such as body tissue.

Many body organs are involved in the process of digestion: the esophagus, stomach, pancreas, gallbladder, liver, small intestine, and colon. Many people have few, if any, digestive problems related to aging. Sometimes there are changes affecting the length of time food travels through the system. For example, digestive muscles might move slower or produce less acid.

Lifestyle changes such as increased use of medicines, reduced exercise, and changes in eating habits can hamper the digestive system.

## *Taking Care of the System*

To keep your digestive system working at its best:

---

This chapter is part of the Age Page series published by the National Institute of Aging, a division of the National Institutes of Health.

- Eat a well-balanced diet that includes a variety of fresh fruits, vegetables, and whole grain breads, cereals, and other grain products
- Eat slowly and try to relax for 30 minutes after each meal
- Exercise regularly
- Drink alcohol in moderation, if at all
- Avoid large amounts of caffeine
- Use caution when taking over-the-counter drugs and always follow your doctor's directions exactly when taking prescribed medications.

## When to See a Doctor

No matter how well your digestive system is treated, there are times when things go wrong. Often the problem will take care of itself. Sometimes, symptoms can be a signal that something more serious is wrong. Some important warning signs are:

- Stomach pains that are severe, last a long time, are recurring, or come with shaking, chills, and cold, clammy skin
- Blood in vomit or recurrent vomiting
- A sudden change in bowel habits or consistency of stools lasting more than a few days (for example, diarrhea for more than 3 days or the sudden onset of constipation)
- Blood in stools or coal-black stools
- Jaundice (a yellowing of the skin and the whites of the eyes) or dark, tea-colored urine
- Pain or difficulty in swallowing food
- Loss of appetite or unexpected weight loss

- Diarrhea that wakes you up at night.

If you have any of these symptoms, see a doctor at once.

## *Digestive Diseases*

Disorders of the digestive tract cause more hospital admissions than any other group of diseases. They occur most often in people who are middle age or older.

Stress, infection, diseases, poisons, and defects present at birth can cause digestion problems. But the causes of many digestive diseases are unknown. There is evidence that diet may be involved in a few of them. For example, eating less fiber (the part of the plant that is not digested) may play a role in constipation, cancer of the colon, and diverticulosis, a condition in which small sacs form in the intestinal wall. Alcoholism has been linked to inflammation of the pancreas (pancreatitis).

Progress is being made in diagnosing many digestive diseases. In addition to the upper and lower gastrointestinal series, which uses x-rays and barium to find trouble spots, doctors can use a flexible instrument called the endoscope to see inside the esophagus, stomach, duodenum, and colon. The endoscope is also used to perform biopsies and some forms of surgery. There are also techniques for getting better images of body organs, such as ultrasound and the CT scan (computer tomographic scan), which takes detailed, three-dimensional x-rays.

Treatment advances include new drugs for peptic ulcers, a vaccine to prevent hepatitis B, and microsurgery to remove gallstones.

Some common digestive disorders are listed below.

*Constipation*. This is a decrease in the number of bowel movements, along with long or hard passing of stools. Older people report this problem much more often than do younger ones. Most cases of constipation can be easily treated. "Regularity" does not necessarily mean one bowel movement every day. Normal bowel habits can range from three movements each day to three each week. Eating a poor diet, drinking too few liquids, changing activities, taking certain prescription medications, or misusing laxatives can lead to constipation. Regularity is usually improved by eating foods high in fiber and staying physically active. (Also see the Age Page "Constipation.")

*Diarrhea*. When body wastes are discharged from the bowel more often than usual in a more or less liquid state, the condition is called diarrhea. There are many possible causes, but many cases are related to infection or improper handling of food. Treatment of the underlying disorder is needed but, most important, replacing lost fluids, even when there is no feeling of thirst, is essential.

*Diverticulosis and diverticulitis*. In diverticulosis, which is common in older people, small sacs form on the wall of the large intestine. Although they usually cause no symptoms, occasionally there is pain in the lower left side of the abdomen. Treatment includes a diet high in fiber and liquids. Diverticulitis develops after the sacs become inflamed and causes a fever. Treatment consists of bed rest and antibiotics.

*Functional disorders*. Sometimes symptoms such as pain, diarrhea, constipation, bloating, and gas are caused by a functional disorder such as irritable bowel syndrome. In these disorders there are no signs of disease and yet the intestinal tract still fails to work properly. A functional disorder may cause discomfort, but it is unlikely to lead to a serious disease. A doctor may prescribe medication to relieve symptoms. Because diet and stress are thought to trigger functional disorders, the same guidelines that help to keep your system running smoothly should help control the symptoms.

*Gallbladder disease*. In this disease, stones (usually composed of cholesterol) form in the gallbladder. These stones are often silent: that is, they cause no symptoms or discomfort, but they sometimes result in problems requiring drug treatment or surgery. Severe pain in the upper abdomen may mean that a gallstone has lodged in one of the tubes leading from the gallbladder.

*Gas*. Some gas is normally present in the digestive tract. It is usually caused by swallowing air, stress, or eating foods such as cauliflower, brussel sprouts, brown beans, broccoli, bran, and cabbage. (Since these foods are good sources of fiber and vitamins, eat smaller amounts rather than removing them from the diet.) The body rids itself of gas by belching or passing gas. However, if gas collects in the digestive tract, it can lead to pain and bloating.

*Gastritis*. An inflammation of the stomach, gastritis can be caused by excess acid production in the stomach, infections, medications, and alcohol. Treatment is aimed at correcting the condition causing the gastritis, such as an infection, too much alcohol, an allergic response, or certain medicines.

*Heartburn*. A burning pain felt behind the breastbone that occurs after meals and lasts for anywhere from a few minutes to several hours is called heartburn. It is caused by stomach acid washing backward up into the tube connecting the mouth and stomach (esophagus). Heartburn can be brought on by eating spicy or rich foods such as tomato products, chocolate, fried foods, or peppermint, or by smoking cigarettes. It is relieved by changing your diet, taking an antacid, sleeping with the head of the bed raised 6 inches, or stopping cigarette smoking. If pain persists, see a doctor.

*Peptic ulcer*. This is a sore on the lining of the stomach or the small intestine just below the stomach (duodenum). An ulcer occurs when the lining is unable to resist the damaging effects of acid and pepsin that are produced by the stomach to digest foods. Antacids, which neutralize acid in the stomach, and drugs that decrease the production of acid or coat the ulcer are very useful in treating peptic ulcer. Continued pain should be checked by a doctor.

*Indigestion*. Known as dyspepsia, this common condition involves painful, difficult, or disturbed digestion. The symptoms include nausea, regurgitation, vomiting, heartburn, abdominal fullness or bloating after a meal, and stomach discomfort or pain. Overeating or eating certain foods can also cause symptoms, but they may also be related to other digestive problems such as peptic ulcer, gallbladder disease, or gastritis. Indigestion usually can be controlled through diet or by treating the specific disorder.

*Hemorrhoids*. When veins in and around the rectum and anus become weakened and enlarged, they are called hemorrhoids. This condition may be caused by pressure in the rectal veins due to constipation, pregnancy, obesity, or other conditions. The veins may become inflamed, develop blood clots, and bleed. Hemorrhoids are treated with frequent warm baths, creams, or suppositories, and if necessary, by injections or surgery. Eating high-fiber foods and drinking fluids may also help.

*Hiatal hernia.* In this condition the esophagus breaks through the opening in a thin muscle separating the abdominal cavity from the chest cavity. Hiatal hernias are common after middleage and usually have no symptoms. But if the lower end of the esophagus becomes weak, stomach acids may flow back to the esophagus and result in a sense of burning. Most problems can be treated without medicines or surgery. For example, a change in eating habits or losing weight may be all that's needed to remove discomfort.

*Milk intolerance.* Also called lactose intolerance, this is the inability to digest milk and milk products properly due to a lack of lactase, the intestinal enzyme that digests the sugar found in milk. Some people develop this problem as they grow older. Symptoms, including cramps, gas, bloating, and diarrhea, appear 15 minutes to several hours after consuming milk or a milk product. Most people manage the problem by mixing milk with food or beverages, eating processed cheeses and yogurt, taking smaller servings more frequently, or adding a special nonprescription preparation such as acidophilus to milk that makes it easy to digest. When eating fewer dairy products, help keep bones strong by consuming calcium rich foods such as dark green leafy vegetables, salmon, and bean curd. Since these foods will not provide as much calcium as dairy products, a doctor may suggest supplements.

*Ulcerative colitis.* This chronic disorder usually develops in young adults, but it also appears in older people. In ulcerative colitis, parts of the large intestine become inflamed causing abdominal cramps and often rectal bleeding. Joint pain and skin rashes may also develop. The symptoms are usually controlled with drugs, but some patients eventually need surgery. Sometimes irritable bowel syndrome (IBS) is incorrectly called "spastic colitis." However, IBS does not cause inflammation and it is not related to ulcerative colitis.

## For More Information

For further information about these and other digestive problems, consult your doctor. You can also write to the National Digestive Diseases Information Clearinghouse, P.O. Box NDDIC, 9000 Rockville Pike, Bethesda, MD 20892.

For a free list of NIH publications, call 1-800-222-2225; or write to the NIH Information Center, P.O. Box 8057, Gaithersburg, MD 20898-8057.

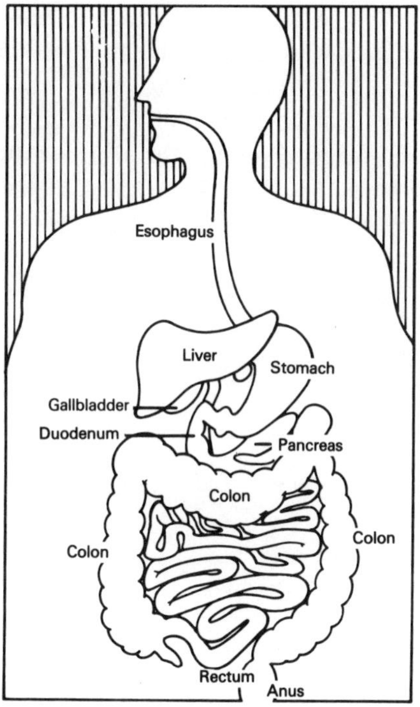


***Figure 3.1.*** *The digestive system.*

## The Digestive System

Digestion begins in the mouth. As you chew, tiny glands give off a fluid (saliva) that moistens food so it can be swallowed easily. Saliva also contains an enzyme that begins to change carbohydrates—like vegetables and breads—into a form the body can absorb. Once the food is swallowed, wavelike (peristaltic) motions push it through the esophagus and into the stomach. Stomach muscles crush and mix the food with enzymes and acids, creating a mixture called chyme. The stomach allows small amounts of the chyme to enter the duodenum, the first part of the small intestine. It is in the duodenum that most digestion takes place. There, juices from the liver and pancreas break down fats, protein, and carbohydrates. As the digested food passes into the last two-thirds of the small intestine, nutrients are absorbed into the blood. The remaining material is pushed into the colon, which is part of the large intestine. This material includes water and waste—the part of food that is not digested, such as fiber from fruit, vegetables, and grains. The lining of the colon absorbs water from the material and, when the waste is solid enough, nerves in the wall of the large intestine signal the urge for a bowel movement.

## Chapter 4

# *Facts and Fallacies About Digestive Diseases*

The digestive tract is a complex system of organs responsible for converting the food we eat into the nutrients we need to live. We would expect a system as well used as the digestive tract to be the source of many problems, and it is. Diseases of the digestive tract are responsible for the hospitalization of more people in the United States than any other group of disorders. Yet, until recently, little was known about the causes, treatment, or prevention of these illness.

In recent years, researchers have begun to shed light on some of the more baffling aspects of digestive diseases. Some studies have indicated that those diseases once thought to have been caused by emotional problems may, in fact, be the result of viruses interacting with the body's immune system or disturbances in the motility patterns of the organs. And doctors now know that an ulcer has more to do with the presence of the bacterium Helicobacter pylori than with the level of stress in one's life. Listed below are facts about common digestive diseases.

## *Hiatal Hernia*

**Fallacy:** Hiatal hernia causes heartburn.

The fact is, while some people who suffer from heartburn also have a hiatal hernia, heartburn is not caused by the hernia. As shown in figure 4.1, a hiatal hernia is the protrusion of a portion of the stomach through a teardrop-shaped hole in the diaphragm where the

---

NIH Pub. 95-2673.

esophagus and the stomach join. The most frequent cause of hiatal hernia is an increased pressure in the abdominal cavity produced by coughing, vomiting, straining at stool, or sudden physical exertion. A majority of people over 60 years have hiatal hernias and, in most cases, the hiatal hernia does not cause problems.

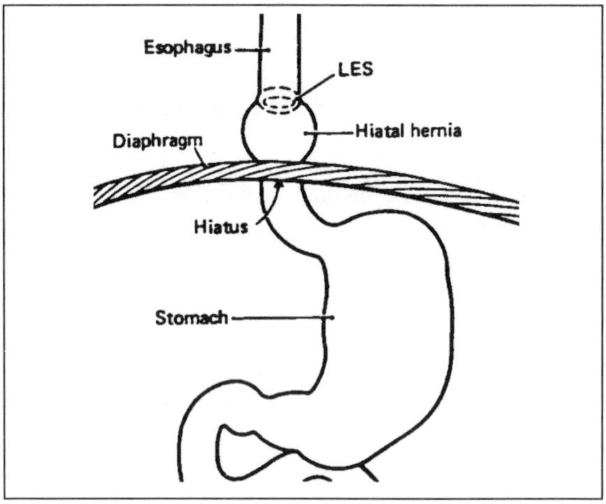


***Figure 4.1.*** *Hiatal hernia.*

## Heartburn

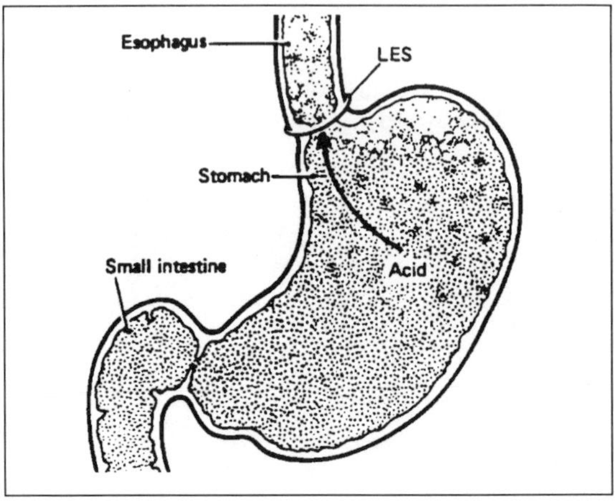


***Figure 4.2.*** *Relaxed or weak lower esophageal sphincter causes heartburn.*

**Fact:** Chocolate and peppermint cause heartburn in many people.

The fact is heartburn occurs when the lower esophageal sphincter (called the LES), located at the junction of the esophagus and the stomach, either relaxes inappropriately or is very weak (figure 4.2). This allows the highly acidic contents of the stomach to back up into the esophagus. Both chocolate and peppermint are thought to cause the LES to relax and allow the contents of the stomach to back up into the esophagus. Other foods associated with heartburn include tomato products, citrus fruits and juices, coffee, and fried or fatty foods.

**Fact:** Cigarette smoking causes heartburn.

The fact is that studies have shown that cigarette smoking dramatically decreases the LES pressure.

**Fact:** Nonprescription antacids relieve heartburn.

The fact is that many people have discovered that nonprescription antacids provide temporary or partial relief from heartburn. Long-term use of antacids can, however, result in side effects like diarrhea, altered calcium metabolism, and magnesium retention. (Magnesium retention can be serious for patients with kidney disease.) As with other nonprescription drugs, if prolonged use (longer than 3 weeks) becomes necessary, consult your doctor.

## Peptic Ulcer Disease

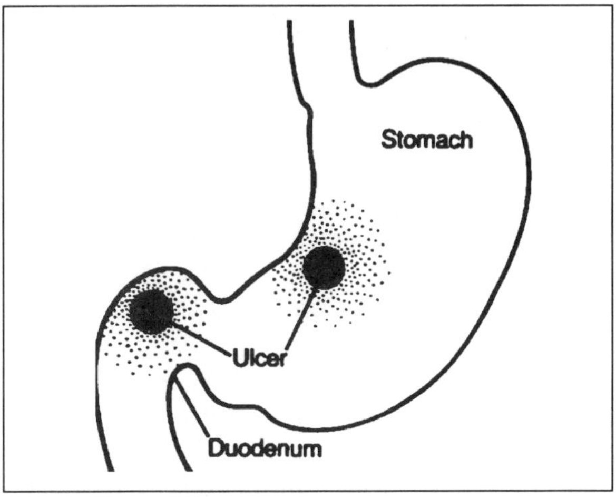


***Figure 4.3.*** *Peptic ulcers occur in the lining of the stomach and the duodenum.*

**Fallacy:** Peptic ulcer disease is most prevalent among persons under stress.

The facts are that peptic ulcers are sores in the lining of the stomach or duodenum (figure 4.3) and occur in many people. According to some studies, ulcers have been found to be more common among people in lower socioeconomic groups.

**Fact:** Cigarette smokers are about twice as likely to have ulcers as nonsmokers.

The fact is that current research indicates an association between smoking cigarettes and peptic ulcer disease. This applies to both gastric (stomach) and duodenal ulcers and to both men and women. Also, ulcers heal slower and recur more often in cigarette smokers than in nonsmokers.

**Fact:** People who take aspirin regularly increase their risk of getting a gastric ulcer.

The fact is that people who take aspirin 4 or more days a week for 3 or more months increase their risk of getting a gastric ulcer. Also, aspirin increases the likelihood of bleeding from an ulcer.

**Fallacy:** Peptic ulcers should be treated with a bland diet.

The fact is that there is little agreement about what the term "bland" means. Also, there is little indication that any particular diet is helpful for all peptic ulcer patients. Although some patients find that coffee or extremely spicy foods are bothersome, each person has to find out for him/herself which foods, if any, cause distress.

## Lactose Intolerance

**Fact:** Many people cannot drink milk.

The fact is that an estimated 50 million Americans have lactose intolerance. Certain racial and ethnic populations are more affected than others. As many as 75 percent of African Americans, Jewish, Mexican Americans, and American Indian adults and 90 percent of Asian American adults have lactose intolerance.

Lactose intolerance is caused by a deficiency of lactase, the intestinal enzyme that digests milk sugar (lactose). Persons with lactose intolerance cannot properly digest milk and milk products when taken in the usual amounts. Some people are even sensitive to extremely small quantities of dairy products. Symptoms of lactose intolerance include cramps, gas, bloating, or diarrhea within 15 minutes to 3 hours after consuming milk or milk products.

## Celiac Sprue

**Fallacy:** A person with celiac sprue (an inherited disorder affecting the lining of the small intestine) may eat small amounts of food containing gluten (a substance found in wheat, rye, barley, and oats) as long as symptoms do not develop.

The fact is that a person with celiac sprue should avoid all foods containing wheat, rye, barley, and oats (foods containing gluten). Severe damage to the intestines can occur even when there are no symptoms. Some experts think that small amounts of gluten can cause damage to the intestines.

## Constipation

**Fallacy:** Bowel regularity means a bowel movement every day.

The facts are that the frequency of bowel movements among normal, healthy people varies from three movements a day to three a week, and perfectly healthy people may fall outside both ends of this range.

**Fallacy:** Nonprescription laxatives are always safe and always cure constipation.

The fact is that, although short-term use of laxatives is usually effective in relieving temporary constipation, long-term use of laxatives impairs the natural muscle actions required to have a bowel movement. Also, overuse of mineral oil, a popular laxative, may reduce the absorption of certain vitamins (A, D, E, and K). Mineral oil also may interact with some drugs, causing undesirable side effects. Consult your doctor if you need to use a laxative for longer than 3 weeks. And, if you are on medication, check with your doctor before taking any laxative.

**Fact:** Habitual use of enemas eventually leads to loss of normal bowel function.

The fact is that habitual use of enemas usually is not necessary and will eventually lead to an inability of the bowels to function normally. As with laxatives, overuse of enemas can impair the natural muscle actions of the bowel.

## Irritable Bowel Syndrome

**Fallacy:** Irritable bowel syndrome (spastic colon, mucous colitis) is a serious disease that often leads to ulcerative colitis.

The fact is that irritable bowel syndrome (IBS) is a common functional disorder characterized by gas, abdominal pain, and diarrhea or constipation or the cyclical occurrence of both. IBS, although often causing considerable discomfort, generally does not lead to other gastrointestinal disorders.

**Fallacy:** IBS frequently leads to cancer of the colon.

The fact is that there is no evidence that IBS is a precursor of cancer.

## Diverticulosis and Diverticulitis

**Fallacy:** Diverticulosis always causes a serious problem.

The fact is that diverticulosis is a condition in which little sacs (diverticula) develop in the wall of the colon. In the United States, the majority of people over the age of 60 years have diverticulosis. Most people do not have symptoms and would not know that they had diverticula unless an x-ray or intestinal examination were done. Only about 20 percent of patients with diverticulosis develop complications such as diverticulitis, bleeding, or perforation.

## Inflammatory Bowel Disease

**Fallacy:** Inflammatory bowel disease (Crohn's disease and ulcerative colitis) is caused by personality disorders.

The fact is that the cause of inflammatory bowel disease (IBD) is not known. IBD is a name for a group of disorders in which various parts of the intestinal tract become inflamed. Currently, researchers speculate that IBD may be caused by a viral or bacterial agent interacting with the body's immune system. There is no evidence to support the theory that IBD is caused by tension, anxiety, or other psychological factors or disorders.

**Fallacy:** Patients with IBD require a special diet.

The fact is that there is no evidence that the inflammation of the intestines is affected by specific foods. Many patients tolerate all varieties of food and require no dietary restrictions. Others, particularly when their disease is active, find a diet low in fiber and spicy foods easier to tolerate. Maintaining good general nutrition, however, is more important than emphasizing or avoiding any particular foods.

## Gallbladder Disease

**Fallacy:** Gallbladder disease always causes severe pain.

The fact is that about 10 percent of the American population has gallstones, but many do not have symptoms. However, when gallbladder pain occurs, it is usually sudden, severe, and steady and is felt in the upper abdomen.

## Pancreatitis

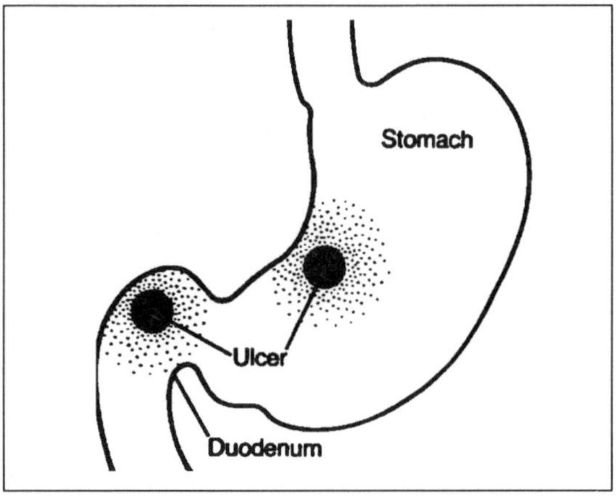


*Figure 4.4. The pancreas is located next to the duodenum.*

**Fact:** The pancreas is a digestive organ.

The fact is that the pancreas, a gland that is located next to the duodenum (see figure 4.4), produces enzymes and hormones that aid in digestion.

**Fallacy:** Pancreatitis (inflammation of the pancreas) is always caused by alcoholism.

The facts are that approximately one-third of all cases of pancreatitis are due to unknown causes, and many attacks of acute pancreatitis are associated with gallstones.

## Cirrhosis

**Fallacy:** Chronic alcoholism is the only cause of cirrhosis of the liver.

The fact is that cirrhosis has many causes. In the United States, three-fourths of the cases are due to chronic alcoholism. In those parts of the world where viral hepatitis is common, hepatitis is the leading cause of cirrhosis. In children, cirrhosis may be caused by a host of inherited disorders including cystic fibrosis, alpha-1 antitrypsin deficiency, biliary atresia, glycogen storage disease, and other rare diseases. In adults, cirrhosis may be caused by hepatitis B or a host of rare diseases, such as primary biliary cirrhosis, abnormal storage of metals by the body, severe reactions to prescribed drugs, and prolonged exposure to environmental toxins.

**Fact:** You may have cirrhosis of the liver and not know it.

The fact is that onset of cirrhosis is often "silent," having few specific symptoms. In fact, cirrhosis may not cause symptoms until the disease is far advanced.

## Hemorrhoids

**Fallacy:** Hemorrhoids are the only cause of bright red bleeding from the rectum.

The fact is that, although most cases of bright red bleeding from the rectum are due to hemorrhoids, polyps and cancer of the rectum also can cause a similar type of bleeding. Any bleeding from the rectum should be evaluated by a doctor.

## Ostomy Surgery

**Fact:** Ostomy surgery is a common procedure.

The fact is that about 100,000 ostomy surgeries are performed each year and about 1 million persons have ostomies. Although ostomies create great changes for the patient, they are rather simple procedures. Ostomy surgery is a procedure in which the affected part of the small or large intestine is removed, an opening (stoma) is created on the body's surface, and a portion of the intestine is brought out through the opening. A pouch is worn to collect the body's waste.

**Fallacy:** Men become impotent following ostomy surgery.

The fact is that men who have ostomy surgery may have full potency (the ability to have an erection and orgasm) or complete impotence (the inability to have an erection).

**Fallacy:** After ostomy surgery, women experience impaired sexual function and cannot become pregnant.

The fact is that, in general, having an ostomy does not lessen a woman's sexual or reproductive capabilities. In a few cases, the condition that necessitates ostomy surgery also may necessitate additional surgery such as hysterectomy. Hysterectomies make it impossible to conceive but have no effect on sexual desire or the ability to have sexual relations.

## *Additional Resources*

American Liver Foundation, 1425 Pompton Avenue, Cedar Grove, NJ 07009; (800) 223-1079 or (201) 256-2550. General information about cirrhosis and other liver diseases.

Crohn's & Colitis Foundation of America, Inc., 386 Park Avenue South, 17th Floor, New York, NY 10016-8804; (800) 932-2423 or (212) 685-3440. Information about inflammatory bowel disease.

United Ostomy Association, 36 Executive Park, Suite 120, Irvine, CA 92714-6744; (800) 826-0862 or (714) 660-8624. Information about ostomy care and management.

**National Digestive Diseases Information Clearinghouse**
2 Information Way
Bethesda, MD 20892-3570
(301) 654-3810

The National Digestive Diseases Information Clearinghouse (NDDIC) is a service of the National Institute of Diabetes and Digestive and Kidney Diseases, part of the National Institutes of Health, under the U.S. Public Health Service. This clearinghouse, authorized by Congress in 1980, provides information about digestive diseases and health to people with digestive diseases and their families, health care professionals, and the public. The NDDIC answers inquiries; develops, reviews, and distributes publications; and works closely with professional and patient organizations and government agencies to coordinate resources about digestive diseases.

Publications produced by the clearinghouse are reviewed carefully for scientific accuracy, content, and readability. Publications produced by other sources are also reviewed for scientific accuracy and are used, along with clearinghouse publications, to answer requests.

## Chapter 5

# *Bleeding in the Digestive Tract*

Bleeding in the digestive tract is a symptom of digestive problems rather than a disease itself. Bleeding can occur as the result of a number of different conditions, many of which are not life threatening. Most causes of bleeding are related to conditions that can be cured or controlled, such as hemorrhoids. The cause of bleeding may not be serious, but locating the source of bleeding is important.

The digestive or gastrointestinal (GI) tract includes the esophagus, stomach, small intestine, large intestine or colon, rectum, and anus. Bleeding can come from one or more of these areas, that is, from a small area such as an ulcer on the lining of the stomach or from a large surface such as an inflammation of the colon. Bleeding can sometimes occur without the person noticing it. This type of bleeding is called occult or hidden. Fortunately, simple tests can detect occult blood in the stool.

## *What Causes Bleeding in the Digestive Tract?*

Stomach acid can cause inflammation that may lead to bleeding at the lower end of the esophagus. This condition is called esophagitis or inflammation of the esophagus. Sometimes a muscle between the esophagus and stomach fails to close properly and allows the return of food and stomach juices into the esophagus, which can lead to esophagitis. In addition, enlarged veins (varices) at the lower end of

---

NIH Pub. 93–1133.

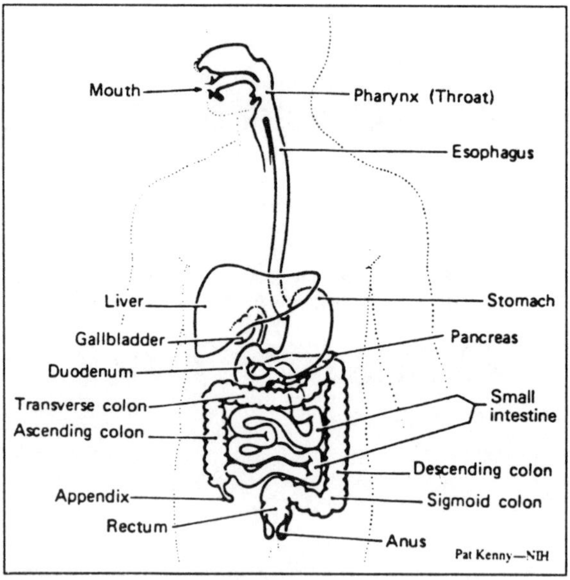


***Figure 5.1.***

the esophagus may rupture and bleed massively. Cirrhosis of the liver is the most common cause of esophageal varices.

Esophageal bleeding can be caused by Mallory-Weiss syndrome, a tear in the lining of the esophagus. Mallory-Weiss syndrome usually results from prolonged vomiting but may also be caused by increased pressure in the abdomen from coughing, hiatal hernia, or childbirth.

The stomach is a frequent site of bleeding. Alcohol, aspirin, aspirin-containing medicines, and various other medicines (particularly those used for arthritis) can cause stomach ulcers or inflammation (gastritis). The stomach is often the site of ulcer disease. Acute or chronic ulcers may enlarge and erode through a blood vessel, causing bleeding. Also, patients suffering from burns, shock, head injuries, or cancer, or those who have undergone extensive surgery may develop stress ulcers. Bleeding can occur from benign tumors or cancer of the stomach, although these disorders usually do not cause massive bleeding.

The most common source of bleeding from the upper digestive tract is ulcers in the duodenum (the upper small intestine). Researchers now believe that these ulcers are caused by excess stomach acid and infection with *Helicobacter pylori* bacteria.

In the lower digestive tract, the large intestine and rectum are frequent sites of bleeding. Hemorrhoids are probably the most common cause of visible blood in the digestive tract, especially blood that appears bright red. Hemorrhoids are enlarged veins in the anal area that can rupture and produce bright red blood, which can show up in the toilet or on toilet paper. If red blood is seen, however, it is essential to exclude other causes of bleeding since the anal area may also be the site of cuts (fissures), inflammation, or tumors.

Benign growths or polyps of the colon are very common and are thought to be forerunners of cancer. These growths can cause either bright red blood or occult bleeding. Colorectal cancer is the second most frequent of all cancers in the United States and usually causes bleeding at some time.

Inflammation from various causes can produce extensive bleeding from the colon. Different intestinal infections can cause inflammation and bloody diarrhea. Ulcerative colitis can produce inflammation and extensive surface bleeding from tiny ulcerations. Crohn's disease of the large intestine can also produce spotty bleeding.

Diverticular disease caused by diverticula (outpouchings of the colon wall) can result in massive bleeding. Finally, as one gets older, abnormalities may develop in the blood vessels of the large intestine, which may result in recurrent bleeding.

## *How Is Bleeding in the Digestive Tract Recognized?*

The signs of bleeding in the digestive tract depend upon the site and severity of bleeding. If blood is coming from the rectum or the lower colon, bright red blood will coat or mix with the stool. The stool may be mixed with darker blood if the bleeding is higher up in the colon or at the far end of the small intestine. When there is bleeding in the esophagus, stomach, or duodenum, the stool is usually black or tarry. Vomited material may be bright red or have a coffee-grounds appearance when one is bleeding from those sites. If bleeding is occult, the patient might not notice any changes in stool color.

If sudden massive bleeding occurs, a person may feel weak, dizzy, faint, short of breath, or have crampy abdominal pain or diarrhea. Shock may occur, with a rapid pulse, drop in blood pressure, and difficulty in producing urine. The patient may become very pale. If bleeding is slow and occurs over a long period of time, a gradual onset of fatigue, lethargy, shortness of breath, and pallor from the anemia will result. Anemia is a condition in which the blood's iron-rich substance, hemoglobin, is diminished.

## How Is Bleeding in the Digestive Tract Diagnosed?

The site of the bleeding must be located. A complete history and physical examination are essential. Symptoms such as changes in bowel habits, stool color (to black or red) and consistency, and the presence of pain or tenderness may tell the doctor which area of the GI tract is affected. Because the intake of iron or foods such as beets can give the stool the same appearance as bleeding from the digestive tract, a doctor must test the stool for blood before offering a diagnosis. A blood count will indicate whether the patient is anemic and also will give an idea of the extent of the bleeding and how chronic it may be.

### *Endoscopy*

Endoscopy is a common diagnostic technique that allows direct viewing of the bleeding site. Because the endoscope can detect lesions and confirm the presence or absence of bleeding, doctors often choose this method to diagnose patients with acute bleeding. In many cases, the doctor can use the endoscope to treat the cause of bleeding as well.

The endoscope is a flexible instrument that can be inserted through the mouth or rectum. The instrument allows the doctor to see into the esophagus, stomach, duodenum (esophago-duodenoscopy), colon (colonoscopy), and rectum (sigmoidoscopy); to collect small samples of tissue (biopsies); to take photographs; and to stop the bleeding.

Small bowel endoscopy, or enteroscopy, is a new procedure using a long endoscope. This endoscope may be introduced during surgery to localize a source of bleeding in the small intestine.

### *Other Procedures*

Several other methods are available to locate the source of bleeding. Barium x-rays, in general, are less accurate than endoscopy in locating bleeding sites. Some drawbacks of barium x-rays are that they may interfere with other diagnostic techniques if used for detecting acute bleeding; they expose the patient to x-rays; and they do not offer the capabilities of biopsy or treatment.

Angiography is a technique that uses dye to highlight blood vessels. This procedure is most useful in situations when the patient is acutely bleeding such that dye leaks out of the blood vessel and identifies the site of bleeding. In selected situations, angiography allows injection of medicine into arteries that may stop the bleeding.

Radionuclide scanning is a noninvasive screening technique used for locating sites of acute bleeding, especially in the lower GI tract. This technique involves injection of small amounts of radioactive material. Then, a special camera produces pictures of organs, allowing the doctor to detect a bleeding site.

In addition, barium x-rays, angiography, and radionuclide scans can be used to locate sources of chronic occult bleeding. These techniques are especially useful when the small intestine is suspected as the site of bleeding since the small intestine may not be seen easily with endoscopy.

## How Is Bleeding in the Digestive Tract Treated?

The use of endoscopy has grown and now allows doctors not only to see bleeding sites but to directly apply therapy as well. A variety of endoscopic therapies are useful to the patient for treating GI tract bleeding.

Active bleeding from the upper GI tract can often be controlled by injecting chemicals directly into a bleeding site with a needle introduced through the endoscope. A physician can also cauterize, or heat treat, a bleeding site and surrounding tissue with a heater probe or electrocoagulation device passed through the endoscope. Laser therapy, although effective, is no longer used regularly by many physicians because it is expensive and cumbersome.

Once bleeding is controlled, medicines are often prescribed to prevent recurrence of bleeding. Medical treatment of ulcers to ensure healing and maintenance therapy to prevent ulcer recurrence can also lessen the chance of recurrent bleeding. Studies are now underway to see if elimination of *Helicobacter pylori* affects the recurrence of ulcer bleeding.

Removal of polyps with an endoscope can control bleeding from colon polyps. Removal of hemorrhoids by banding or various heat or electrical devices is effective in patients who suffer hemorrhoidal bleeding on a recurrent basis. Endoscopic injection or cautery can be used to treat bleeding sites throughout the lower intestinal tract.

Endoscopic techniques do not always control bleeding. Sometimes angiography may be used. However, surgery is often needed to control active, severe or recurrent bleeding when endoscopy is not successful.

## Symptoms of Bleeding in the Digestive Tract

### How Do You Recognize Blood in the Stool and Vomit?

- Bright red blood coating the stool
- Dark blood mixed with the stool
- Black or tarry stool
- Bright red blood in vomit
- Coffee-grounds appearance of vomit

### What Are the Symptoms of Acute Bleeding?

- Weakness
- Dizziness
- Faintness
- Shortness of breath
- Crampy abdominal pain
- Diarrhea

### What Are the Symptoms of Chronic Bleeding?

- Fatigue
- Shortness of breath
- Lethargy
- Pallor

## Common Causes of Bleeding in the Digestive Tract

### Esophagus

- Inflammation (esophagitis)
- Enlarged veins (varices)
- Mallory-Weiss syndrome

### *Stomach*

- Ulcers
- Inflammation (gastritis)

### *Small Intestine*

- Duodenal ulcer

### *Large Intestine and Rectum*

- Hemorrhoids
- Inflammation (ulcerative colitis)
- Colorectal polyps
- Colorectal cancer
- Diverticular disease

## *Additional Readings*

Bowden, PR, Glombicki, AP, Smith, JL. "Diagnosis of Lower GI Bleeding." *Hospital Medicine* 1992; 28(2): 50–70. General review article for health care professionals. Available in medical libraries.

Clayman, CB, ed. *The American Medical Association Encyclopedia of Medicine*. New York: Random House, 1989. General medical guide with sections on common disorders that cause digestive tract bleeding. Available in libraries and bookstores.

Larson, DE, editor. *Mayo Clinic Family Health Book*. New York: William Morrow and Company, Inc., 1990. General medical guide with sections on common disorders that cause digestive tract bleeding. Available in libraries and bookstores.

Marshall, JB. "Bleeding Esophagogastric Varices: Ways to Treat Active Episodes and Prevent Recurrence." *Postgraduate Medicine* 1991; 89(6): 147–50, 155–57.

*Therapeutic Endoscopy and Bleeding Ulcers*. National Institutes of Health. Consensus Development Conference Statement. 7(6): March 1989.

**National Digestive Diseases Information Clearinghouse**
Box NDDIC
9000 Rockville Pike
Bethesda, MD 20892
(301) 468-4344

The National Digestive Diseases Information Clearinghouse is a service of the National Institute of Diabetes and Digestive and Kidney Diseases, part of the National Institutes of Health, under the U.S. Public Health Service. The clearinghouse was authorized by Congress to focus a national effort on providing information to the public, patients and their families, and doctors and other health care professionals. The clearinghouse works with organizations to educate people about digestive health and disease. The clearinghouse answers inquiries; develops, reviews, and distributes publications; and coordinates informational resources about digestive diseases.

Publications produced by the clearinghouse are reviewed carefully for scientific accuracy, appropriateness of content, and readability. Publications produced by sources other than the clearinghouse also are reviewed for scientific accuracy and are used, along with clearinghouse publications, to answer requests.

## Chapter 6

# *Smoking and Your Digestive System*

Cigarette smoking causes a variety of life-threatening diseases, including lung cancer, emphysema, and heart disease. An estimated 400,000 deaths each year are caused directly by cigarette smoking. Smoking is responsible for changes in all parts of the body, including the digestive system. This fact can have serious consequences because it is the digestive system that converts foods into the nutrients the body needs to live.

Current estimates indicate that about one-third of all adults smoke. And, while adult men seem to be smoking less, women and teenagers of both sexes seem to be smoking more. How does smoking affect the digestive system of all these people?

### *What Are Some of the Harmful Effects of Smoking on the Digestive System?*

Smoking has been shown to have harmful effects on all parts of the digestive system, contributing to such common disorders as heartburn and peptic ulcers. The effects of smoking on the liver often are not discussed, but studies show that smoking may alter the way in which the liver handles drugs and alcohol. In addition, smoking apparently changes the way in which food is processed by the body. In fact, there seems to be enough evidence to stop smoking solely on the basis of digestive distress.

---

NIH Pub. 92–949.

## How Does Smoking Contribute to Heartburn?

Heartburn is a very common disorder among Americans. Heartburn is especially common among pregnant women, with 25 percent reporting daily heartburn and more than 50 percent experiencing occasional distress.

Most people will experience heartburn if the lining of the esophagus comes into contact with too much stomach juice for a long period of time. This stomach juice consists of acid produced by the stomach, as well as bile salts and digestive enzymes that may have washed into the stomach from the intestine.

Normally, a muscular valve at the lower end of the esophagus, the lower esophageal sphincter (LES), keeps the acid solution in the stomach and out of the esophagus. Sometimes the LES is weak and allows stomach juice to reflux, or flow backward into the esophagus.

Many people have occasional reflux episodes. Persons with heartburn usually have frequent episodes or fail to return the refluxed material to the stomach promptly. The prolonged contact of acid stomach juice with the esophageal lining injures the esophagus and produces burning pain. Smoking decreases the strength of the esophageal valve, thereby allowing more refluxed material into the esophagus.

Smoking also seems to promote the movement of bile salts from the intestine to the stomach to produce a more harmful reflux material. Finally, smoking may directly injure the esophagus, making it less able to resist further damage because of contact with refluxed material from the stomach.

## Does Smoking Cause Peptic Ulcers?

An ulcer is an open sore in the lining of the stomach or duodenum, the first part of the small intestine. The exact cause of ulcers is not known. A relationship between smoking cigarettes and ulcers, especially duodenal ulcers, does exist. The 1989 Surgeon General's Report stated that ulcers are more likely to occur, less likely to heal, and more likely to cause death in smokers than in nonsmokers.

Why is this so? Doctors are not really sure, but smoking does seem to be one of several factors that work together to promote the formation of ulcers.

Stomach acid is important in producing ulcers. Normally, most of this acid is buffered by the food we eat. Most of the unbuffered acid that enters the duodenum is quickly neutralized by sodium bicarbonate, a naturally occurring alkali produced by the pancreas. Some studies show that smoking reduces the bicarbonate produced by the pancreas, interfering with the neutralization of acid in the duodenum. Other studies suggest that chronic cigarette smoking may increase the amount of acid secreted by the stomach. There also is some evidence suggesting that smoking increases the speed at which the stomach empties its acid contents into the small intestine. Although the evidence is inconclusive on some of these issues, all are possible explanations for the higher rate and slower healing of ulcers among smokers.

Whatever causes the link between smoking and ulcers, two points have been repeatedly demonstrated: persons who smoke are more likely to develop an ulcer, especially a duodenal ulcer, and ulcers are less likely to heal quickly among smokers in response to otherwise effective treatment. This research tracing the relationship between smoking and ulcers strongly suggests that a person with an ulcer should stop smoking.

## How Does Smoking Affect the Liver?

The liver is a very important organ that has many tasks. Among other things, the liver is responsible for processing drugs, alcohol, and other toxins to remove them from the body. There is evidence that smoking alters the ability of the liver to handle these substances. In some cases, this may influence the dose of medication necessary to treat an illness. One theory, based on current evidence also suggests that smoking can aggravate the course of liver disease caused by excessive alcohol intake.

## Does Smoking Help Control Weight?

A common belief is that smoking helps to control weight. Smokers do, indeed, weigh less, on the average, than nonsmokers. And those who quit smoking are more likely to gain weight. Most people think this is because smokers eat less than nonsmokers.

Some researchers have found, however, that smokers actually eat more than nonsmokers. How can they weigh less? What happens to the extra calories? Scientists are not really sure about the answers to these questions, but they caution smokers not to think that just because they weigh less, they are healthier than if they didn't smoke. Research shows that the bodies of smokers use food less efficiently than nonsmokers. Scientists are still studying what implications this has on the long-range health of smokers.

## Can the Damage to the Digestive System Be Reversed?

Some of the effects of smoking on the digestive system appear to be of short duration. For example, the effect of smoking on bicarbonate production by the pancreas does not appear to last. Within a half-hour after smoking, the production of bicarbonate returns to normal. The effects of smoking on how the liver handles drugs also disappear when a person stops smoking. While doctors suspect that most other digestive abnormalities caused by smoking would also disappear soon after stopping smoking, this question has received little study.

## Summary

While all the evidence is not yet available, it seems clear that smoking cigarettes plays an important role in causing some digestive diseases. The relationship between heartburn and smoking is very clear. The link between smoking and ulcers, especially duodenal ulcers, seems indisputable. Studies showing that cigarettes affect the way the liver processes drugs, alcohol, and other substances suggest more problems for smokers.

Not all the effects of smoking on the digestive system are understood clearly. However, the evidence that is available makes a powerful statement that smoking is bad for digestive health.

## Additional Readings

Office on Smoking and Health, Public Information Branch. Publishes and distributes materials on smoking and health, including the Surgeon General's annual reports. Park Building, Room 1-18, 5600 Fishers Lane. Rockville, MD 20857 (301) 443-5287.

National Digestive Diseases Information Clearinghouse. Provides information about digestive diseases, including heartburn and peptic ulcer. Box NDDIC, 9000 Rockville Pike, Bethesda, MD 20892 (301) 468-6344.

National Digestive Diseases Information Clearinghouse is a service of the National Institute of Diabetes and Digestive and Kidney Diseases, part of the National Institutes of Health, under the U.S.

Public Health Service. The clearinghouse was authorized by Congress to focus a national effort on providing information to the public, patients and their families, and doctors and other health care professionals. The clearinghouse works with organizations to educate people about digestive health and disease. The clearinghouse answers inquiries; develops, reviews, and distributes publications; and coordinates informational resources about digestive diseases.

Publications produced by the clearinghouse are reviewed carefully for scientific accuracy, appropriateness of content, and readability. Publications produced by sources other than the clearinghouse are also reviewed for scientific accuracy and are used, along with clearinghouse publications, to answer requests.

Chapter 7

# Gas in the Digestive Tract

Gas in the digestive tract is not a subject that most people like to talk about, but the truth is that all of us have it and must get rid of it in some way. Normally, the gas passes out through the rectum or is belched through the mouth. These are both necessary functions of the body that allow us to eliminate gas.

When gas does not pass out of the body easily, it can collect in some part of the digestive tract, causing bloating and discomfort. Even normal amounts of gas in the body can bother people who are sensitive to this pressure. Although gas usually is not a sign of a medical problem, it can be. So if you have persistent or extreme gassiness (flatulence), mention it to your doctor when you have a checkup.

## What Causes Gas?

A common source of upper intestinal gas is swallowed air. Each time we swallow, small amounts of air enter the stomach. This gas in the stomach is usually passed into the small intestine where part of it is absorbed. The rest travels into the colon (large intestine) to be passed out through the rectum.

In some people, part of the gas is belched out instead of being passed from the stomach into the intestine. This happens for several reasons. People under a lot of stress often swallow large amounts of air. Some people swallow air frequently because they have postnasal drip, chew gum, or smoke. Rapid eating or poorly fitting dentures also

---

NIH Pub. 92-883.

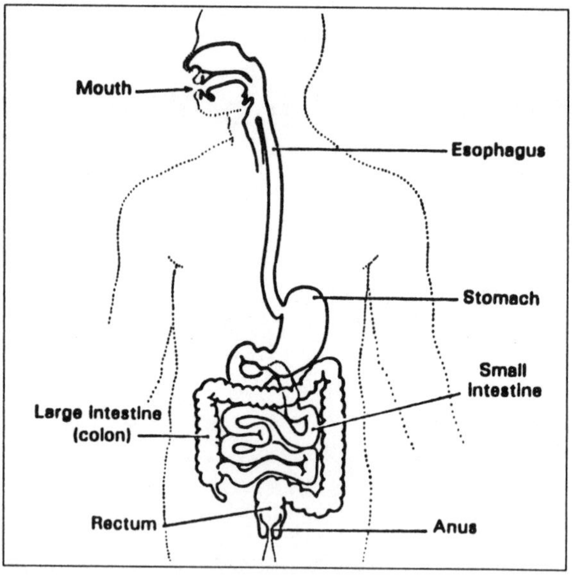


***Figure 7.1.*** *The Digestive System.*

may cause too much air to be swallowed. Also, drinking beverages that contain carbonated water may increase gas in the digestive tract. These drinks contain carbon dioxide, which can produce large amounts of gas when warmed in the stomach. People with a gas problem should avoid carbonated or "sparkling" drinks.

## What Causes Repetitive Belching?

Some people experience frequent belching. This might occur after a person has swallowed air without realizing it. Sometimes belching accompanies movement of stomach material back up (reflux) into the esophagus (swallowing tube). To clear material from the esophagus, a person may swallow frequently, which leads to more intake of air and further belching.

Another cause of repeated belching is gastritis (inflammation of the stomach). There are many causes of acute or chronic gastritis, but the most common cause is infection with a bacterium called *Helicobacter pylori*. When this organism gets into the stomach, it can produce bloating. This condition usually can be diagnosed by a specialist in digestive diseases (gastroenterologist). The doctor may detect the infection with a breath test or a blood test. The doctor also may take a sample of tissue (biopsy) from the stomach, using a lighted, flexible tube (endoscope) that is inserted through the mouth. *Helicobacter pylori* infection usually is treated with antibiotics and a bismuth preparation.

## Do Any Foods Cause Gas?

The foods we eat can be a factor in the production of gas in the lower intestine. Some foods such as cauliflower, brussel sprouts, dried beans, broccoli, cabbage, and bran are not completely digested in the small intestine. When the undigested bits of food reach the colon, they are fermented by the bacteria that live in the colon, causing gas.

Today many people are trying to improve their nutrition and health by eating more fiber. However, some people discover that adding large amounts of fiber to their diets causes gassiness. This can happen when someone begins eating more whole grain cereals such as whole bran, oatmeal, or oat bran, or whole grain breads or fresh fruits, and vegetables. They get a feeling of being bloated when they first begin the high-fiber diet, but within 3 weeks or so, they may adapt to it. Some people, however, don't adapt, and the bloating from eating a lot of fiber can be a permanent problem.

A common cause of excess lower intestinal gas is that a person's body may not have enough lactase, an enzyme normally found in the small intestine. Lactase is needed to digest lactose, the sugar found in milk and other dairy products. When this sugar passes undigested into the colon, it is fermented by bacteria, and gas forms. This can be a cause of excessive flatulence.

If lactase deficiency is suspected of causing your gas, your doctor may tell you to stop eating dairy products for a while to see if you will have less gas. The doctor also may give you a blood test or a breath test to find out if you are lactose intolerant. The breath test detects hydrogen that is released by the bacteria as the undigested lactose ferments in the colon.

## How Much Gas Does the Body Produce?

The amounts of gas that people produce vary. Most people produce between a pint and a half gallon of gas each day. Oxygen, carbon dioxide, and nitrogen from swallowed air make up large part of flatus. Fermenting foods in the colon produce hydrogen and methane as well as carbon dioxide and oxygen. All of these components of flatus (gas) are odorless. The unpleasant odor of some flatus is the result of trace gases, such as hydrogen sulfide, indole, and skatole, which are produced when foods decompose in the colon.

## What Causes the Abdominal Pain and Bloating?

Eating a lot of fatty food can cause bloating and discomfort because the fat delays stomach emptying, allowing gas to build up there. This problem can be avoided by eating less fatty meals. The feeling of bloating in the abdomen may increase during the day and become most severe after a large meal. Many people think the bloated feeling after eating is caused by large amounts of gas. Researchers, however, have not found any connection between this symptom and the total amount of gas in the abdomen. Studies show that in some people even modest amounts (1 ounce to ½ pint) of gas in the intestine can cause spasms there, especially after eating.

Gas in the upper abdomen often is relieved by belching. Sometimes people try to swallow air to make themselves belch. This doesn't work, however, because it only adds to the amount of gas in the stomach and does not reduce the discomfort.

Gas can collect anywhere in the lower intestine. Often it collects on the left side of the colon, and the pain can be confused with heart disease. When gas collects on the right side of the colon, the pain can be like that caused by gallbladder disease or even appendicitis.

A bloated feeling is probably not anything to be concerned about, but it can be a symptom of a more serious problem, such as an intestinal obstruction. If your problem is chronic, or if you are experiencing a severe increase in gassiness, you should talk to your doctor.

## Is Gassiness Caused by a Disease?

If excess gas is your only symptom, it is probably not caused by a disease. The problem may occur simply because you swallow air or digest food incompletely. It could be that your intestines have the kind of bacteria that produce a lot of gas. You could have a sluggish bowel that does not get rid of air readily. You might have an irritable bowel, often called spastic colon, which means that you cannot tolerate gas accumulation inside of the intestines, so even small amounts of air feel uncomfortable.

## Do Over-the-Counter Drugs Relieve Gas?

Many claims are made for over-the-counter drugs intended to relieve gassiness. Often people find that these drugs do not help much, but some of them do help some people. Simethicone, activated charcoal, and digestive enzymes, such as the lactose supplement lactase, are among those doctors often recommend. Sometimes doctors prescribe drugs called gastrointestinal stimulants that help move gas through the intestines more readily and that may help gassiness in some cases.

## Some Suggestions on How to Reduce Gas in the Digestive Tract

If you are bothered by excessive belching or flatus, and your physician has determined that you have no serious disease, the following suggestions may be helpful:

- Check with a dentist to make sure dentures fit properly.
- Avoid chewing gum or sucking on hard candies (especially sugarless gum or dietetic candies that contain sorbitol).
- Eliminate carbonated beverages from your diet.
- Avoid milk and milk products if you have lactose intolerance.
- Eat fewer gas-producing foods such as cauliflower, brussels sprouts, bran, beans, broccoli, and cabbage.
- Walking, jogging, calisthenics, and other exercises help to stimulate the passage of gas through the digestive tract.

If your symptoms persist or worsen, see your doctor to make sure that the condition is not caused by abnormalities in your digestive tract.

## Additional Readings

Clayman, CB, ed. *The American Medical Association Encyclopedia of Medicine*. New York: Random House, 1989. Reference guide with sections on digestive tract gas and other digestive problems. Available in libraries and bookstores.

Jain, NK, Vela, JS, Pitchumoni, CS. "Intestinal Gas: Insights into an Ancient Malady." *Practical Gastroenterology* 1987; 11(6): 32–44. Review article for physicians discusses the causes and treatments of gas. Available in medical libraries.

Levitt, MD. "Intestinal Gas: What Do We Offer the Patient?" *Endoscopy Review* 1991; 8(5): 43–46. Article for physicians discusses the causes, evaluations, and treatments for gas. Available in medical libraries.

Larson, DE, editor. *Mayo Clinic Family Health Book*. New York: William Morrow and Company, Inc., 1990. General medical guide with section on intestinal gas. Available in libraries and bookstores.

**National Digestive Diseases Information Clearinghouse**
Box NDDIC
9000 Rockville Pike
Bethesda, MD 20892
(301) 468-6344

The National Digestive Diseases Information Clearinghouse is a service of the National Institute of Diabetes and Digestive and Kidney Diseases, part of the National Institutes of Health, under the U.S. Public Health Service. The clearinghouse was authorized by Congress to focus a national effort on providing information to the public, patients and their families, and doctors and other health care professionals. The clearinghouse works with organizations to educate people about digestive health and disease. The clearinghouse answers inquiries; develops, reviews, and distributes publications; and coordinates informational resources about digestive diseases.

Publications produced by the clearinghouse are reviewed carefully for scientific accuracy, appropriateness of content, and readability. Publications produced by sources other than the clearinghouse also are reviewed for scientific accuracy and are used, along with clearinghouse publications, to answer requests.

## Chapter 8

# *Hazards of Laxative Overuse*

If you reach for a laxative every time your bowels refuse to move, you could be headed for trouble. Laxatives are, after all, drugs, the Food and Drug Administration warns. And, like other drugs, they pose the risk of side effects and habituation. Moreover, use of a laxative at the onset of constipation could delay treatment for a serious underlying problem that's causing the irregularity.

"If you have a change of bowel habits, it's really important for you to see your doctor," says Stephen Fredd, M.D., FDA's director of gastrointestinal and coagulation drug products. "Later, if you do take laxatives, make sure you follow instructions carefully and don't overuse them. Overuse can lead to a worsening of the patient's condition. People who think they need laxatives frequently shouldn't take them on their own. They should see their doctor."

FDA announced in a Federal Register notice on Nov. 7, 1990, a ban on 23 laxative ingredients due to lack of proof of their effectiveness. After the ban takes effect in May, manufacturers wishing to continue using any of these ingredients in over-the-counter (OTC) products must prove the ingredient is safe and effective and obtain FDA approval.

The FDA Advisory Panel on Over-the-Counter Laxatives, Antidiarrheal, Emetic, and Anti-emetic Drugs in 1975 analyzed the ingredients in most OTC oral and rectal laxatives available in the United

---

DHHS Pub. (FDA) 92-1182. This article originally appeared as "Overuse Hazardous: Laxatives Rarely Needed" in *FDA Consumer*, the magazine of the U.S. Food and Drug Administration. For a sample copy of *FDA Consumer* write to: Food and Drug Administration, HFI-40, Rockville, MD 20857.

States. It approved some ingredients as safe and effective for temporary use (category I), some as unsafe and ineffective (category II), and some as lacking sufficient data on safety and effectiveness, needing further testing (category III). A key finding of the advisory panel was that overuse of laxatives was common. This continues to be a problem.

Many people are under the impression that serious health-endangering consequences will occur if the bowel is not evacuated daily. According to the report, in most cases, this isn't true; there is no evidence to suggest that a daily bowel movement is a must.

In fact, the normal range varies from as many as three bowel movements a day to as few as three a week. Even when constipation does develop, sufferers can usually relieve their symptoms by increasing their fiber and fluid intake, or simply by altering their daily routines to allow more time on the commode to relax and let nature take its course.

## Avoid the Quick Fix

"The public should get out of the habit of taking a quick laxative fix," says William H. Lipshutz, M.D., clinical professor of medicine at the University of Pennsylvania and head of gastroenterology at Pennsylvania Hospital in Philadelphia. "True, laxatives are of value before a patient undergoes a test or a procedure which requires us to look inside the bowels. But frequent or habitual use of laxatives to promote evacuation can lead to addiction and the ultimate destruction of neurological and muscular control of the large intestine."

Prolonged laxative use can also deplete the body of fluids, salts, and essential vitamins and minerals and inhibit the absorption or effectiveness of other drugs. Furthermore, it can cause dizziness, confusion, fatigue, skin irritation, diarrhea, irregular heartbeat, belching, and a range of other side effects, depending on the laxative used.

For these reasons, the panel stated that OTC laxative drug products should bear labels with a warning to consumers not to use laxatives for more than one week except on the advice of a physician. The agency's proposed labeling claim for laxatives is "For relief of occasional constipation (irregularity)."

In addition, consumers should also be warned not to use laxatives in the presence of abdominal pain, nausea or vomiting unless directed by a doctor. The greatest danger here is taking a laxative during an attack of appendicitis, because the action of the drug can cause the appendix to rupture.

FDA expanded the panel's recommendations by proposing in the Federal Register of January 15, 1985, that the labeling for laxatives inform consumers how the product works, how to use it, and how long it takes to achieve its effect. The agency also proposed that the label advise the patient to see a doctor if the recommended dose of the laxative has had no effect after one week, if rectal bleeding develops, or if a sudden change of bowel habits lasts two weeks or more. In addition, FDA proposed that the words "regular" and "regularity" (to imply a daily bowel movement is normal and desirable) not be used in the labeling of OTC laxative drug products.

Other proposed labeling caveats depend on the laxative ingredients present in the product and on the age of the patient. Special restrictions have been proposed for laxative use by small children. Therefore, FDA cautions consumers to read all label warnings and instructions before taking or administering a laxative.

Prolonged laxative use without consulting a physician is not advisable because:

- An underlying problem or condition such as stress, depression, lack of exercise, an underactive thyroid gland, kidney failure, and colon or rectal cancer may be causing the irregularity.

- Diet may be playing a role. Quite often, constipation results from lack of sufficient fiber or liquids in the diet. Sometimes it develops from eating too many foods that promote constipation, such as processed cheese and eggs.

- Drugs the patient is taking may be causing the irregularity: Antacids, antidepressants, antihistamines, and calcium-channel blockers are some drugs that can interfere with regularity.

## Lifestyle Changes

In most cases, patients can alleviate constipation with dietary and lifestyle changes.

For example, if the constipation results from a lack of dietary fiber, which is necessary to form easily passed stools, patients can increase their intake of fiber-rich foods such as potatoes, beans (kidney, navy, lima, pinto), whole-grain breads, bran cereals, and fresh fruits, along with vegetables such as asparagus, brussel sprouts, cabbage, carrots, cauliflower, corn, peas, kale, and parsnips. They can also limit the amount of foods they eat that have little or no fiber, such as ice cream, soft drinks, cheese, white bread, and meat.

If lack of exercise or a fast-paced daily routine is at fault, patients may be able to take the necessary steps to rectify the problem. Sometimes the solution lies in combining lifestyle and dietary changes. Talking with a psychotherapist may be advisable for patients who become preoccupied with their bowel habits.

For persons in relatively good health, laxatives should be a last resort. Persons suffering from heart disease, high blood pressure, hemorrhoids, hernia, and stroke-related conditions may take laxatives according to a physician's instructions to reduce straining. In addition, pregnant women, bedridden constipated patients, surgery patients, and patients preparing for rectal or intestinal exams may take laxatives under a physician's supervision.

Patients should read labels and avoid products that might affect them adversely. Kidney patients, for example, should steer clear of saline laxatives containing potassium, magnesium or phosphates. Bedridden patients should avoid taking mineral oil orally; it can cause pneumonia if accidentally inhaled.

## Be Alert to Adverse Effects

Patients should discontinue use and consult their doctors immediately if laxative use causes asthma, skin rash, dizziness, irregular heartbeat, dehydration, muscle cramps, nausea, or other side effects. Unless advised otherwise by a physician, consumers should avoid prolonged laxative use because of the potential for habituation.

"Habitual use and abuse of laxatives (especially stimulant laxatives) can damage the nerves and muscles of the bowel to the point that the patient can't evacuate at all," warns Lipshutz. "So, in attempting to relieve irregularity, the patient actually starts creating it. In other words, the laxatives eventually do the direct opposite of what they're supposed to do."

Moreover, laxatives can react adversely with other drugs and hamper the body's ability to absorb nutrients. Mineral oil, for example, can limit the effectiveness of other medicines and inhibit absorption of vitamins A, D, E, and K.

Furthermore, if a laxative-induced evacuation empties the bowels completely (which can happen when large laxative doses are taken), several days may pass before new stools form. In the interim, the user may mistakenly conclude that he or she is constipated again and decide to resume a laxative regimen. If this pattern continues, the bowels may eventually stop functioning.

Although the makers of some laxatives have promoted the ingredients in their products as "natural" enhancers of bowel movements, the FDA advisory panel found such claims unacceptable and recommended against including them on labels as indications of safety or effectiveness. Manufacturers may, however, indicate that an ingredient came from a natural source.

The panel also disapproved of claims for effectiveness on the basis of gender, age, and other demographic characteristics, although FDA has no objections to promotional efforts aimed at particular groups. The panel also said a pleasing taste cannot be used to support claims for effectiveness or to promote regular use.

To allow manufacturers enough time to revise formulas and labels, the final regulation for laxative drug products will become effective 12 months after its publication in the Federal Register. However, the deadline may come sooner for specially designated products, including those that may compromise public safety.

## Types of Laxatives

Laxatives now available over the counter come in liquid, tablet, gum, powder, granule, suppository, and enema dosage forms. They work in different ways to promote stool evacuation.

### Stimulant Laxatives

Stimulant laxatives agitate or excite intestinal walls, causing waves of muscular contractions that expel fecal matter. Product names include Carter' s Little Pills, Castor Oil, Dulcolax, Ex-Lax, Feen-A-Mint, Fletcher's Castoria, and Modane. FDA has banned the following stimulant-laxative ingredients beginning in May [1992]: calomel, colocynth, elaterin resin, gamboge, ipomea, jalap, podophyllum resin, aloin, bile salts, bile acids, calcium pantothenate, frangula, ox bile, prune concentrate, prune powder, rhubarb-Chinese, and sodium oleate.

### Lubricants

Lubricant laxatives "grease" stools, facilitating excretion. Mineral oil and mineral oil emulsion are the most common forms of lubricants. Among them are Agoral Plain and Fleet Mineral Oil Enema.

### Saline Laxatives

Saline laxatives act like a sponge to draw water into the bowel, thereby promoting easier passage of stools. Loss of body salts is a key risk of long term use of these products. Among laxatives in this group are Milk of Magnesia, Citrate of Magnesia, and Epsom Salts. The recent ban forbids the use of tartaric acid as a saline-laxative ingredient.

### Stool Softeners

Stool softeners, or emollients, soften hard stools by enabling them to absorb more liquids. They are often given to women after childbirth and to patients recovering from surgery. Brands include Colace, Dialose, Regutol, and Surfak. Stool softeners should never be taken within two hours of a mineral oil dose because the combination can result in excessive buildup of mineral oil in body tissues. Polaxarner 188 is now banned as a stool softener ingredient.

### Hyperosmotics

Hyperosmotic laxatives mimic the action of saline laxatives but pose less risk of salt depletion. OTC hyperosmotics such as glycerin are available for rectal use only. Oral hyperosmotics must be prescribed by a physician. Overuse of hyperosmotics can cause continuing diarrhea.

### Carbon Dioxide Releasing Agents

Carbon dioxide releasing suppositories produce carbon dioxide in the bowels. The gas pushes stubborn stools toward excretion. The suppositories are available over the counter under the brand name Ceo-Two.

### Bulk Laxatives

Bulk-forming laxatives absorb water in the intestine and swell the stool into an easily passed soft mass. Each dose should be taken with an eight ounce glass of liquid. Although bulk agents are generally regarded as the safest form of laxative, users should be aware that the products can interfere with the absorption of certain drugs, including aspirin, digitalis, antibiotics, and anticoagulants. People with the genetic disorder phenylketonuria should not take any sugar-free bulk laxative containing phenylalanine, because it can damage their brain tissue.

Bulk laxatives include FiberCon, Metamucil, and Serutan. Although bran is considered a bulk agent, FDA has said that bran cereals marketed solely as food products will not be subject to laxative regulations. However, any bran product marketed as a laxative will be regarded as a drug and, therefore, must conform with FDA rules.

The following bulk-laxative ingredients are now banned: carrageenan (degraded), agar, carrageenan (native), and guar gum. Many bulk-laxative products contain water-soluble gums as their active ingredients—for example, karaya, methylcellulose, plantago seed, psyllium, and polycarbophil. Recognizing that water-soluble gums taken without adequate water can cause problems, FDA proposed in the Federal Register of October 30, 1990, that products containing water-soluble gums have the following warning on their labels:

> "Warning: (Select one of the following, as appropriate: Take or Mix) this product with at least 8 ounces (a full glass) of water or other fluid. Taking this product without adequate fluid may cause it to swell and block your throat or esophagus and may cause choking. Do not take this product if you have ever had difficulty in swallowing or have any throat problems. If you experience chest pain, vomiting, or difficulty in swallowing or breathing after taking this product, seek immediate medical attention."

## *Combination Laxatives and Bowel Cleansing Systems*

Some products contain a combination of laxatives that act together to promote evacuation. These drugs may carry a higher risk of side effects. A combination laxative drug with more than two active ingredients will be permitted only if it can be shown that the combination is equal to or better than each of the active ingredients used alone at its therapeutic dose and presents no additional safety risk.

Although bowel cleansing systems contain a number of ingredients, these ingredients are used sequentially at specified intervals and are not true combination drug products. Bowel cleansing systems are used to evacuate the bowel before surgery or diagnostic exams. But such products are not intended for general laxative use and will be labeled for use only as directed by a doctor.

*—by Mike Cummings*

## Chapter 9

# *When Do You Need an Antacid?*

You can't believe you ate the whole thing. But you did. All seven courses. Then you had two helpings of dessert. Then, to be sociable, you had a couple of drinks. Or maybe three or four.

And now you're paying for it. You've got a "burning sensation" in your stomach or your chest, or maybe you feel all knotted up inside.

Your first reaction may be to reach for your favorite antacid to make the hurting go away. And if you do, you won't be alone.

Americans are currently spending close to $1 billion per year on these popular, over-the-counter drugs. Used according to directions and in moderation, they can quickly relieve the symptoms associated with occasional heartburn and indigestion. But these useful products may not always be necessary, and they have their dark side if used improperly.

"Improperly" means taking too much of an antacid over a short period, or using antacids frequently over a long period (weeks, months or years). Frequent and prolonged use of these products can cause irreparable harm to your heart, kidneys or bones.

Even if used occasionally and in moderation, antacids can mean bad news for people with special medical conditions.

Hugo Gallo-Torres, M.D., a medical officer with FDA's Center for Drug Evaluation and Research, said it's a good idea to consult your doctor before using antacids if you:

---

DHHS Pub. (FDA) 92–3179. This article originally appeared in *FDA Consumer,* the magazine of the U.S. Food and Drug Administration. For a sample copy of *FDA Consumer* write to: Food and Drug Administration, HFI-40, Rockville, MD 20857.

- are on any kind of medication
- are pregnant or breast-feeding
- have kidney problems
- have chronic constipation, diarrhea or colitis
- have stomach or intestinal bleeding
- have an irregular heartbeat
- have any kind of chronic illness
- have symptoms that may indicate appendicitis.

Though they cause problems for some, most people can take antacids without worrying. Consumers who use them only once in a while, and as directed, are unlikely to experience significant side effects.

But, like most everything else in life, moderation is the key.

"Antacids are useful drugs; they serve a purpose," said Gallo-Torres. "Ideally, though, it's always better to try dealing with heartburn and indigestion, at least initially, without taking any medications at all, or by avoiding trouble in the first place."

Gallo-Torres said there are some simple steps you can take that may help prevent heartburn or indigestion.

- Don't eat big meals. Your stomach has to work long and hard to process them, which means it has to produce a lot of acid. It helps to eat smaller, more frequent meals.

- Eat slowly. Downing a lot of food in a hurry can overwhelm your stomach, which responds by producing extra digestive acids.

- After you eat, don't lie down right away. If you do, you're more likely to have heartburn, because gravity is now preventing food from going speedily to the intestines. It's also a good idea to eat your last big meal at least three hours before bedtime. When you go to sleep, everything slows down, including your digestive system, so food you've eaten right before bedtime will stay in your stomach longer. It won't feel good.

- Don't wear tight-fitting garments. They can literally compress your stomach, making it more likely that the stomach's acid contents will enter your esophagus and cause a burning sensation.

- Cut down on caffeine; it makes your stomach produce more acid. Caffeine-heavy items include coffee, tea, chocolate, and some sodas.

- Avoid foods that contain a lot of acid, such as citrus fruits and tomatoes, and any other food that gives you problems.

- Cut back on alcohol and smoking. Both irritate the lining of your stomach and both tend to lower esophageal sphincter pressure. When this happens, it's easier for the contents of your stomach to shoot back up into your esophagus.

- Sleep with your head and shoulders propped up six to eight inches, so that your body is at a slight angle. This gets gravity working for you and not against you, and the digestive juices in your stomach are more likely to head south, for your intestine, instead of back up into your esophagus.

"If you do take an antacid, remember that what you're taking is a drug," Gallo-Torres said. "It is a drug that, in the vast majority of cases, should be used only for occasional relief of mild heartburn or indigestion. Antacids are fast-acting. They should bring relief within minutes. If you're taking antacids and there's no relief, then something else may be going on, something that requires a physician's evaluation."

Igor Cerny, a pharmacist with FDA's Center for Drug Evaluation and Research, agreed. "If you find yourself taking antacids frequently," he said, "you need to say to yourself: 'Wait a minute, I wasn't doing this before, so why am I doing it now? Something might be wrong with me.'"

"If your symptoms last more than two weeks, go see your doctor," he recommended. "Two weeks is the general rule of thumb. Beyond that, taking antacids can actually mask a more serious medical problem."

Cerny said it's a good idea to see your doctor even sooner—preferably right away—if you're experiencing any symptoms severe enough to interfere with your lifestyle, symptoms such as continuous vomiting or diarrhea, extreme discomfort or pain in your gastrointestinal (GI) tract, vomiting of blood or material that looks like coffee grounds (but which is actually digested blood), or any of these accompanied by fever.

"Using antacids to alleviate serious symptoms like these is like trying to put out a building fire with a hand-held extinguisher," Cerny said. "Serious symptoms require professional evaluation and treatment."

## A Quick Look Inside

Your entire digestive system is called the alimentary canal, or GI tract. About 30 feet from beginning to end, it includes your mouth (where digestion actually begins), esophagus, stomach, small intestine, and colon (also called the large intestine). Antacids do most of their work in the stomach.

The stomach serves as a kind of "holding tank" for food before it moves on to the intestines, where the major part of digestion takes place. But the stomach does more than just hold food. It helps with digestion, too. It secretes pepsin and hydrochloric acid, which work together to break down proteins into simpler compounds.

Under normal conditions, the digestive process rolls along quietly and efficiently, unnoticed. But every once in a while something happens down there that catches your attention: a burning sensation, a cramped or bloated feeling, or other unpleasant phenomena that tell you something is not quite right.

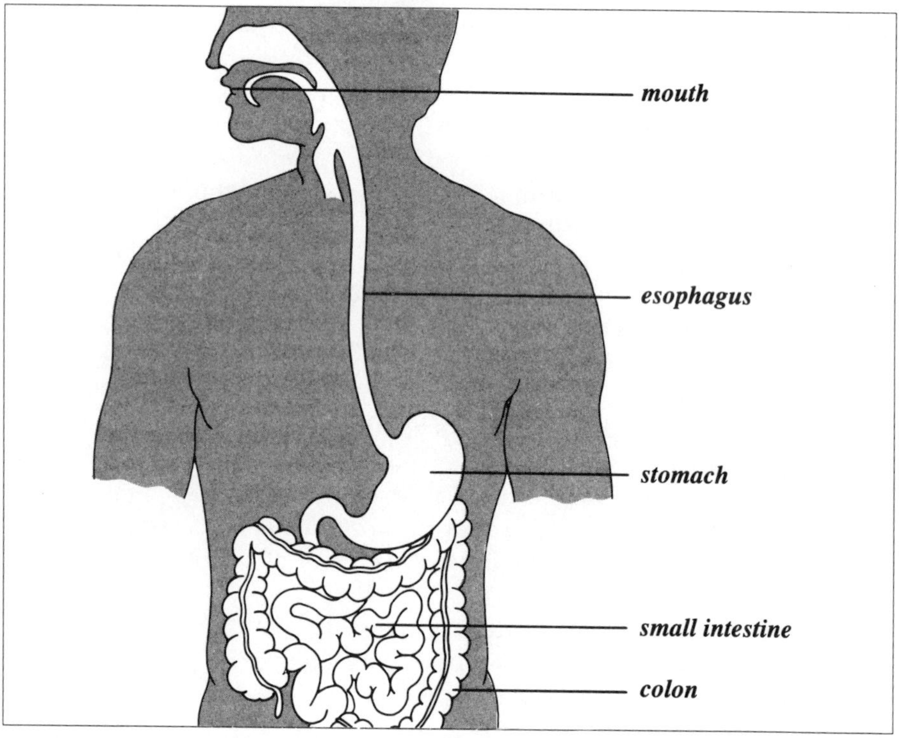


**Figure 9.1.** *The Digestive System.*

## The pH Factor

Antacids make you feel better by increasing the pH balance in your stomach. The pH system is a scale for measuring the acidity or alkalinity of a given environment (in this case, your stomach). The scale goes from zero to 14.

Seven is neutral. Below seven is acid. Above seven is alkaline.

Normally, the acid level in your stomach is about 2 or 3. Trouble may start when your pH drops below those numbers.

To make you feel better, an antacid need not bring the pH level all the way up to 7 (neutral), which would be a highly unnatural state for your stomach anyway. In order to work, all the antacid has to do is get you to 3 or 4. It does this by neutralizing some of the excess acid.

## So What's Wrong with Me Anyway?

The world of gastrointestinal disorders is a complex and sometimes baffling one. If you're feeling pain or discomfort in your GI tract, it could be something as unworrisome as simple indigestion, or maybe a stress ulcer.

Or it could be cancer.

In between these extremes are a billion other possibilities (a slight exaggeration, but you get the idea).

For example, your doctor may say you're suffering from non-ulcer dyspepsia. According to the Handbook of Nonprescription Drugs (ninth edition), non-ulcer dyspepsia "refers to intermittent [on and off] upper abdominal discomfort, the cause of which is not clearly defined."

In other words, when you get right down to it, non-ulcer dyspepsia is a catch-all term used for all sorts of stomach upset problems. Some symptoms include upper abdominal pain, nausea, vomiting, bloating, and indigestion.

Indigestion is another fuzzy word. Some people like to call it sour stomach, or acid indigestion, or upset stomach, or acid stomach.

It could mean that you have a touch of gastritis (when your stomach lining becomes inflamed by too much acid secretion). Or it could mean you've simply eaten too much at once, and all that food is sitting heavy in your stomach, like a bowling ball, trying to get digested (as in the case of the massive overindulgence described at the beginning of this article).

Then there's heartburn, which is another matter.

Heartburn happens when the stomach's contents, along with all its corrosive digestive juices, goes into reverse and shoots back up into the esophagus (the tube that extends from the pharynx, or throat, into the stomach). Normally, the pressure in your stomach is lower than the pressure in your esophagus, which helps prevent food from re-entering the esophagus. But once in a while the delicate pressure system can break down.

This unsettling event, called gastroesophageal reflux (heartburn), may sometimes announce itself with an embarrassing belch.

But whether you make a noise or not, you feel the burning. The lining of your stomach is fairly accustomed to an acid environment, but your esophagus definitely isn't, so even a little acid in there will sometimes be enough to get your attention.

If gastroesophageal reflux is happening to you all the time, then you may have something called gastroesophageal reflux disease. It could be that your esophageal sphincter (the "door" between your esophagus and your stomach) is weak, chronically allowing the stomach's contents to push back out into the esophagus, burning it.

If the burning sensation is a little lower, and stays around for more than a few days, you could have another problem altogether: a peptic ulcer. An ulcer is simply a sore in your stomach that keeps getting irritated by all the acid swirling around down there.

Antacids can be used to treat all these GI problems. But most people who experience occasional discomfort somewhere along the GI tract, are likely not dealing with an ulcer, or stomach cancer, or anything else major.

Chances are it's run-of-the-mill heartburn or indigestion.

You don't need to see a doctor for occasional heartburn or indigestion. The hurting will disappear on its own. If you want some relief in the meantime, antacids will fit the bill nicely.

Again, it should be emphasized that if you experience unpleasant GI symptoms for more than two weeks, or if your symptoms are severe, it may be more than something run-of-the-mill.

Get it checked out.

## Recipe For Relief

FDA requires that every antacid on the market be safe (which means the antacid won't cause serious side effects, provided you take it in the proper dosage over the recommended period of time) and effective (which means the antacid will do what it's supposed to do).

Drug manufacturers must make and label their antacids according to specific guidelines in FDA's monograph on antacids. If manufacturers don't follow this federal antacids "recipe," they are not allowed to market their products.

According to FDA's monograph, an antacid is safe and effective if it meets the following conditions:

- It must contain at least one of the antacid active ingredients (acid neutralizers) approved by the agency. (All the approved ingredients are listed in the antacid monograph.)

- It must contain a sufficient amount of the active ingredients. Specifically, each active ingredient included in the antacid product must contribute at least 25 percent to the product's total neutralizing capacity.

- In a laboratory test, the antacid must neutralize a specific amount of acid and keep it neutralized for at least 10 minutes.

- The label on the antacid must state that the product is good only for relieving the symptoms of "heartburn," "sour stomach," "acid indigestion," and "upset stomach associated with these symptoms." The label can't make any other medical claims.

- The label must contain certain warnings concerning proper dosage, side effects (such as constipation or diarrhea), and how much sodium the product contains.

- The label must warn about the product's possible interactions with other drugs. Antacids can increase or decrease the speed at which some medications are eliminated from the body. For example, antacids can block the body's absorption of tetracycline, an antibiotic.

- The label must give directions for using the product, and it must carry a warning not to use the product for more than two weeks except under the supervision of a physician.

## What's In an Antacid?

The opposite of an acid is a base, and that's exactly what antacids are.

But a base all by itself can't neutralize the acid inside you. For reasons that are best explained on a blackboard in chemistry class, a base needs some chemical "helpers," or ingredients, to accompany it on its neutralizing mission into your stomach.

All antacids contain at least one of the four primary "helpers" or ingredients: sodium, calcium, magnesium, and aluminum.

Here's a brief rundown of the composition and some potential side effects of various antacids:

### Sodium (Alka-Seltzer, Bromo Seltzer, and others)

Sodium bicarbonate or baking soda, perhaps the best known of the sodium-containing antacids, is potent and fast-acting. As its name suggests, it's heavy in sodium. If you're on a salt-restricted diet, and especially if the diet is intended to treat high blood pressure, take a sodium-containing antacid only under a doctor's orders.

### Calcium (Tums, Alka-2, Titralac, and others)

Antacids in the form of calcium carbonate or calcium phosphate are potent and fast-acting.

Regular or heavy doses of calcium (more than five or six times per week) can cause constipation. Heavy and extended use of this product may clog your kidneys and cut down the amount of blood they can process, and can also cause kidney stones.

### Magnesium (Maalox, Mylanta, Camalox, Riopan, Gelusil, and others)

Magnesium salts come in many forms: carbonate, glycinate, hydroxide, oxide, trisilicate, and aluminosilicates. Magnesium has a mild laxative effect; it can cause diarrhea. For this reason, magnesium salts are rarely used as the only active ingredients in an antacid, but are combined with aluminum, which counteracts the laxative effect. (The brand names listed above all contain magnesium-aluminum combinations.)

Like calcium, magnesium may cause kidney stones if taken for a very prolonged period, especially if the kidneys are functioning improperly to begin with. A serious magnesium overload in the bloodstream (hypermagnesemia) can also cause blood pressure to drop, leading to respiratory or cardiac depression (a potentially dangerous decrease in lung or heart function).

### *Aluminum (Rolaids, AlternaGEL, Amphojel, and others)*

Salts of aluminum (hydroxide, carbonate gel, or phosphate gel) can also cause constipation. For these reasons, aluminum is usually used in combination with the other three primary ingredients.

Used heavily over an extended period, antacids containing aluminum can weaken bones, especially in people who have kidney problems. Aluminum can cause dietary phosphates, calcium and fluoride to leave the body, eventually causing bone problems such as osteomalacia or osteoporosis.

It should be emphasized that aluminum-containing antacids present virtually no danger to people with normal kidney function who use these products only occasionally and as directed.

### *Simethicone*

Some antacids contain an ingredient called simethicone, a gastric defoaming agent that breaks up gas bubbles, making them easier to eliminate from your body.

FDA says simethicone is safe and effective in combination with antacids for relief of gas associated with heartburn. But not all antacids contain this ingredient.

If you're looking for relief of symptoms associated with gas, read the antacid's label carefully to make sure it contains simethicone.

*—by Tom Cramer*

Tom Cramer is a staff writer for *FDA Consumer*.

# Chapter 10

# *Harmful Effects of Medicines on the Adult Digestive System*

Many medicines taken by mouth may affect the digestive system. These medicines include prescription (those ordered by a doctor and dispensed by a pharmacist) and nonprescription or over-the-counter (OTC) products. A glossary at the end of this fact sheet describes some common prescription and nonprescription medicines discussed below that may affect the digestive system.

Although these medicines usually are safe and effective, harmful effects may occur in some people. OTCs typically do not cause serious side effects when taken as directed on the product's label. It is important to read the label to find out the ingredients, side effects, warnings, and when to consult a doctor.

Always talk with your doctor before taking a medicine for the first time and before adding any new medicines to those you already are taking. Tell the doctor about all other medicines (prescription and OTCs) you are taking. Certain medicines taken together may interact and cause harmful side effects. In addition, tell the doctor about any allergies or sensitivities to foods and medicines and about any medical conditions you may have such as diabetes, kidney disease, or liver disease.

Be sure that you understand all directions for taking the medicine, including dose and schedule, possible interactions with food, alcohol, and other medicines, side effects, and warnings. If you are an older adult read all directions carefully and ask your doctor questions about

---

NIH Pub. No. 92–3421.

the medicine. As you get older, you may be more susceptible to drug interactions that cause side effects.

People with a food intolerance such as gluten intolerance should make sure their medicines do not contain fillers or additives with gluten.

Check with your doctor if you have any questions or concerns about your medicines. Follow the doctor's orders carefully, and immediately report any unusual symptoms or the warning signs described below.

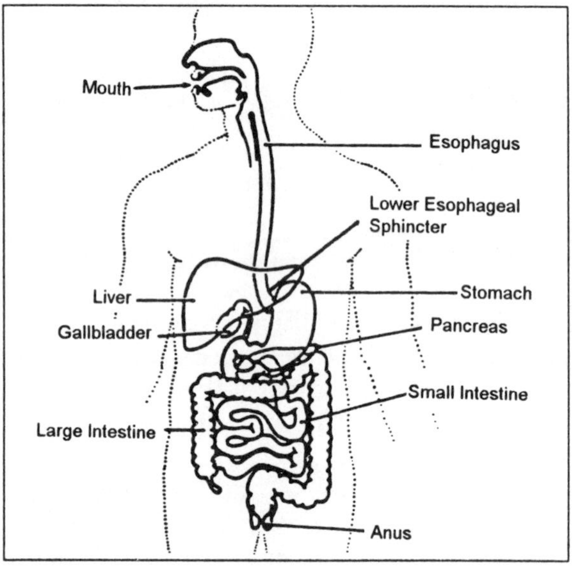


***Figure 10.1.*** *The Digestive System.*

## The Esophagus

### *Irritation*

Some people have difficulty swallowing medicines in tablet or capsule form. Tablets or capsules that stay in the esophagus may release chemicals that irritate the lining of the esophagus. The irritation may cause ulcers, bleeding, perforation (a hole or tear), and strictures (narrowing) of the esophagus. The risk of pill-induced injuries to the esophagus increases in persons with conditions involving the esophagus, such as strictures, scleroderma (hardening of the skin), achalasia (irregular muscle activity of the esophagus, which delays the passage of food), and stroke.

Some medicines can cause ulcers when they become lodged in the esophagus. These medicines include aspirin, several antibiotics such as tetracycline, quinidine, potassium chloride, vitamin C, and iron.

**Warning signs**

- Pain when swallowing food or liquid.
- Feeling of a tablet or capsule "stuck" in the throat.
- Dull, aching pain in the chest or shoulder after taking medicines.

**Precautions**

- Swallow tablets or capsules while you are in an upright or sitting position.
- Before taking a tablet or capsule, swallow several sips of liquid to lubricate the throat, then swallow the tablet or capsule with at least a full glass (8 ounces) of liquid.
- Do not lie down immediately after taking medicines to ensure that the pills pass through the esophagus into the stomach.
- Tell your doctor if painful swallowing continues or if pills continue to stick in the throat.

### *Esophageal Reflux*

The lower esophageal sphincter (LES) muscle is between the esophagus and the stomach. The muscle allows the passage of food into the stomach after swallowing. Certain medicines interfere with the action of the sphincter muscle, which increases the likelihood of backup or reflux of the highly acidic contents of the stomach into the esophagus.

Medicines that can cause esophageal reflux include nitrates, theophylline, calcium channel blockers, anticholinergics, and birth control pills.

**Warning Signs**

- Heartburn or indigestion.
- Sensation of food coming back up into the throat.

### Precautions

- Avoid foods and beverages that may worsen reflux, including coffee, alcohol, chocolate, and fried or fatty foods.
- Cut down on, or preferably quit, smoking.
- Do not lie down immediately after eating.

## The Stomach

### *Irritation*

One of the most common drug-induced injuries is irritation of the lining of the stomach caused by nonsteroidal anti-inflammatory drugs (NSAIDs) .

NSAIDs can irritate the stomach by weakening the ability of the lining to resist acid made in the stomach. Sometimes this irritation may lead to inflammation of the stomach lining (gastritis), ulcers, bleeding, or perforation of the lining. In addition, you should be aware that stomach irritation may occur without having any of the symptoms below.

Older people are especially at risk for irritation from NSAIDs because they are more likely to regularly take pain medicines for arthritis and other chronic conditions. Also at risk are individuals with a history of peptic ulcers and related complications or gastritis. These individuals should tell their doctor about any of these previous conditions. Special medicines may be needed to protect the stomach lining.

#### Warning Signs

- Severe stomach cramps or pain or burning in the stomach or back.
- Black, tarry, or bloody stools.
- Bloody vomit.
- Severe heartburn or indigestion.
- Diarrhea.

#### Precautions

- Use coated tablets, which may lessen stomach irritation.
- Avoid drinking alcoholic beverages while taking medicines.

- Take medicines with a full glass of water or milk or with food, which may reduce irritation.

### *Delayed Emptying of the Stomach*

Some medicines cause nerve and muscle activity to slow down in the stomach. This slowing down causes the contents of the stomach to empty at a slower rate than normal.

Drugs that may cause this delay include anticholinergics and drugs used to treat Parkinson's disease and depression.

#### Warning Signs

- Nausea.
- Bloating.
- Feeling of fullness.
- Vomiting of food eaten many hours earlier.
- Pain in mid-abdomen.
- Heartburn or indigestion.
- Sensation of food coming back up into the throat.

#### Precautions

- Eat frequent, small meals.
- Do not lie down for about 30 minutes after eating.
- Tell your doctor if symptoms continue. Your doctor may consider changing your dosage of your medicine or trying a new medicine.

## *The Intestine*

### *Constipation*

Constipation can be caused by a variety of medicines. These medicines affect the nerve and muscle activity in the large intestine (colon). This results in the slow and difficult passage of stool. Medicines also may bind intestinal liquid and make the stool hard.

Medicines that commonly cause constipation include antihypertensives, anticholinergics, cholestyramine, iron, and antacids that contain mostly aluminium.

### Warning Signs

- Constipation that is severe or disabling or that lasts several weeks.

### Precautions

- Drink plenty of fluids.
- Eat a well-balanced diet that includes whole grains, fruits, and vegetables.
- Exercise regularly.
- Take laxatives only under a doctor's supervision.

## *Diarrhea*

Diarrhea is a common side effect of many medicines. Diarrhea is often caused by antibiotics, which affect the bacteria that live normally in the large intestine.

Antibiotic-induced changes in intestinal bacteria allow overgrowth of another bacteria, Clostridium (C. difficile), which is the cause of a more serious antibiotic-induced diarrhea.

The presence of C. difficile can cause colitis, an inflammation of the intestine in which the bowel "weeps" excess water and mucus, resulting in loose, watery stools. Almost any antibiotic may cause C. difficile-induced diarrhea, but the most common are ampicillin, clindamycin, and the cephalosporins. Antibiotic-induced colitis is treated with another antibiotic that acts on C. difficile.

Diarrhea also can be a side effect of drugs that do not cause colitis but that alter the movements or fluid content of the colon. Colchicine is a common cause of drug-induced diarrhea. Magnesium-containing antacids can have the effect of laxatives and cause diarrhea if overused. In addition, the abuse of laxatives may result in damage to the nerves and muscles of the colon and cause diarrhea.

### Warning signs

- Blood, mucus, or pus in the stool.
- Pain in the lower abdomen.
- Fever.
- If diarrhea lasts for several days, consult your doctor.

## *The Liver*

The liver processes most medicines that enter the bloodstream and governs drug activity throughout the body. Once a drug enters the bloodstream, the liver converts the drug into chemicals the body can use and removes toxic chemicals that other organs cannot tolerate. During this process, these chemicals can attack and injure the liver.

Drug-induced liver injury can resemble the symptoms of any acute or chronic liver disease. The only way a doctor can diagnose drug-induced liver injury is by stopping use of the suspected drug and excluding other liver diseases through diagnostic tests. Rarely, long term use of a medicine can cause chronic liver damage and scarring (cirrhosis).

Medicines that can cause severe liver injury include large doses of acetaminophen (and even in small doses when taken with alcohol), anticonvulsants such as phenytoin and valproic acid, the antihypertensive methyldopa, the tranquilizer chlorpromazine, antituberculins used to treat tuberculosis such as isoniazid and rifampin, and vitamins such as vitamin A and niacin.

### Warning signs (for liver injury)

- Severe fatigue.
- Abdominal pain and swelling.
- Jaundice (yellow eyes and skin, dark urine).
- Fever.
- Nausea or vomiting.

### Precautions

- If you have ever had a liver disease or gallstones, you should discuss this with your doctor before taking any medicines that may affect the liver or the gallbladder.

- Take these medicines only in the prescribed or recommended doses.

## *Glossary of Medicines*

The following glossary is a guide to medicines used to treat many medical conditions. The glossary does not include all medicines that may affect the digestive system. If a medicine you are taking is not listed here, check with your doctor.

*Acetaminophen.* Acetaminophen relieves fever and pain by blocking pain centers in the central nervous system.

—Examples of brand names include Tylenol, Panadol, and Datril.

*Antacids.* Antacids relieve heartburn, acid indigestion, sour stomach, and symptoms of peptic ulcer. They work by neutralizing stomach acid.

—Aluminum hydroxide antacids include AluTab and Amphojel; calcium carbonate antacids include Tums, Alka Mints and Rolaids Calcium Rich; magnesium antacids include Mylanta and Maalox.

*Antibiotics.* Antibiotics destroy or block the growth of bacteria that cause infection.

—Hundreds of antibiotics are available, including penicillins (Amoxil, Amcil, and Augmentin), clindamycin, cephalosporins (Keflex and Ceclor), tetracyclines (Minocin, Sumycin, and Vibramycin), quinolones (Cipro), and sulfa drugs (Bactrim).

*Anticholinergics.* This class of medicines affects the nerve cells or nerve fibers and includes drugs for depression, anxiety, and nervousness.

—Examples of anticholinergics include propantheline (Probanthine) and dicyclomine (Bentyl). Examples of antidepressants include amitriptyline (Elavil and Endep), and nortriptyline (Aventyl and Pamelor).

—Medicines for relieving the symptoms of Parkinson's disease also are in this category. Examples include levodopa (Dopar), and carbidopa and levodopa combination (Sinemet).

*Anticonvulsants.* These medicines control epilepsy and other types of seizure disorders. They act by lessening overactive nerve impulses in the brain.

—Examples of this class of medicines include phenytoin (Dilantin) and valproic acid (Dalpro).

*Antihypertensives.* Antihypertensives lower high blood pressure. They act by relaxing blood vessels, which makes blood flow more easily.

—Examples of antihypertensives include methyldopa (Aldomet) and clonidine hydrochloride (Catapres).

*Antituberculins.* These drugs for tuberculosis limit the growth of bacteria or prevent tuberculosis from developing in people who have a positive tuberculin skin test.

—Brand names include INH, Dow-Isoniazid, Rifadin, and Rimactane.

*Calcium channel blockers.* These medicines for angina (chest pain) and high blood pressure affect the movement of calcium into the cells of the heart and blood vessels, relax blood vessels, and increase the flow of blood and oxygen to the heart.

—Examples of calcium channel blockers include diltiazem (Cardizem), nifedipine (Procardia), and verapamil (Isoptin).

*Chlorpromazine.* This tranquilizer relieves anxiety or agitation.

—Examples of brand names include Thorazine and Ormazine.

*Colchicine.* This medicine eases the inflammation from gout and prevents attacks from recurring.

*Iron.* Iron is a mineral the body needs to produce red blood cells. Iron supplements are used to treat iron deficiency or iron-deficiency anemia.

*Laxatives.* Many forms of laxatives are available for relieving constipation.

—Common brand names of laxatives include Phillips' Milk of Magnesia, Citroma, Epsom salts, Correctol, and ExLax.

*Nitrates.* These drugs for angina (chest pain) relax blood vessels and increase the flow of blood to the heart.

—Examples of generic and brand names include isosorbide dinitrate (Iso-Bid and Isonate) and nitroglycerin (Nitro-Bid and Nitrocap).

*Nonsteroidal anti-inflammatory drugs* (NSAIDs). These drugs block the body's production of prostaglandins, substances that mediate pain and inflammation. NSAIDs relieve the pain from chronic and acute inflammatory conditions, including arthritis and other rheumatic conditions, and pain associated with injuries, bursitis, tendinitis, and dental problems. NSAIDs also relieve pain associated with noninflammatory conditions.

—Generic and brand names of NSAIDs include aspirin (Bayer and Bufferin), ibuprofen (Advil, Nuprin, and Motrin), tometin (Tolectin), naproxen (Naprosyn), and piroxicam (Feldene).

*Potassium chloride.* Potassium is a vital element in the body. Potassium supplements help prevent and treat potassium deficiency in people taking diuretics.

*Quinidine.* This medicine often is used to correct irregular heartbeat.
—Brand names of quinidine include Quinalan and Quiniglute.

*Theophylline.* This medicine eases breathing difficulties associated with emphysema, bronchitis, and bronchial asthma. The medicine works by relaxing the muscles of the respiratory tract, which allows an easier flow of air into the lungs.
—Examples of brand names include TheoDur, Theophyl and Bronkodyl.

*Vitamins.* Vitamins serve as nutritional supplements in people with poor diets, in people recovering from surgery, or in people with special health problems.
—Niacin helps the body break down food for energy and is used to treat niacin deficiency and to lower levels of fats and cholesterol.
—Vitamin A is necessary for normal growth and for healthy eyes and skin.
—Vitamin C is necessary for healthy function of cells.

## Additional Readings

*AARP Pharmacy Service Prescription Drug Handbook.* Glenview, Illinois: Scott, Foreman and Company, 1988. General reference book for the public by the American Association of Retired Persons that provides information about medicines most frequently prescribed for persons over 50 years of age.

*Advice for the Patient: Drug Information in Lay Language,* USP DI, 12th edition. Rockville, Maryland: The United States Pharmacopeial Convention, 1992. Guide for the patient that provides information about medicines by brand and generic names in sections on dosage forms, proper use directions, precautions, and side effects.

*Drug Information for the Health Care Professional,* USP DI, 12th edition. Rockville, Maryland: The United States Pharmacopeial

Convention, 1992. Guide for health care professionals that provides information about medicines by brand and generic names in sections on pharmacology, indications, precautions, side effects, general dosing, dosage forms, and patient consultation.

Kimmey, MG. "Gastroduodenal Effects of Nonsteroidal Anti-inflammatory Drugs." *Postgraduate Medicine*, 1989; 85(5): 65–71. General review article for primary care physicians.

*Physicians' Desk Reference*, 46th edition. Montvale, New Jersey: Medical Economics Company, Inc., 1992. Reference book for health care professionals that includes information about 2,800 pharmaceutical products in sections on pharmacology, indications, contraindications, precautions, adverse reactions, and dosage and administration.

Stehlin, D. "How to Take Your Medicine: Nonsteroidal Anti-inflammatory Drugs." *FDA Consumer*, 1990; 24(5): 33–35. General review article for the public.

## *Additional Resources*

*National Council on Patient Information and Education.* 666 11th Street, NW, Suite 810, Washington, DC 20001; (202) 347-6711. Distributes resources to the public and health care professionals about prescription medicines.

The United States Pharmacopeial Convention, Inc. 12601 Twinbrook Parkway, Rockville, MD 20852; (301) 881-0666. Distributes information about drug use and drug standards to health professionals and the public.

**National Digestive Diseases Information Clearinghouse**
Box NDDIC
9000 Rockville Pike
Bethesda, MD 20892
(301) 468-6344

The National Digestive Diseases Information Clearinghouse is a service of the National Institute of Diabetes and Digestive and Kidney Diseases, part of the National Institutes of Health, under the U.S.

Public Health Service. The clearinghouse was authorized by Congress to focus a national effort on providing information to the public, patients and their families, and doctors and other health care professionals. The clearinghouse works with organizations to educate people about digestive health and disease. The clearinghouse answers inquiries; develops, reviews, and distributes publications; and coordinates informational resources about digestive diseases.

Publications produced by the clearinghouse are reviewed carefully for scientific accuracy, appropriateness of content, and readability. Publications produced by sources other than the clearinghouse also are reviewed for scientific accuracy and are used, along with clearinghouse publications, to answer requests.

# Chapter 11

# Directories of Digestive Diseases: Organizations for Patients and Professionals

## Directory of Digestive Diseases Organizations for Patients

This directory lists voluntary and private organizations involved in digestive diseases-related activities for patients. The organizations offer educational materials and other services.

**Alagille Syndrome Alliance**
**10630 S.W. Garden Park Place**
**Tigard, OR 97223**
**(503) 639-6217**

*Purpose*: Provides a support network for children, their parents, and others with Alagille syndrome.

*Materials*: Newsletter—*LiverLink*.

**American Celiac Society-Dietary Support Coalition**
**58 Musano Court**
**West Orange, NJ 07052**
**(201) 325-8837**

*Purpose:* Provides practical assistance to members and individuals with celiac disease and information about the disease to the public.

*Materials*: Newsletter—*Whooo's Report*.

---

This chapter is composed of two separate unnumbered publications of the National Institutes of Health, *Directory of Digestive Diseases Organizations for Patients* and *Directory of Digestive Diseases Organizations for Professionals.*

**American Liver Foundation (ALF)**
**1425 Pompton Avenue**
**Cedar Grove, NJ 07009**
**(800) 223-0179 or (201) 256-2550**

*Purpose:* Promotes awareness and supports research on liver disease; disseminates information about liver wellness, liver diseases, and prevention of liver disease with audiovisual and printed materials, seminars, and training programs; promotes organ donation; encourages vaccination against hepatitis B; serves as trustee of transplant funds; and offers support groups through local chapters.

*Materials:* Member newsletter—*Progress*; clinical newsletter for physicians—*Liver Update*; and pamphlets and fact sheets about liver diseases, transplantation, organ donation, and prevention of liver diseases.

**American Porphyria Foundation**
**P.O. Box 22712**
**Houston, TX 77227**
**(713) 266-9617**

*Purpose:* Advances awareness, research, and treatment of the porphyrias; provides self-help services for members; provides referrals to porphyria treatment specialists.

*Materials:* Informational brochures—*Common Questions About Porphyria, Acute Intermittent Porphyria, Porphyria Cutanea Tarda (PCT), Diet and Nutrition in Porphyria, Hematin, Erythropoietic Protoporphyria (EPP),* and *EPP In Children*; and newsletter.

**American Pseudo-obstruction and Hirschsprung's Disease Society, Inc. (APHS)**
**P.O. Box 772**
**Medford, MA 02155**
**(617) 395-4255**

*Purpose:* An international support organization that promotes public awareness of gastrointestinal motility disorders, in particular intestinal pseudo-obstruction and Hirschsprung's disease; provides education and support to individuals and families of children who have been diagnosed with these disorders through person-to-person contact, publications, and annual educational symposia; and encourages and supports medical research in the area of gastrointestinal motility disorders.

*Materials:* Member newsletter—*APHS Newsletter*, informational brochures about intestinal pseudo-obstruction and Hirschsprung's disease; GI Tract video and fun book for children ages 4-10 years; and additional audiovisual materials.

**American Society of Adults with Pseudo-Obstruction, Inc. (ASAP)**
**International Corporate Headquarters**
**19 Carroll Road**
**Woburn, MA 01801**
**(617) 935-9776**

*Purpose:* Advocacy group that educates the public and medical community about the existence of chronic intestinal pseudo-obstruction (CIP); provides support for adults affected with the disease; serves as resource for physicians for information about CIP as it affects adults; supplies information about disability, social security, medical insurance, drug protocols, and practical strategies for dealing with the many components of CIP; maintains a reference library of pertinent articles from recognized medical journals for patients and physicians; maintains close contact with physicians at major medical institutions who treat adults with CIP; and provides referral lists of physicians willing to diagnose and treat adults with CIP.

*Materials:* Member newsletter—*ASAP Forum*.

**Celiac Disease Foundation**
**(CDF) 13251 Ventura Blvd. #3**
**Studio City, CA 91604**
**(818) 990-2354**

*Purpose:* Non-profit corporation that provides services and support to persons with celiac disease and dermatitis herpetiformis, through programs of awareness, education, advocacy and research; telephone information and referral services; medical advisory board; and special educational seminars and quarterly meetings.

*Materials:* Member newsletter—*Celiac Disease Foundation Newsletter*; brochure; gluten-free food sources; and special announcements.

**Celiac Sprue Association/USA, Inc.**
**P.O. Box 31700**
**Omaha, NE 68131-0700**
**(402) 558-0600**

*Purpose:* National support organization that provides information and referral services for persons with celiac sprue and dermatitis herpetiformis and parents of celiac children. Made up of six regions in the United States with 42 chapters and 78 resource units.

*Materials:* Information sheets—*Celiac Sprue, Basics for the Gluten-free Diet, Gluten-free Commercial Products*; new patient packet; handbook—*On the Celiac Condition*; quarterly newsletter for celiacs—*Lifeline*; membership forms; chapter information; resource unit information; and promotion brochure.

**Center for Digestive Disorders**
**Central DuPage Hospital**
**25 North Winfield Road**
**Winfield, IL 60190-1295**
**(708) 682-1600 Ext. 6493**

*Purpose:* Multifaceted program to meet the needs of people who suffer from gastrointestinal problems; offers literature, videotapes, and educational meetings; and if medical care is needed, appropriate referrals are made.

*Materials:* Individual packets of information sent based on complaints, diseases, or symptoms; and videotapes for viewing on many topics.

**Crohn's & Colitis Foundation of America, Inc.**
**386 Park Avenue South, 17th floor**
**New York, NY 10016-8804**
**(800) 932-2423 or (212) 685-3440**

*Purpose:* Supports basic and clinical research on a cure and treatment for Crohn's disease and ulcerative colitis; conducts professional education activities; produces public service programs and a wide variety of literature about inflammatory bowel disease for patients and their families, professionals, and the public; and sponsors more than 97 chapters and satellite groups.

*Materials:* Patient education and instructional materials about all aspects of Crohn's disease and ulcerative colitis, including emotional factors and issues specific to women and children; resource guides; three full-length books; and magazine for foundation supporters—*Foundation Focus*.

**Cyclic Vomiting Syndrome Association (CVSA)**
**13180 Caroline Court**
**Elm Grove, WI 53122**
**(414) 784-6842**

*Purpose:* Provides patients, families, and professionals opportunities to offer and receive support and share knowledge about cyclic vomiting syndrome; actively promotes and facilitates medical research; increases worldwide public and professional awareness; and serves as a resource center for information.

*Materials:* Member newsletter—*Code V* and patient education publications.

**Digestive Disease National Coalition**
**711 2nd Street, NE, Suite 200**
**Washington, DC 20002**
**(202) 544-7497**

*Purpose:* Informs the public and the health care community about digestive diseases; seeks Federal funding for research, education, and training; and represents members' interests regarding Federal and state legislation that affects digestive diseases research, health care, and education.

*Materials:* Brochures and newsletter.

**Gastro-Intestinal Research Foundation**
**70 East Lake Street, Suite 1015**
**Chicago, IL 60601**
**(312) 332-1350**

*Purpose:* Supports research and training programs at the University of Chicago Medical Center, Section of Gastroenterology; sponsors educational activities for the public.

*Materials:* Newsletter and patient education pamphlet—*Inflammatory Bowel Disease.*

**Gluten Intolerance Group of North America**
**P.O. Box 23053**
**Seattle, WA 98102-0353**
**(206) 325-6980**

*Purpose:* Provides instructional and general information materials, as well as counseling and access to gluten-free products and ingredients to persons with celiac sprue and their families; operates telephone information and referral service; conducts educational seminars for health professionals; conducts and supports research; and offers leadership and assistance to 14 affiliates and local member contacts.

*Materials:* Cookbook; dietary recommendations; fact sheets; member newsletter—*GIG Newsletter;* videotapes; patient packets for celiac sprue and dermatitis herpetiformis; and dietary guidelines for hospitalized persons with celiac sprue and dermatitis herpetiformis.

**The Greater New York Pull-thru Network**
**62 Edgewood Avenue**
**Wyckoff, NJ 07481**
**(201) 891-5977**

*Purpose:* A national support network providing emotional support and information to patients and families of children who have had or will have a pull-thru type surgery to correct an imperforate anus or associated malformation, Hirschsprung's or other fecal incontinence problems. Support group meetings held quarterly. A chapter of United Ostomy Association.

*Materials:* Quarterly publication—*Pull-thru Network News.*

**Help for Incontinent People, Inc. (HIP)**
**P.O. Box 544**
**Union, SC 29379**
**(800) BLADDER or (803) 579-7900**

*Purpose:* A leading source of education, advocacy, and support to the public and to the health profession about the causes, prevention, diagnosis, treatments, and management alternatives for incontinence.

*Materials:* Quarterly newsletter—*The HIP Report; Resource Guide of Continence Products and Services*; and other educational materials, including books and audiovisuals.

**The Hemochromatosis Foundation, Inc.**
**P.O. Box 8569**
**Albany, NY 12208**
**(518) 489-0972**

*Purpose:* Through publications, symposia, and meetings provides information to the public, hemochromatosis families, and professionals about hereditary hemochromatosis (HH); conducts and raises funds for research; encourages early screening for HH; and offers genetic counseling along with support for patients and professionals.

*Materials:* Informational booklets for the public, affected families and professionals; and audiovisual materials for the public and professionals.

**Hepatitis B Coalition**
**1573 Selby Avenue, Suite 229**
**Saint Paul, MN 55104-6328**
**(612) 647-9009**

*Purpose:* Works to prevent transmission of hepatitis B in high-risk groups; to achieve vaccination of all infants, children and adolescents;

and to promote education and treatment for the hepatitis B carrier.

*Materials:* Newsletter—*Hepatitis B Coalition News* brochures, articles, videotapes, audiocassette tapes, and manuals for different ethnic populations.

**International Foundation For Bowel Dysfunction (IFBD)**
**P.O. Box 17864**
**Milwaukee, WI 53217**
**(414) 964-1799**

*Purpose:* Provides support and educational information for people affected by the various forms of functional bowel disorders, including irritable bowel syndrome (IBS), constipation, diarrhea, pain, and incontinence.

*Materials:* Quarterly newsletter—*Participate*; educational pamphlets; and fact sheets.

**Intestinal Disease Foundation, Inc.**
**1323 Forbes Avenue, Suite 200**
**Pittsburgh, PA 15219**
**(412) 261-5888**

*Purpose:* Provides one-on-one telephone support, educational programs and materials, and self-help groups for people with irritable bowel syndrome (IBS) and inflammatory bowel diseases primarily in the Pennsylvania/Ohio/West Virginia area; sponsors medical seminars and educational meetings; and provides a speakers bureau, research updates, and physician referral lists.

*Materials:* Member newsletter—*Intestinal Fortitude*; brochures; and books.

**Iron Overload Diseases Association, Inc.**
**433 Westwind Drive**
**N. Palm Beach, FL 33408**
**(407) 840-8512**

*Purpose:* Conducts programs, including professional education through symposia and exhibits at medical meetings; serves and counsels hemochromatosis patients and families; offers doctor referrals; promotes patient advocacy concerning insurance, Medicare, blood banks, and the Food and Drug Administration; encourages research; maintains international consortium; offers public information through the media; develops chapters and self-help groups; and sponsors annual symposium and annual IOD Awareness Week.

*Materials:* Booklet—*Overload: An Ironic Disease*; bimonthly newsletter—*Ironic Blood*; informational brochure—*Iron Overload Alert*; and fact sheet.

**National Center for Nutrition and Dietetics (NCND) of The American Dietetic Association**
**216 W. Jackson Boulevard**
**Chicago, IL 60606-6995**
**Consumer Nutrition Hot Line: (800) 366-1655**

*Purpose:* Provides consumers with direct and immediate access to reliable nutrition information. Callers may speak with a registered dietitian directly, may listen to regularly updated recorded nutrition messages in English and Spanish, or may be referred to a dietitian in their local area.

**National Organization for Rare Disorders (NORD®)**
**P.O. Box 8923**
**New Fairfield, CT 06812-1783**
**(800) 999-6673 or (203) 746-6518**

*Purpose:* Acts as a clearinghouse for information about rare disorders and brings together families with similar disorders for mutual support; fosters communication among rare disease voluntary agencies, government bodies, industry, scientific researchers, academic institutions, and concerned individuals; and encourages and promotes research and education on rare disorders and Orphan Drugs.

*Materials:* Fact sheets and reprints on rare disorders and newsletter—*Orphan Disease Update*.

**The Oley Foundation, Inc.**
**214 Hun Memorial A-23**
**Albany Medical Center**
**Albany, NY 12208**
**(800) 776-OLEY or (518) 445-5079**

*Purpose:* Promotes and advocates education and research in home parenteral and enteral nutrition; provides support and networking to patients through information clearinghouse and regional volunteer network; sponsors meetings and conferences, including annual patient/clinician conference; maintains consumers' representative speakers bureau; manages the North American Home Parenteral and Enteral Nutrition Patient Registry, formerly known as OASIS, which is a voluntary database of patient outcome information from across the

United States and Canada; and publishes annual summaries of results and basic statistics.

*Materials:* Newsletters—*Lifeline Letter* and *Lifeline p.s.*, published monthly; *North American HPEN Patient Registry Report*, published annually, containing summaries of results and basic statistics on home parenteral and enteral nutrition patient outcomes; and audiovisual materials on psychosocial issues.

**Pediatric Crohn's & Colitis Association, Inc.**
**P.O. Box 188**
**Newton, MA 02168**
**(617) 244-6678**

*Purpose:* Focuses on all aspects of pediatric and adolescent Crohn's disease and ulcerative colitis, including medical, nutritional, psychological, and social factors. Activities include information sharing, educational forums, newsletters, and hospital outreach program as well as support of research.

*Materials:* Information pamphlets: *The ABC's of Pediatric Inflammatory Bowel Disease; Crohn's Disease, Ulcerative Colitis, and School*; PCCA newsletter; video material; and membership forms.

**Reach Out for Youth with Ileitis and Colitis, Inc.**
**15 Chemung Place**
**Jericho, NY 11753**
**(516) 822-8010**

*Purpose:* Non-profit organization providing educational seminars and both individual and group support to patients and their families. Sponsor of The Center for Pediatric Ileitis and Colitis at North Shore University Hospital Cornell University Medical College. Fund-raising efforts support the Center's programs, clinical and laboratory research, and purchase of state-of-the-art equipment.

*Materials:* Newsletter—*The Inner Circle* and educational brochure—*The Inside Story.*

**TEF/VATER Support Network**
**15301 Grey Fox Road**
**Upper Marlboro, MD 20772**
**(301) 627-2131**

*Purpose:* Dedicated to the support of children and adults born with tracheoesophageal fistula, esophageal atresia, or VATER (V: vertebral defects, A: imperforate anus, TE: tracheoesophageal defects, R: radial and renal dysplasia).

*Materials:* Newsletter—*TEF/VATER SUPPORT Newsletter* and general information.

**The Simon Foundation for Continence**
**P.O. Box 835**
**Wilmette, IL 60091**
**(800) 23-SIMON or (708) 864-3913**

*Purpose:* Seeks to bring the topic of incontinence out of the closet and remove the stigma associated with it; provides educational materials to patients, their families, and the health care professionals who provide their care.

*Materials:* Quarterly newsletter—*The Informer*; hardbound 122-page book—*Managing Incontinence: A Guide to Living with Loss of Bladder Control*; video—*The Solution Starts with You*; I WILL MANAGE program director's kit—a community outreach program led by professionals; and additional patient education materials.

**United Ostomy Association, Inc. (UOA)**
**36 Executive Park, Suite 120**
**Irvine,CA 92714-6744**
**(800) 826-0826 or (714) 660-8624**

*Purpose:* Produces and distributes materials about ostomy care and management; through trained UOA members, offers practical assistance and emotional support to ostomy patients; sponsors annual youth rally and state and regional conferences for local affiliates; and 650 chapters serve people locally.

*Materials:* Journal—*Ostomy Quarterly*; patient education pamphlets; self-care handbooks; and audiovisual program.

**Wilson's Disease Association**
**P.O. Box 75324**
**Washington, DC 20013**
**(703) 636-3003**

*Purpose:* Serves as a communications and support network for individuals affected by Wilson's disease and related disorders of copper metabolism; and distributes information to professionals and the public.

*Materials:* Fact sheets about Wilson's disease and member newsletter.

## Directory of Digestive Diseases Organizations for Professionals

This directory lists organizations that represent health professionals involved in the study and treatment of digestive diseases. The organizations do not provide medical services or advice.

**American Association for the Study of Liver Diseases**
**c/o SLACK Inc.**
**6900 Grove Road**
**Thorofare, NJ 08086**
**(609) 848-1000**

*Purpose:* Provides a forum for ongoing research in liver disease.
*Materials:* Journal—*Hepatology*; member roster; newsletter.

**American College of Gastroenterology**
**4900-B South 31st Street**
**Arlington, VA 22206-1656**
**(703) 820-7400**

*Purpose:* Serves clinical and scientific information needs of member physicians and surgeons, who specialize in digestive and related disorders. Emphasis is on scholarly practice, teaching, and research.
*Materials:* Journal—*American Journal of Gastroenterology* and member newsletter.

**American Dietetic Association (ADA)**
**216 W. Jackson Boulevard**
**Chicago, IL 60606-6995**
**(312) 899-0040**

*Purpose:* Provides direction and leadership for dietetic practice, education, and research; offers scholarships and awards through the ADA foundation; and sponsors affiliated state groups.
*Materials:* Journal—*Journal of the American Dietetic Association*; and patient education publications, including three-part Food Sensitivity Series containing meal plans for lactose and gluten intolerant individuals.

**American Gastroenterological Association National Office**
**7910 Woodmont Avenue, Suite 914**
**Bethesda, MD 20814**
**(301) 654-2055**

*Purpose:* Fosters the development and application of the science of gastroenterology by providing leadership and aid, including patient care, research, teaching, continuing education, scientific communication, and matters of national health policy pertaining to gastroenterology.

*Materials:* Journals—*Gastroenterology* and *Gastrointestinal Disease Today* and member newsletter—*AGA News*.

**American Motility Society**
**c/o Sidney F. Phillips, M.D.,**
**President Gastroenterology Unit,**
**Mayo Clinic Rochester, MN 55905**
**(507) 255-6028**

*Purpose:* Promotes research and sponsors professional education seminars about gastro-intestinal motility topics, including disorders of esophageal, gastric, small intestinal, and colonic function; and sponsors biennial meeting (even years), symposia, and courses.

**American Pancreatic Association**
**c/o Howard A. Reber, M.D.**
**UCLA School of Medicine**
**10833 LeConte Avenue 72-215 CHS**
**Los Angeles, CA 90024-6904**
**(310) 825-4976**

*Purpose:* Provides forum for presentation of scientific research related to the pancreas.

*Material:* Journal—*PANCREAS*.

**American Society for Gastrointestinal Endoscopy**
**13 Elm Street**
**Manchester, MA 01944**
**(508) 526-8330**

*Purpose:* Provides information, training, and practice guidelines about gastrointestinal endoscopic techniques.

*Materials:* Journal—*Gastrointestinal Endoscopy; Clinical Update* (quarterly); clinical guidelines; member newsletter; and patient information brochures.

**American Society for Parenteral and Enteral Nutrition**
**8630 Fenton Street, Suite 412**
**Silver Spring, MD 20910-3805**
**(301) 587-6315**

*Purpose:* Offers information and continuing medical education to professionals involved in the care of parenterally and enterally fed patients.

*Materials:* Journals—*Journal of Parenteral and Enteral Nutrition* and *Nutrition in Clinical Practice*; member newsletter; product resource manual and monographs; nutrition support team resource kit; and standards for clinical guidelines.

**American Society of Abdominal Surgeons**
**675 Main Street**
**Melrose, MA 02176**
**(617) 665-6102**

*Purpose:* Sponsors extensive continuing education program for physicians in the field of abdominal surgery; maintains library.

*Materials:* Journal—*Journal of Abdominal Surgery* and member newsletter.

**American Society of Colon and Rectal Surgeons**
**85 West Algonquin Road, Suite 550**
**Arlington Heights, IL 60005**
**(708) 290-9184**

*Purpose:* Serves as information network for surgeons specializing in the diagnosis and treatment of colorectal disorders.

*Material:* Journal—*Diseases of the Colon and Rectum.*

**International Academy of Proctology**
**c/o George Donnally, M.D.**
**2209 John R. Wooden Drive**
**P.O.Box 1716**
**Martinsville, IN 46151**
**(317) 342-3686**

*Purpose:* Encourages study of diseases of the colon and accessory organs of digestion, and conducts seminars.

*Materials:* Journals—*Gastroenterology* and *Colon and Rectal Surgery.*

**National Center for the Study of Wilson's Disease, Inc.**
**432 W. 58th Street, Suite 614**
**New York, NY 10019**
**(212) 523-8717**

*Purpose:* Conducts genetic, pathological, biochemical, and clinical research about Wilson's and Menkes' diseases; and the interactions of copper, zinc, and iron and the genetic regulation of their metabolism; provides clinical care to patients with Wilson's and Menkes' diseases and related disorders; performs quantitative analyses of copper and zinc in body tissues and fluids, and of ceruloplasmin in serum for physicians and medical institutions; and disseminates information to professionals and the public.

*Material:* Brochure.

**North American Society for Pediatric Gastroenterology and Nutrition**
**c/o SLACK Inc.**
**6900 Grove Road**
**Thorofare, NJ 08086**
**(609) 848-1000**

*Purpose:* Promotes research and provides a forum for professionals in the areas of pediatric GI liver disease, gastroenterology, and nutrition. Associated with fellow organizations in Europe and Australia (ESPGAN, AUSPGAN).

*Materials:* Journal—*Journal of Pediatric Gastroenterology and Nutrition* and member newsletter.

**The Society for Surgery of the Alimentary Tract**
**c/o David Fromm, M.D., Secretary**
**4201 Saint Antoine**
**University Health Center, 6C**
**Detroit, MI 48201**
**(313) 577-5017**

*Purpose:* Provides forum for exchange of information among physicians specializing in alimentary tract surgery.

*Materials:* Journal—*American Journal of Surgery* and member newsletter.

**Society of American Gastrointestinal Endoscopic Surgeons**
**2716 Ocean Park Blvd., Suite 3000**
**Santa Monica, CA 90405**
**(310) 314-2404**

*Purpose:* Encourages study and practice of gastrointestinal endoscopy as integral part of surgery.

*Materials:* Guidelines and position statements.

**Society of Gastroenterology Nurses and Associates, Inc.**
**401 N. Michigan Avenue**
**Chicago, Il 60611**
**(800) 245-SGNA (312) 644-6610**

*Purpose:* Provides members with continuing education opportunities, practice and training guidelines, and information about trends and developments in the field of gastroenterology.

*Materials:* Journal—*Gastroenterology Nursing*, professional instructional and resource materials; and member newsletter—*SGNA News.*

**UNOS (United Network for Organ Sharing)**
**1100 Boulders Parkway, Suite 500**
**P.O. Box 13770**
**Richmond, VA 23225-8770**
**(800) 24-DONOR or (804) 330-8500**

*Purpose:* Improves the effectiveness of human organ donation, procurement, distribution, and transplantation; and maintains scientific registry of transplant data.

*Materials:* Journal—*UNOS Update* and other educational materials.

**Wound, Ostomy and Continence Nurses Society**
**2755 Bristol Street, Suite 110**
**Costa Mesa, CA 92626**
**(714) 476-0268**

*Purpose:* A professional nursing society that supports its members by promoting educational, clinical, and research opportunities to guide the delivery of expert health care to individuals with wounds, ostomies, and incontinence.

*Materials:* Journal—*Journal of Wound, Ostomy and Continence Nursing; Standards of Care*; member newsletter—*WOCN News*; ET nurse brochure; and professional education and resource materials.

**National Digestive Diseases Information Clearinghouse**
**2 Information Way**
**Bethesda, MD 20892-3570**
**(301)654-3810**

The National Digestive Diseases Information Clearinghouse (NDDIC) is a service of the National Institute of Diabetes and Digestive and Kidney Diseases, part of the National Institutes of Health, under the U.S. Public Health Service. The clearinghouse, authorized by Congress in 1980, provides information about digestive diseases and health to people with digestive diseases and their families, health care professionals, and the public. The NDDIC answers inquiries; develops, reviews, and distributes publications; and works closely with professional and patient organizations and government agencies to coordinate resources about digestive diseases.

Publications produced by the clearinghouse are reviewed carefully for scientific accuracy, content, and readability. Publications produced by other sources are also reviewed for scientific accuracy and are used, along with clearinghouse publications, to answer requests.

Chapter 12

# Digestive Diseases and the National Digestive Diseases Information Clearinghouse

## What Are Digestive Diseases?

The digestive tract is a complex system of organs that converts the food we eat into the nutrients we need to sustain our bodies.

Some conditions such as gas, heartburn, and indigestion may cause occasional discomfort but usually do not indicate a serious problem. However, digestive diseases such as pancreatitis, inflammatory bowel disease, hepatitis, ulcers, and gallstones are serious and potentially life-threatening illnesses.

Digestive diseases affect an estimated 60 million Americans. These diseases and their associated long-term complications have catastrophic social and economic consequences. They are responsible for approximately 13 percent of all admissions to hospitals in the United States and about 200,000 deaths each year. Digestive diseases cost the nation more than $60 billion annually, of which $45 billion are direct medical costs such as hospitalizations and medications.

## What is the National Digestive Diseases Information Clearinghouse?

The National Digestive Diseases Information Clearinghouse (NDDIC) is an information and referral service of the National Institute

---

This publication is an unnumbered publication of the National Institutes of Health.

of Diabetes and Digestive and Kidney Diseases (NIDDK), National Institutes of Health. The clearinghouse, authorized by Congress in 1980, is designed to increase knowledge and understanding about digestive diseases and health among people with digestive diseases and their families, health care professionals, and the general public. To carry out this mission, NDDIC works closely with professional, patient, and voluntary associations; Government agencies; and other digestive diseases organizations forming a unique network that identifies and responds to informational needs about these diseases.

## How Can the Clearinghouse Help You?

The NDDIC provides the following information products and services:

- Response to requests for information about digestive diseases—from information about available patient and professional education materials to statistical data about a variety of common diseases.

- Publications, including patient fact sheets and brochures, conference proceedings, monographs, article reprints, and materials developed by NDDIC and NIDDK about specific digestive diseases.

- The Digestive Diseases subfile of the Combined Health Information Database (CHID), which contains thousands of references to materials produced for patients and health care professionals, including fact sheets, brochures, books, articles, audiovisual materials, and other educational materials. The subfile is available to the public through BRS Online, a division of InfoPro Technologies, a national database vendor.

- DD Notes, the NDDIC newsletter that features news about digestive diseases research, special events, professional and patient organizations, and publications available from NDDIC and other organizations.

## How Can You Help Us?

The NDDIC's key sources of information are the individuals and organizations involved in providing informational and educational services related to digestive diseases. By informing the clearinghouse of your educational materials and programs, you expand the information base of products and services available through NDDIC. Please inform the clearinghouse about your resources and needs and add us to your mailing list.

You may write or call:

National Digestive Diseases Information Clearinghouse
Box NDDIC
9000 Rockville Pike
Bethesda, MD 20892
(301) 654-3810

# *Part Two*

# *Esophageal Problems*

Chapter 13

# Gastroesophageal Reflux Disease (Hiatal Hernia and Heartburn)

Gastroesophageal reflux disease (GERD) is a digestive disorder that affects the lower esophageal sphincter (LES), the muscle connecting the esophagus with the stomach. Many people, including pregnant women, suffer from heartburn or acid indigestion caused by GERD. Doctors believe that some people suffer from GERD due to a condition called hiatal hernia. In most cases, heartburn can be relieved through diet and lifestyle changes; however, some people may require medication or surgery. This fact sheet provides information on GERD: its causes, symptoms, treatment, and long-term complications.

## *What Is Gastroesophageal Reflux?*

Gastroesophageal refers to the stomach and esophagus. Reflux means to flow back or return. Therefore, gastroesophageal reflux is the return of the stomach's contents back up into the esophagus.

In normal digestion, the LES opens to allow food to pass into the stomach and closes to prevent food and acidic stomach juices from flowing back into the esophagus. Gastroesophageal reflux occurs when the LES is weak or relaxes inappropriately allowing the stomach's contents to flow up into the esophagus. Figure 13.1 shows the location of the LES between the esophagus and the stomach.

The severity of GERD depends on LES dysfunction as well as the type and amount of fluid brought up from the stomach and the neutralizing effect of saliva.

---

NIH Pub. 94–882.

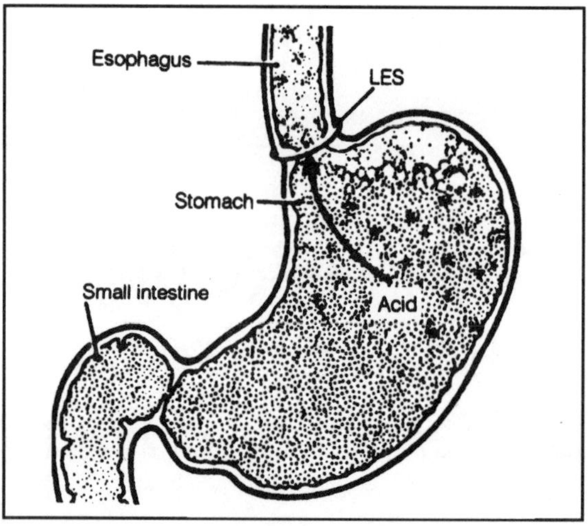


*Figure 13.1.*

## What Is the Role of Hiatal Hernia?

Some doctors believe a hiatal hernia may weaken the LES and cause reflux. Hiatal hernia occurs when the upper part of the stomach moves up into the chest through a small opening in the diaphragm (diaphragmatic hiatus). The diaphragm is the muscle separating the stomach from the chest. (See Figure 13.2.) Recent studies show that the opening in the diaphragm acts as an additional sphincter around the lower end of the esophagus. Studies also show that hiatal hernia results in retention of acid and other contents above this opening. These substances can reflux easily into the esophagus.

Coughing, vomiting, straining, or sudden physical exertion can cause increased pressure in the abdomen resulting in hiatal hernia. Obesity and pregnancy also contribute to this condition. Many otherwise healthy people age 50 and over have a small hiatal hernia. Although considered a condition of middle age, hiatal hernias affect people of all ages.

Hiatal hernias usually do not require treatment. However, treatment may be necessary if the hernia is in danger of becoming strangulated (twisted in a way that cuts off blood supply, i.e., paraesophageal hernia) or is complicated by severe GERD or esophagitis (inflammation of the esophagus). The doctor may perform surgery to reduce the size of the hernia or to prevent strangulation.

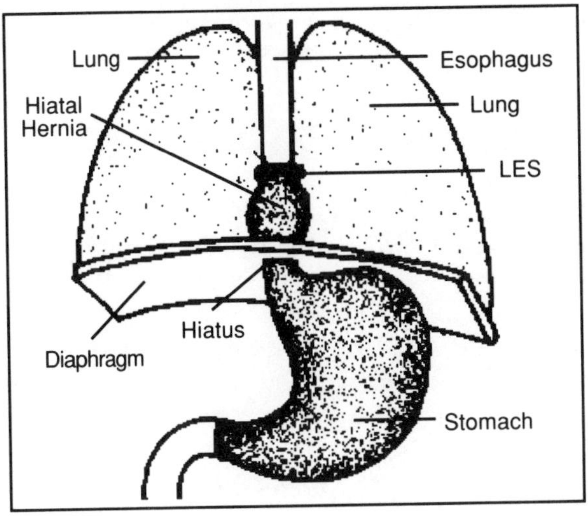


*Figure 13.2.*

## What Other Factors Contribute to GERD?

Dietary and lifestyle choices may contribute to GERD. Certain foods and beverages, including chocolate, peppermint, fried or fatty foods, coffee, or alcoholic beverages, may weaken the LES causing reflux and heartburn. Studies show that cigarette smoking relaxes the LES. Obesity and pregnancy can also cause GERD.

## What Does Heartburn Feel Like?

Heartburn, also called acid indigestion, is the most common symptom of GERD and usually feels like a burning chest pain beginning behind the breastbone and moving upward to the neck and throat. Many people say it feels like food is coming back into the mouth leaving an acid or bitter taste.

The burning, pressure, or pain of heartburn can last as long as 2 hours and is often worse after eating. Lying down or bending over can also result in heartburn. Many people obtain relief by standing upright or by taking an antacid that clears acid out of the esophagus.

Heartburn pain can be mistaken for the pain associated with heart disease or a heart attack, but there are differences. Exercise may aggravate pain resulting from heart disease, and rest may relieve the pain. Heartburn pain is less likely to be associated with physical activity.

## How Common Is Heartburn?

More than 60 million American adults experience GERD and heartburn at least once a month, and about 25 million adults suffer daily from heartburn. Twenty-five percent of pregnant women experience daily heartburn, and more than 50 percent have occasional distress. Recent studies show that GERD in infants and children is more common than previously recognized and may produce recurrent vomiting, coughing and other respiratory problems, or failure to thrive.

## What Is the Treatment for GERD?

Doctors recommend lifestyle and dietary changes for most people with GERD. Treatment aims at decreasing the amount of reflux or reducing damage to the lining of the esophagus from refluxed materials.

Avoiding foods and beverages that can weaken the LES is recommended. These foods include chocolate, peppermint, fatty foods, coffee, and alcoholic beverages. Foods and beverages that can irritate a damaged esophageal lining, such as citrus fruits and juices, tomato products, and pepper, should also be avoided.

Decreasing the size of portions at mealtime may also help control symptoms. Eating meals at least 2 to 3 hours before bedtime may lessen reflux by allowing the acid in the stomach to decrease and the stomach to empty partially. In addition, being overweight often worsens symptoms. Many overweight people find relief when they lose weight.

Cigarette smoking weakens the LES. Therefore, stopping smoking is important to reduce GERD symptoms.

Elevating the head of the bed on 6-inch blocks or sleeping on a specially designed wedge reduces heartburn by allowing gravity to minimize reflux of stomach contents into the esophagus.

Antacids taken regularly can neutralize acid in the esophagus and stomach and stop heartburn. Many people find that nonprescription antacids provide temporary or partial relief. An antacid combined with a foaming agent such as alginic acid helps some people. These compounds are believed to form a foam barrier on top of the stomach that prevents acid reflux from occurring.

Long-term use of antacids, however, can result in side effects, including diarrhea, altered calcium metabolism (a change in the way the body breaks down and uses calcium), and buildup of magnesium in the body. Too much magnesium can be serious for patients with kidney disease. If antacids are needed for more than 3 weeks, a doctor should be consulted.

For chronic reflux and heartburn, the doctor may prescribe medications to reduce acid in the stomach. These medicines include $H_2$ blockers, which inhibit acid secretion in the stomach. Currently, four $H_2$ blockers are available: cimetidine, famotidine, nizatidine, and ranitidine. Another type of drug, the proton pump (or acid pump) inhibitor omeprazole inhibits an enzyme (a protein in the acid-producing cells of the stomach) necessary for acid secretion. The acid pump inhibitor lansoprazole is currently under investigation as a new treatment for GERD.

Other approaches to therapy will increase the strength of the LES and quicken emptying of stomach contents with motility drugs that act on the upper gastrointestinal (GI) tract. These drugs include cisapride, bethanechol, and metoclopramide.

## What If Symptoms Persist?

People with severe, chronic esophageal reflux or with symptoms not relieved by the treatment described above may need more complete diagnostic evaluation. Doctors use a variety of tests and procedures to examine a patient with chronic heartburn.

An *upper GI series* may be performed during the early phase of testing. This test is a special x-ray that shows the esophagus, stomach, and duodenum (the upper part of the small intestine). While an upper GI series provides limited information about possible reflux, it is used to rule out other diagnoses, such as peptic ulcers.

*Endoscopy* is an important procedure for individuals with chronic GERD. By placing a small lighted tube with a tiny video camera on the end (endoscope) into the esophagus, the doctor may see inflammation or irritation of the tissue lining the esophagus (esophagitis). If the findings of the endoscopy are abnormal or questionable, biopsy (removing a small sample of tissue) from the lining of the esophagus may be helpful.

The *Bernstein test* (dripping a mild acid through a tube placed in the mid-esophagus) is often performed as part of a complete evaluation. This test attempts to confirm that the symptoms result from acid in the esophagus. *Esophageal manometric studies* (pressure measurements of the esophagus) occasionally help identify critically low pressure in the LES or abnormalities in esophageal muscle contraction.

For patients in whom diagnosis is difficult, doctors may measure the acid levels inside the esophagus through pH testing. Testing pH monitors the acidity level of the esophagus and symptoms during meals, activity, and sleep. Newer techniques of long-term pH monitoring are improving diagnostic capability in this area.

## Does GERD Require Surgery?

A small number of people with GERD may need surgery because of severe reflux and poor response to medical treatment. Fundoplication is a surgical procedure that increases pressure in the lower esophagus. However, surgery should not be considered until all other measures have been tried.

## What Are the Complications of Long-Term GERD?

Sometimes GERD results in serious complications. Esophagitis can occur as a result of too much stomach acid in the esophagus. Esophagitis may cause esophageal bleeding or ulcers. In addition, a narrowing or stricture of the esophagus may occur from chronic scarring. Some people develop a condition known as Barrett's esophagus, which is severe damage to the skin-like lining of the esophagus. Doctors believe this condition may be a precursor to esophageal cancer.

## Conclusion

Although GERD can limit daily activities and productivity, it is rarely life-threatening. With an understanding of the causes and proper treatment most people will find relief.

### Tips To Control Heartburn

- Avoid foods and beverages that affect LES pressure or irritate the esophagus lining, including fried and fatty foods, peppermint, chocolate, alcohol, coffee, citrus fruit and juices, and tomato products.

- Lose weight if overweight.
- Stop smoking.
- Elevate the head of the bed 6 inches.
- Avoid lying down 2 to 3 hours after eating.
- Take an antacid.

## Additional Readings


Cramer T. "A Burning Question: When Do You Need an Antacid?" *FDA Consumer* 1992; 26(1): 19–22. This article for consumers provides general information about antacids.

Larson DE, Editor-in-chief. *Mayo Clinic Family Health Book*. New York: William Morrow and Company, Inc., 1990. This general medical guide includes sections about esophageal reflux and hiatal hernia.

Richter JE. "Why Does Surgery Work for GERD?" *Practical Gastroenterology* 1993; XVII(10): 10–18. This article for physicians describes antireflux surgery.

Sutherland JE. "Gastroesophageal Reflux Disease: When Antacids Aren't Enough." *Postgraduate Medicine* 1991; 89(7): 45–53. This article for primary care physicians provides guidelines to determine if a patient has reflux disease and offers treatment methods.

# Chapter 14

# *Gastroesophageal Reflux Diet*

## *Introduction*

### *What Is Gastroesophageal Reflux?*

Gastroesophageal reflux is a term used to describe the backwash of stomach contents up into the esophagus. This occurs when the lower esophageal sphincter (a ring-shaped muscle between the esophagus and the stomach) becomes very weak or, more common, when it relaxes inappropriately.

### *What Are the Symptoms?*

Heartburn, usually described as a burning sensation, is the most classic symptom. Often, there is also a sensation of food coming back into the mouth, accompanied by an acid or bitter taste.

### *What Is the Treatment?*

It is important to remember that any chest pain (even a burning sensation that may be heartburn) necessitates a medical evaluation by a doctor. If gastroesophageal reflux is diagnosed, treatment usually

---

This diet plan was developed by New England Deaconess Hospital and published in the *Dietitian's Patient Education Manual*, Vol. 1, published by Aspen Publishers, Gaithersburg, MD. Reprinted by permission.

includes the following: dietary modifications, antacids, and smoking cessation (if indicated). If you must take meals in bed, you will also be advised to elevate the head of the bed at mealtime.

This fact sheet addresses the dietary modifications that can help to relieve the symptoms of gastroesophageal reflux. Be sure to discuss any other treatments that you may need with your doctor.

## General Dietary Guidelines

- If you are overweight, weight loss can have a dramatic effect on improving esophageal reflux symptoms.
- Eat small meals that are high in protein and low in fat at equal intervals throughout the day.
- Do not eat within 3 hours of going to bed, and do not lie down after eating.
- Avoid the following foods since they can relax the lower esophageal sphincter and contribute to reflux: fried or fatty foods; garlic, onions, radishes, and peppers; chocolate; spearmint and peppermint; alcohol; coffee, tea, cola, and other caffeine-containing beverages (substitute decaffeinated beverages if well tolerated).
- Avoid the following foods since they may irritate the lining of the esophagus: citrus fruits and juices (such as orange, grapefruit, and lemon) and tomato products.
- Individual tolerance varies; therefore, you need to avoid any other foods that regularly give you heartburn.
- Try to relax, especially at mealtimes, because stress can increase gastric acid secretion and thereby worsen heartburn symptoms.
- Since citrus products are to be avoided on this diet, your vitamin C intake may be low. There are other good sources of vitamin C, including cantaloupes, potatoes, and strawberries, which should be included in your diet. Your dietitian may also recommend a multivitamin supplement.

- Aim for a well-balanced diet. Choose a variety of foods daily from the basic four food groups.

## Basic Four Food Groups and Examples

**Protein**
*2 Servings Daily*
Meat
Poultry
Fish
Eggs
Cheese, low fat
Dried beans

**Milk**
*2 Servings Daily*
Low-fat selection of each of the following:
- milk
- yogurt
- cheese
- pudding
- milk-based soup

**Grain**
*4 Servings Daily*
Bread
Cereal
Rice
Noodles
Potato

**Fruit & Vegetable**
*4 Servings Daily*
Banana
Prune juice
Spinach
Green beans
Squash
Cantaloupe

## Sample Meal Plan

**Breakfast**
1 banana
1-1/2 cups dry cereal
1 cup low-fat milk
1 cup decaffeinated tea

**Midmorning Snack**
1/2 cup low-fat cottage cheese
6 crackers
1/2 fruit cocktail

**Lunch**
3 oz. turkey breast
2 slices bread
Carrot and celery sticks
Lettuce slices
1 tsp reduced-fat mayonnaise
1/4 cantaloupe
1/2 cup low-fat

**Midafternoon Snack**
1 cup low-fat yogurt

**Dinner**
3 oz. baked fish
1/2 cup rice pilaf
1/2 cup broccoli
1 tsp margarine
1/2 cup sherbet
1/2 cup low-fat milk
1 cup decaffeinated tea

## Chapter 15

# *Chronic Pulmonary Aspiration in Children*


## *Abstract*

According to established diagnostic and therapeutic guidelines for chronic pulmonary aspiration, clinical suspicion is raised by coughing and choking with feeding, coughing during deep, recurrent pneumonia, failure to thrive, and radiologic signs of chronic lung injury. The upper gastrointestinal series accurately defines anatomy and function, can differentiate between direct and reflux aspiration, and identifies conditions that predispose to aspiration. Gastroesophageal scintigraphy lacks anatomic detail but increases observation time, may differentiate between direct and reflux aspiration, and identifies delayed gastric emptying and gastroesophageal reflux. The lipid-laden macrophage[1] index improves identification of aspiration, but cannot differentiate between direct and reflux aspiration. The esophageal pH probe identifies gastroesophageal reflux. Treatment options include medical therapy (thickened feedings, prone positioning, and metoclopramide) and surgical intervention (gastrostomy, fundoplication, and definitive correction of predisposing conditions). Therapy is determined by severity of illness and results of diagnostic evaluation.


Chronic Pulmonary Aspiration is frequently encountered in the differential diagnosis of pulmonary diseases in children. Unfortunately,


This article originally appeared in *Southern Medical Journal*, Vol. 86, No. 7, July 1993. Reprinted with permission from Martin L. Bauer, MD, Pediatric Pulmonology, Children's Mercy Hospital, 24th and Gillham Rd., Kansas City, MO 64108.

current diagnostic techniques do not provide sufficient positive and negative predictive value to consistently identify or rule out aspiration. The lack of a "gold standard" leads to delayed diagnosis ant complicates the evaluation of therapeutic intervention.

In recognition of the frustration encountered in the evaluation of chronic pulmonary aspiration in children, this article will review the pathophysiology of chronic pulmonary aspiration, discuss the strengths, weaknesses, and interpretation of currently available diagnostic tests, and present treatment options.

## Pathophysiology

Pulmonary aspiration may be direct (also known as primary), with oral flora and food entering the airways during the act of swallowing, or it may occur as a result of gastroesophageal reflux, spilling gastric content into the airways and producing reflux, or secondary, pulmonary aspiration. Reflux aspiration adds gastric acid and enzymes to the contamination of the lungs. The result of aspiration is desquamation of tracheal mucosa, damage to alveolar lining cells and capillaries, and acute neutrophilic inflammation followed by foreign-body reaction consisting of mononuclear cell inflammation with granuloma formation. Aspiration events are sporadic and intermittent, and though they may be infrequent, the recurrent contamination of the lung can lead to progressive bronchiectasis and ultimately to respiratory failure.

The lungs are normally protected from aspiration by the larynx. The epiglottis diverts material laterally into the pyriform fossae, away from the glottic opening. Swallowing lifts the larynx proximally, allowing the bolus to move inferior as well as lateral to the glottic opening. The aryepiglottic folds further direct the food bolus away from the glottic opening. The true vocal cords appose to act as the final barrier preventing solid and liquid from entering the airways.

Any process interfering with normal laryngeal protection of the airway will predispose to aspiration. Aspiration occurs with increased frequency in the neurologically impaired because of inadequate control of reflex laryngeal protection of the airways. Nasogastric, endotracheal, and tracheostomy tubes mechanically hamper the normal protective function of the larynx, leading to an increased incidence of aspiration. Anatomic abnormalities such as laryngomalacia inhibit efficient protection of the airways. Dysmotility disorders of the esophagus, such as esophageal atresia or stricture, and vascular rings cause pooling of material in the vicinity of the glottic opening, setting the stage for aspiration. Tracheoesophageal fistulas bypass the protective mechanism of the larynx.

Aspiration of refluxed gastric content may occur with or without apparent laryngeal dysfunction. Gastroesophageal reflux results from impaired lower esophageal sphincter function or delayed gastric emptying, which in turn may be the result of gastritis, duodenal ulcer, pyloric channel ulcer, pyloric stenosis, or malrotation. Reflux of gastric content to the level of the larynx predisposes to aspiration. Chronic reflux into the distal esophagus can also cause esophageal stricture, which may in turn lead to pooling of the swallowed bolus and ultimate aspiration.

Clearly, aspiration is not a primary pathologic process, but rather the result of many other abnormalities. This multifactorial origin of chronic pulmonary aspiration and its sporadic, intermittent occurrence contribute to the difficulties encountered in diagnosis.

## Diagnostic Procedures

Intermittent aspiration of food, oral flora, and gastric content into the lungs and the resultant injury by this contamination produce symptoms and/or signs that may be initially diagnosed as pneumonia, cystic fibrosis, asthma, failure to thrive, bronchopulmonary dysplasia, stridor, chronic cough, apparent life-threatening events (ALTE), interstitial lung disease, or congestive heart failure. Suspicion of chronic pulmonary aspiration is reinforced by observation of coughing and choking with feeding, a history of frequent vomiting with choking, or coughing and choking while supine. Diagnostic tools available for evaluation of chronic aspiration are imaging techniques (chest x-ray, upper gastrointestinal series, and gastroesophageal scintigraphy), flexible fiberoptic bronchoscopy with lipid-laden macrophage index, and the esophageal pH study.

### *Imaging Techniques*

Plain film examination of the chest, including anteroposterior (AP) and lateral views of the chest, provide the initial imaging study for the diagnosis of aspiration. Classically, patients with a history of aspiration have radiographic features of pneumonia. These can be airspace or interstitial infiltrates in the basilar or superior segments of the lower lobes or in the posterior segments of the upper lobes. In infants less than 1 year of age, features of bronchiolitis (ie, slight peribronchial thickening and generalized air trapping) may be seen. Recurrent radiologic evidence of pulmonary infection should suggest aspiration.

The upper gastrointestinal examination using fluoroscopy is a more specific diagnostic imaging study. With this examination, initial airway fluoroscopy can be done with AP and lateral imaging of the trachea and primary bronchi. Magnification imaging using rapid sequence spot filming or video taping can record the appearance of these structures. Barium can then be administered for evaluation of deglutition and detection of primary transglottic aspiration, which may appear as tiny amounts of barium passing through the vocal cords into the cervical trachea.

The upper GI series includes examination of the esophagus, stomach, and duodenum to the duodenojejunal junction. Many abnormalities that predispose to aspiration can be identified, including dysmotility disorder of the upper part of the esophagus, vascular ring, esophageal atresia, tracheoesophageal fistula, esophageal stricture, distal esophageal dysmotility, gastroesophageal reflux, duodenal ulcer, pyloric channel ulcer, pyloric stenosis, and malrotation.

If tracheoesophageal fistula is suspected, but not detected by routine techniques, a feeding catheter can be passed into the esophagus to instill barium directly into the esophagus. This provides excellent distention of the esophagus and may elucidate a tiny fistula undetected by other means.

Although the upper GI series will frequently identify conditions that predispose to aspiration, the sporadic and intermittent nature of aspiration reduces the likelihood of routine demonstration of an aspiration event during an upper GI examination. If aspiration is observed, differentiation between direct and reflux aspiration can be documented. If an aspiration event is not observed, differentiation can be inferred by observation of conditions that predispose to either reflux or direct aspiration.

A second diagnostic imaging study that has proved useful is gastroesophageal scintigraphy with determination of gastric emptying. Small tracer quantities of technetium Tc 99m sulfur colloid can be mixed with a milk or formula feeding and given to the patient by mouth. Gamma camera imaging of the esophagus, stomach, and chest can be obtained at intervals for up to 24 hours. The detection of radioactivity in the lung fields indicates aspiration. Early detection suggests direct aspiration, while late detection suggests reflux aspiration. Delayed imaging increases observation time during which an aspiration event may be documented.

Gastroesophageal scintigraphy also allows evaluation for gastroesophageal reflux over a longer period by showing multiple waves of repetitious reflux of gastric content into the esophagus. Focus on a region of interest allows measurement of tracer within the stomach and calculation of gastric emptying time. This can be particularly useful before planned fundoplication to determine necessity for pyloromyotomy.

A modification of the conventional gastroesophageal scintigram is the salivagram. Using this technique, small amounts of tracer can be dropped into the patient's oral cavity for detection of small quantities of aspirate. Another variation of this technique is the night-time administration of tracer-laden formula. Delayed imaging the following morning can show aspiration events that occurred during sleep.

Aspiration events continue to be difficult to detect by imaging techniques that are currently available. These techniques frequently fail to demonstrate pathologically significant aspiration.

### *Lipid-Laden Macrophage Index*

Aspirated food is foreign material in the lung. The pulmonary alveolar macrophage maintains clean distal airspaces by phagocytizing foreign material and metabolizing or physically carrying it out of the lung. Flexible fiberoptic bronchoscopy with bronchoalveolar lavage provides safe and simple access to the alveolar macrophage. The lipid component of the phagocytized food can be identified within the macrophage by oil-red-O stain.

The lipid-laden macrophage index is obtained by quantifying the lipid content of each macrophage on a scale of 0 to 4 (0 for no lipid and 4 for cytoplasm completely full of lipid) and totalling the lipid scores of the 100 cells. This provides scores ranging from 0 to 400. Colombo and Hallberg reported that a lipid-laden macrophage index greater than 85 is diagnostic of aspiration, whereas a score less than 73 rules out aspiration.

The lipid-laden macrophage index provides a wider window of opportunity for identification of aspiration, but cannot differentiate between primary and secondary aspiration. Several factors may limit the positive and negative predictive value of this index. First, the definition of recurrent aspiration in the study by Colombo and Hallberg was, "... observation [in the hospital] of coughing or gagging on multiple occasions while swallowing liquid or solid food." Confirmation of aspiration by another study (upper GI series) was obtained for only 23% of patients considered to have aspiration. Response to therapy was not presented. Second, no study has prospectively evaluated this diagnostic technique. Third, clearance time of phagocytized lipid is not known. The rate of macrophage intracellular metabolism of ingested lipid is unknown, as is the timing of macrophage egress from the lung, either via the mucociliary escalator or the interstitial lymphatics, after ingestion of lipid. Rapid clearance of lipid by the macrophage would restrict the effective time frame of the lipid-laden macrophage index.

Therefore, while bronchoscopy provides accurate anatomic and functional definition of the airways and their protective structures, and the lipid-laden macrophage index provides another technique for identifying aspiration, the positive and negative predictive values of this study are unknown.

### *pH Probe*

The most reliable method of evaluating gastroesophageal reflux is the pH probe. After a 2-hour fasting period, the pH probe is placed in the distal esophagus, its position is verified by roentgenogram, a portable recording unit is connected, and the esophageal pH is recorded continuously for 24 hours. The primary caretaker, usually the mother, records the child's position, state of wakefulness, feedings, coughing, crying, and essentially all activity during the 24 hours. Infant feeding is scheduled every 4 hours.

After the study, the record is reviewed for pH below 4.0, evidence of reflux of gastric acid into the esophagus. The number and duration of reflux episodes are tabulated and correlated with the diary. No reflux episodes occurring within 2 hours after feeding are counted.

Reflux episodes are observed by upper GI series in well over 60% of normal infants and are found by esophageal pH studies in most patients during the first 2 hours after feeding. Therefore, the reflux observed by pH probe must be quantified to differentiate pathologic from insignificant reflux. The definition of pathologic reflux identified by pH probe varies among institutions. Significant observations include the number of reflux episodes, the clearance time of each reflux episode, the total reflux time, the pattern of reflux episodes, and association of reflux episodes with symptoms as recorded by the mother. In general, if reflux occurs for more than 5% of the observation time, it is abnormal. Reflux pattern may provide prognostic information.

Although association between gastroesophageal reflux and pulmonary symptoms has been well documented, identification of reflux by pH probe does not establish a causal relationship with pulmonary disease. Furthermore, a relationship between reflux and respiratory symptoms does not necessarily imply aspiration. Respiratory symptoms may be due to reflex bronchospasm caused by gastric acid irritation of esophageal mucosa rather than entry of gastric content into the airways. The identification of reflux by pH probe, at best, suggests the existence of a condition that may predispose to aspiration. The absence of reflux does not rule out aspiration, though it does reduce the likelihood of several predisposing conditions.

Of the diagnostic tests available, only the upper GI series and the gastroesophageal scintigram have accepted positive predictive value. Whether the lipid-laden macrophage index will consistently identify aspiration remains to be seen. None of the studies available, with the possible but unproven exception of the lipid-laden macrophage index, has any negative predictive value. Therefore, the diagnosis of chronic pulmonary aspiration and selection of therapy is usually based on clinical criteria alone. These clinical observations include observed coughing and choking with feeding, coughing at night or during sleep, history of recurrent pneumonia, history of failure to thrive, and radiologic changes consistent with chronic lung injury, though a normal chest film does not rule out aspiration. These criteria easily fit several of the differential diagnostic entities mentioned earlier, leading to frequent delayed or missed diagnosis of chronic pulmonary aspiration.

## Treatment

Therapy for aspiration is determined by acuteness of presentation, underlying disease, and whether aspiration is direct or reflux. Aspiration causing an apparent life-threatening event necessitates aggressive diagnostic and therapeutic intervention. Surgical correction of conditions predisposing to aspiration, such as pyloric stenosis, malrotation, esophageal stricture, or tracheoesophageal fistula, will usually resolve the aspiration without further intervention. Direct aspiration is frequently not correctable, and the swallowing mechanism must be bypassed. Reflux aspiration frequently responds to medical treatment, but may require surgical intervention.

### *Reflux Aspiration*

In most cases, chronic pulmonary aspiration is due to gastroesophageal reflux. Therefore, treatment of reflux will frequently eliminate aspiration. In the absence of underlying disease or serious secondary effects (apparent life-threatening event), most reflux can be managed medically. Medical management of reflux is initiated with thickening of feedings by adding 1 tablespoon of rice cereal to each ounce of formula. The hole in the nipple must be enlarged to allow flow of the gruel-like formula. Prone position should be maintained when the infant is not upright. The head of the bed may be elevated 30° but this is of debatable value because infants invariably scoot to a head-down position at the foot of the crib. Elaborate restraints have been devised to maintain a head-up, prone position. Infant seats and car seats contribute to reflux by increasing intra-abdominal pressure. This is not to discourage the use of car seats, but to suggest that time in the seats, and therefore travel, be kept to a minimum. Attention to feeding and position will frequently resolve the problem of reflux and secondary aspiration.

A trial of medical therapy is warranted if symptoms persist after thickened feedings and attention to positioning, if the infant shows significant failure to thrive or has respiratory symptoms, or if the mother becomes frustrated. Metoclopramide (Reglan), 0.1 mg/kg/dose tid to qid 30 to 40 minutes before feeding, is the medication of choice. It increases lower esophageal sphincter tone, enhances gastric emptying, and promotes pyloric relaxation. Five to fifteen percent of children treated with metoclopramide will become very irritable. A few patients may have extrapyramidal symptoms, opisthotonos, torticollis, or oculogyric crisis, but these are reversed by diphenhydramine (Benadryl) and discontinuance of metoclopramide therapy.

Bethanechol also improves lower esophageal sphincter tone and gastric emptying, but it can stimulate bronchospasm in patients with reactive airways. The histamine $H_2$ blockers ranitidine (Zantac) and cimeditine (Tagamet) mitigate the consequences of reflux by decreasing acid production and preventing esophagitis, but they do nothing to reduce reflux. In the intensive care unit setting there is evidence that $H_2$ blockers contribute to the development of pneumonia by alteration of microbial flora as a result of increasing gastric pH. There is no evidence that this occurs in the ambulatory patient. Sucralfate (Carafate) is useful in the intensive care unit setting because it protects the gastric and esophageal mucosa without changing the pH of the stomach.

[If medical management has failed after six weeks of treatment, this is an indication that antireflux surgery may be necessary.] Surgical intervention without medical trial is indicated for obvious surgical conditions, such as pyloric stenosis or distal esophageal stricture due to esophagitis, or for life-threatening complications of reflux, such as severe aspiration or ALTE.

The two general types of antireflux procedures for gastroesophageal reflux in children are partial fundoplication [a surgical procedure that increases the pressure in the lower esophagus] and complete fundoplication. The most popular complete fundoplication is the Nissen fundoplication, which involves mobilizing the esophagus at the hiatus, pulling the mobilized distal portion of the esophagus down into the abdomen, and wrapping the fundus of the stomach completely around the intra-abdominal part of the esophagus. The longer the wrapped segment of distal esophagus, the more effective the reflux prevention. Unfortunately, a long wrap tends to prevent belching and reduces stomach reservoir capacity, leading to some of the complications of fundoplication. The Thal fundoplication is the most common partial fundoplication technique used in children. The distal segment of the esophagus is brought down into the abdomen, as with the complete fundoplication, but the fundus of the stomach is sutured around only one half to two thirds of the distal esophagus. This partial wrap provides a sharp angle of His, which prevents reflux. The Nissen fundoplication provides more competent antireflux properties than the Thal and is usually the preferred procedure for patients with reflux-induced pulmonary aspiration.

Nissen fundoplication is effective in preventing reflux and the symptoms of vomiting. However, it is less consistent in relief of respiratory symptoms, suggesting that other subtle processes interfering with protection of the airways may coexist in these patients.

Complications of Nissen fundoplication should be anticipated in 20% of patients. The gas bloat syndrome is related to the length of the wrap, a longer wrap reducing the ability to belch. A tight fundoplication, or even a loose fundoplication in association with esophageal dysmotility, leads to symptoms of partial obstruction of the distal esophagus. Bowel obstruction due to abdominal adhesions also occurs occasionally. Wound infection is not uncommon. Morbidity associated with the Nissen fundoplication is usually attributed to other pathologic conditions contributing to the reflux and aspiration.

Gastric retention is fairly common in children with gastroesophageal reflux, especially in the neurologically impaired. For this reason, every patient considered for fundoplication should have a gastric emptying study before the operative procedure. Delayed gastric emptying mandates a procedure to improve gastric emptying, pyloroplasty being the most common technique used to improve gastric emptying in these patients. Pyloroplasty is not recommended as an adjunct to every fundoplication because of the high frequency of subsequent dumping.

### Direct Aspiration

No medical management is available for direct aspiration. The swallowing mechanism must be bypassed by gastrostomy and tube feeding. The term "gastrostomy" refers to a wide variety of surgical procedures. The most common technique is the Stamm gastrostomy, which can be done as an open, endoscopic, or laparoscopic surgical procedure. Purse-string sutures are placed around the prospective ostomy site in the stomach, and the gastrostomy tube is passed through the abdominal wall and into the stomach inside the boundaries of the purse-string sutures. The balloon or mushroom tip of the catheter is distended inside the stomach and is pulled firmly against the anterior abdominal wall. The gastrostomy tube usually tends to be pointed superiorly toward the gastroesophageal junction and can be inadvertently advanced into the esophagus. A Stamm gastrostomy directed toward the pylorus averts this problem and allows the gastrostomy tube to be advanced through the pylorus intermittently for transpyloric feeding once the gastrostomy site has matured.

The Stamm gastrostomy tube must remain in place. The ostomy stoma will constrict by scar contraction within 8 to 12 hours if the tube is removed. Commercially available gastrostomy "buttons" can be placed in the stoma after the gastrostomy tract is mature. These buttons have a skin level profile and are cosmetically superior to the much longer gastrostomy tubes. These buttons have a constellation of complications of their own. The three most common complications of the button are uncontrolled leaking of gastric content, granulation tissue formation around the button, and migration of the button mushroom into the ostomy tract, creating a perigastrostomy abscess. Most buttons must be replaced yearly because their antireflux valves become incontinent.

The Janeway gastrostomy provides a permanent ostomy by mobilizing a full-thickness flap of stomach that is formed into a tube and brought out through the abdominal wall. The feeding tube can be removed between feedings without stoma contraction. The Janeway gastrostomy tends to leak gastric content onto the abdominal wall, irritating the skin. A directed Janeway gastrostomy may decrease this acid leak, and it provides access for transpyloric gastrostomy feeding. The use of sucralfate around the gastrostomy stoma reduces skin irritation due to acid leak. Ambulatory patients have more gastric leak problems from a Janeway gastrostomy than flaccid, bedridden patients.

As with any surgical procedure, there are many potential complications of gastrostomy. Separation of the stomach from the anterior abdominal wall in the first 7 to 14 days after the operative procedure, before the gastrostomy tract seals, may lead to contamination of the peritoneal cavity with acid and pepsin, causing peritonitis. Wound separation and dehiscence occurs in an occasional patient if the gastrostomy tube is pulled through the abdominal surgical wound. Hemorrhage results from pulling the tube through an abdominal wall vessel or from inflammatory erosion into an abdominal wall vessel. Infection is usually caused by bacterial contamination of skin macerated by gastric acid leak. Skin irritation and granulation tissue are common problems. These problems related to gastrostomy leakage are best handled by keeping the gastrostomy tube balloon or mushroom tip pulled up firmly against the abdominal wall. Blow drying the perigastrostomy site frequently with a hair dryer, the use of 10% silver nitrate as an astringent, and sucralfate powder placed around the gastrostomy stoma will frequently ameliorate these skin irritation problems. Esophageal perforation can result from inadvertent catheterization of the esophagus and can be avoided by not passing the gastrostomy tube into the stomach more than 2 inches before insufflating the balloon. When the gastrostomy tube is removed, a persistent gastrocutaneous fistula may develop in gastrostomies present for more than 6 months. Sometimes these fistulas must be closed surgically.

Gastroesophageal reflux frequently develops in gastrostomy-fed infants. Placement of the tube into the stomach near the greater curvature tends to pull down on the fundus and straighten the angle of His, creating a mechanical advantage for reflux. Bolus feeding batters the gastroesophageal junction, ultimately breaking down the functional gastroesophageal sphincter and predisposing the patient to reflux. Placing the gastrostomy tube into the stomach near the lesser curvature tends to preserve the angle of His and seems to lessen the incidence of postgastrostomy reflux. Anticipation of long-term gastrostomy feedings warrants consideration of an antireflux procedure, especially if the child is neurologically impaired.

Many of the problems attributed to fundoplication are actually complications of tube feeding. Diarrhea and constipation are commonly seen in tube-fed infants. Changing the patient to a more suitable, better tolerated formula usually resolves these symptoms.

Retching is common in tube-fed children. It is usually caused by one of four mechanisms. Dumping is by far the most common cause and can be ameliorated by dividing the bolus feedings into two smaller parts given at 30-minute intervals or by drip feeding the patient at night and using smaller bolus feedings during the day. Hyperdistention, another cause of retching, is usually due to a long Nissen wrap resulting in a small gastric reservoir. These patients can best be treated by distending the stomach with water or air to enlarge the size of the reservoir. Hypersatiety, or overfeeding, occurs frequently in patients with respiratory or cardiac distress who require increased caloric intake.

Hypersatiety-induced retching responds to diphenhydramine in some cases. Delayed gastric emptying is another important cause of retching. This problem usually necessitates metoclopramide or bethanechol therapy and in unrelenting cases, a pyloroplasty.

## Conclusion

Clinical evaluation, with emphasis on history, all too often remains the only evidence for diagnosis of chronic pulmonary aspiration. Although the gold standard for diagnosis of chronic pulmonary aspiration is not established, thoughtful application of diagnostic studies currently available should increase the frequency of objective confirmation of aspiration.

The upper gastrointestinal series, providing anatomic and functional definition of the upper gastrointestinal tract and airway, is clearly the first study. Most conditions predisposing to aspiration can be identified by the upper GI series, and direct and reflux aspiration may be differentiated. If neither aspiration nor predisposing disease is demonstrated on the upper GI series, 2 technetium-sulfur colloid gastroesophageal scintigram may be done. This test not only differentiates between direct and reflux aspiration, but also identifies reflux and delayed gastric emptying, conditions that could predispose to aspiration.

When imaging techniques fail to confirm or rule out aspiration, flexible fiberoptic bronchoscopy with bronchoalveolar lavage for lipid-laden macrophage index may document aspiration. It will not differentiate between primary and secondary aspiration. Finally, 24-hour pH probe study may show association between respiratory symptoms and gastroesophageal reflux, suggesting aspiration.

Appropriate therapy will be determined by apparent acuteness of illness and results of evaluation. Further investigation of the diagnosis and treatment of chronic aspiration is needed. Prospective evaluation of the relative positive and negative predictive values of existing diagnostic procedures would be invaluable. Perhaps markers that might be identified by bronchoalveolar lavage will allow a clear distinction between children who have pathologic chronic pulmonary aspiration and those who do not. Until such a tool becomes available, the evaluation and treatment of chronic pulmonary aspiration remains as much art as science.

*—by Martin L. Bauer, MD,*
*Reinaldo Figueroa-Colon, MD,*
*Keith Georgeson, MD,*
*and Daniel W. Young, MD,*
*Birmingham, Alabama.*

[[1]A macrophage is a type of cell that characteristically engulfs foreign material and consumes debris and foreign bodies. It is derived from a monocyte and it helps protect the body against infection and noxious substances.]

# *Part Three*

# *Stomach Problems*

Chapter 16

# *Stomach and Duodenal Ulcers*

## *What Is an Ulcer?*

During normal digestion, food moves from the mouth down the esophagus into the stomach. The stomach produces hydrochloric acid and an enzyme called pepsin to digest the food. From the stomach, food passes into the upper part of the small intestine, called the duodenum, where digestion and nutrient absorption continue.

An ulcer is a sore or lesion that forms in the lining of the stomach or duodenum where acid and pepsin are present. Ulcers in the stomach are called gastric or stomach ulcers. Those in the duodenum are called duodenal ulcers. In general, ulcers in the stomach and duodenum are referred to as peptic ulcers. Ulcers rarely occur in the esophagus or in the first portion of the duodenum, the duodenal bulb.

## *Who Has Ulcers?*

About 20 million Americans develop at least one ulcer during their lifetime. Each year:

- Ulcers affect about 4 million people.
- More than 40,000 people have surgery because of persistent symptoms or problems from ulcers.

---

NIH Publication No. 95–38.

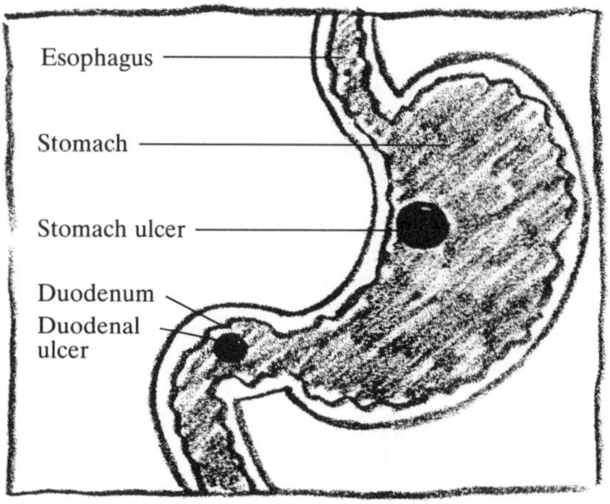


***Figure 16.1.*** *Ulcers frequently occur in the stomach and duodenum.*

- About 6,000 people die of ulcer-related complications.

Ulcers can develop at any age, but they are rare among teenagers and even more uncommon in children. Duodenal ulcers occur for the first time usually between the ages of 30 and 50. Stomach ulcers are more likely to develop in people over age 60. Duodenal ulcers occur more frequently in men than women; stomach ulcers develop more often in women than men.

## What Causes Ulcers?

For almost a century, doctors believed lifestyle factors such as stress and diet caused ulcers. Later, researchers discovered that an imbalance between digestive fluids (hydrochloric acid and pepsin) and the stomach's ability to defend itself against these powerful substances resulted in ulcers.

Today, research shows that most ulcers develop as a result of infection with bacteria called *Helicobacter pylori* (*H. pylori*). While all three of these factors—lifestyle, acid and pepsin, and *H. pylori*—play a role in ulcer development, *H. pylori* is now considered the primary cause.

## Lifestyle

While scientific evidence refutes the old belief that stress and diet cause ulcers, several lifestyle factors continue to be suspected of playing a role. These factors include cigarettes, foods and beverages containing caffeine, alcohol, and physical stress.

*Smoking*

Studies show that cigarette smoking increases one's chances of getting an ulcer. Smoking slows the healing of existing ulcers and also contributes to ulcer recurrence.

*Caffeine*

Coffee, tea, colas, and foods that contain caffeine seem to stimulate acid secretion in the stomach, aggravating the pain of an existing ulcer. However, the amount of acid secretion that occurs after drinking decaffeinated coffee is the same as that produced after drinking regular coffee. Thus, the stimulation of stomach acid cannot be attributed solely to caffeine.

*Alcohol*

Research has not found a link between alcohol consumption and peptic ulcers. However, ulcers are more common in people who have cirrhosis of the liver, a disease often linked to heavy alcohol consumption.

*Stress*

Although emotional stress is no longer thought to be a cause of ulcers, people with ulcers often report that emotional stress increases ulcer pain. Physical stress, however, increases the risk of developing ulcers particularly in the stomach. For example, people with injuries such as severe burns and people undergoing major surgery often require rigorous treatment to prevent ulcers and ulcer complications.

*Acid and pepsin*

Researchers believe that the stomach's inability to defend itself against the powerful digestive fluids, acid and pepsin, contributes to ulcer formation. The stomach defends itself from these fluids in several ways. One way is by producing mucus—a lubricant-like coating that shields stomach tissues. Another way is by producing a chemical called bicarbonate. This chemical neutralizes and breaks down digestive fluids into substances less harmful to stomach tissue. Finally, blood circulation to the stomach lining, cell renewal, and cell repair also help protect the stomach.

Nonsteroidal anti-inflammatory drugs (NSAIDs) make the stomach vulnerable to the harmful effects of acid and pepsin. NSAIDs such as aspirin, ibuprofen, and naproxen sodium are present in many nonprescription medications used to treat fever, headaches, and minor aches and pains. These, as well as prescription NSAIDs used to treat a variety of arthritic conditions, interfere with the stomach's ability to produce mucus and bicarbonate and affect blood flow to the stomach and cell repair. They can all cause the stomach's defense mechanisms to fail, resulting in an increased chance of developing stomach ulcers. In most cases, these ulcers disappear once the person stops taking NSAIDs.

## Helicobacter pylori

*H. pylori* is a spiral-shaped bacterium found in the stomach. Research shows that the bacteria (along with acid secretion) damage stomach and duodenal tissue, causing inflammation and ulcers. Scientists believe this damage occurs because of *H. pylori*'s shape and characteristics.

*H. pylori* survives in the stomach because it produces the enzyme urease. Urease generates substances that neutralize the stomach's acid—enabling the bacteria to survive. Because of their shape and the way they move, the bacteria can penetrate the stomach's protective mucous lining. Here, they can produce substances that weaken the stomach's protective mucus and make the stomach cells more susceptible to the damaging effects of acid and pepsin.

The bacteria can also attach to stomach cells further weakening the stomach's defensive mechanisms and producing local inflammation. For reasons not completely understood, *H. pylori* can also stimulate the stomach to produce more acid.

Excess stomach acid and other irritating factors can cause inflammation of the upper end of the duodenum, the duodenal bulb. In some people, over long periods of time, this inflammation results in production of stomach-like cells called duodenal gastric metaplasia. *H. pylori* then attacks these cells causing further tissue damage and inflammation. which may result in an ulcer.

Within weeks of infection with *H. pylori*, most people develop gastritis—an inflammation of the stomach lining. However, most people will never have symptoms or problems related to the infection. Scientists do not yet know what is different in those people who develop *H. pylori*-related symptoms or ulcers. Perhaps, hereditary or environmental factors yet to be discovered cause some individuals to develop problems. Alternatively, symptoms and ulcers may result from infection with more virulent strains of bacteria. These unanswered questions are the subject of intensive scientific research.

Studies show that *H. pylori* infection in the United States varies with age, ethnic group, and socioeconomic class. The bacteria are more common in older adults, African Americans, Hispanics, and lower socioeconomic groups. The organism appears to spread through the fecal-oral route (when infected stool comes into contact with hands, food, or water). Most individuals seem to be infected during childhood, and their infection lasts a lifetime.

## What Are the Symptoms of Ulcers?

The most common ulcer symptom is a gnawing or burning pain in the abdomen between the breastbone and the naval. The pain often occurs between meals and in the early hours of the morning. It may last from a few minutes to a few hours and may be relieved by eating or by taking antacids.

Less common ulcer symptoms include nausea, vomiting, and loss of appetite and weight. Bleeding from ulcers may occur in the stomach and duodenum. Sometimes people are unaware that they have a bleeding ulcer, because blood loss is slow and blood may not be obvious in the stool. These people may feel tired and weak. If the bleeding is heavy, blood will appear in vomit or stool. Stool containing blood appears tarry or black.

## How Are Ulcers Diagnosed?

The NIH Consensus Panel emphasized the importance of adequately diagnosing ulcer disease and *H. pylori* before starting treatment. If the person has an NSAID-induced ulcer, treatment is quite different from the treatment for a person with an *H. pylori*-related ulcer. Also, a person's pain may be the result of nonulcer dyspepsia (persistent pain or discomfort in the upper abdomen including burning, nausea, and bloating), and not at all related to ulcer disease. Currently, doctors have a number of options available for diagnosing ulcers, such as performing endoscopic and x-ray examinations, and for testing for *H. pylori*.

### *Locating and monitoring ulcers*

Doctors may perform an upper GI series to diagnose ulcers. An upper GI series involves taking an x-ray of the esophagus, stomach, and duodenum to locate an ulcer. To make the ulcer visible on the x-ray image, the patient swallows a chalky liquid called barium.

An alternative diagnostic test is called an endoscopy. During this test, the patient is lightly sedated and the doctor inserts a small flexible instrument with a camera on the end through the mouth into the esophagus, stomach, and duodenum. With this procedure, the entire upper GI tract can be viewed. Ulcers or other conditions can be diagnosed and photographed, and tissue can be taken for biopsy, if necessary.

Once an ulcer is diagnosed and treatment begins, the doctor will usually monitor clinical progress. In the case of a stomach ulcer, the doctor may wish to document healing with repeat x-rays or endoscopy. Continued monitoring of a stomach ulcer is important because of the small chance that the ulcer may be cancerous.

### *Testing for* **H. pylori**

Confirming the presence of *H. pylori* is important once the doctor has diagnosed an ulcer because elimination of the bacteria is likely to cure ulcer disease. Blood, breath, and stomach tissue tests may be performed to detect the presence of *H. pylori*. While some of the tests for *H. pylori* are not approved by the U.S. Food and Drug Administration (FDA), research shows these tests are highly accurate in detecting the bacteria. However, blood tests on occasion give false positive results, and the other tests may give false negative results in people who have recently taken antibiotics, omeprazole (Prilosech), or bismuth (Pepto-Bismol®).

*Blood tests*

Blood tests such as the enzyme-linked immunosorbent assay (ELISA) and quick office-based tests identify and measure *H. pylori* antibodies. The body produces antibodies against *H. pylori* in an attempt to fight the bacteria. The advantages of blood tests are their low cost and availability to doctors The disadvantage is the possibility of false positive results in patients previously treated for ulcers since the levels of *H. pylori* antibodies fall slowly. Several blood tests have FDA approval.

*Breath tests*

Breath tests measure carbon dioxide in exhaled breath. Patients are given a substance called urea with carbon to drink. Bacteria break down this urea and the carbon is absorbed into the blood stream and lungs and exhaled in the breath. By collecting the breath, doctors can measure this carbon and determine whether *H. pylori* is present or absent. Urea breath tests are at least 90 percent accurate for diagnosing the bacteria and are particularly suitable to follow-up treatment to see if bacteria have been eradicated. These tests are awaiting FDA approval.

*Tissue tests*

If the doctor performs an endoscopy to diagnose an ulcer, tissue samples of the stomach can be obtained. The doctor may then perform one of several tests on the tissue. A rapid urease test detects the bacteria's enzyme urease. Histology involves visualizing the bacteria under the microscope. Culture involves specially processing the tissue and watching it for growth of *H. pylori* organisms.

## How Are Ulcers Treated?

### Lifestyle changes

In the past, doctors advised people with ulcers to avoid spicy, fatty, or acidic foods. However, a bland diet is now known to be ineffective for treating or avoiding ulcers. No particular diet is helpful for most ulcer patients. People who find that certain foods cause irritation should discuss this problem with their doctor. Smoking has been shown to delay ulcer healing and has been linked to ulcer recurrence; therefore, persons with ulcers should not smoke.

### Medicines

Doctors treat stomach and duodenal ulcers with several types of medicines including $H_2$ blockers, acid pump inhibitors, and mucosal protective agents. When treating *H. pylori*, these medications are used in combination with antibiotics.

*$H_2$-blockers*

Currently, most doctors treat ulcers with acid-suppressing drugs known as $H_2$-blockers. These drugs reduce the amount of acid the stomach produces by blocking histamine, a powerful stimulant of acid secretion.

$H_2$-blockers reduce pain significantly after several weeks. For the first few days of treatment, doctors often recommend taking an antacid to relieve pain.

Initially, treatment with $H_2$-blockers lasts 6 to 8 weeks. However, because ulcers recur in 50 to 80 percent of cases, many people must continue maintenance therapy for years. This may no longer be the case if *H. pylori* infection is treated. Most ulcers do not recur following successful eradication. Nizatidine (Axid®) is approved for treatment of duodenal ulcers but is not yet approved for treatment of stomach ulcers. $H_2$-blockers that are approved to treat both stomach and duodenal ulcers are:

- Cimetidine (Tagamet®)
- Ranitidine (Zantac®)
- Famotidine (Pepcid®).

*Acid pump inhibitors*

Like $H_2$-blockers, acid pump inhibitors modify the stomach's production of acid. However, acid pump inhibitors more completely block stomach acid production by stopping the stomach's acid pump—the final step of acid secretion. The FDA has approved use of omeprazole for short-term treatment of ulcer disease. Similar drugs, including lansoprazole, are currently being studied.

*Mucosal protective medications*

Mucosal protective medications protect the stomach's mucous lining from acid. Unlike $H_2$-blockers and acid pump inhibitors, protective agents do not inhibit the release of acid. These medications shield the stomach's mucous lining from the damage of acid. Two commonly prescribed protective agents are:

- *Sucralfate (Carafate®).* This medication adheres to the ulcer, providing a protective barrier that allows the ulcer to heal and inhibits further damage by stomach acid. Sucralfate is approved for short-term treatment of duodenal ulcers and for maintenance treatment.

- *Misoprostol (Cytotec®).* This synthetic prostaglandin, a substance naturally produced by the body, protects the stomach lining by increasing mucus and bicarbonate production and by enhancing blood flow to the stomach. It is approved only for the prevention of NSAID-induced ulcers.

Two common non-prescription protective medications are:

- *Antacids.* Antacids can offer temporary relief from ulcer pain by neutralizing stomach acid. They may also have a mucosal protective role. Many brands of antacids are available without prescription.

- *Bismuth Subsalicylate.* Bismuth subsalicylate has both a protective effect and an antibacterial effect against *H. pylori*.

*Antibiotics*

The discovery of the link between ulcers and *H. pylori* has resulted in a new treatment option. Now, in addition to treatment aimed at decreasing the production of stomach acid, doctors may prescribe antibiotics for patients with *H. pylori*. This treatment is a dramatic medical advance because eliminating *H. pylori* means the ulcer may now heal and most likely will not come back.

The most effective therapy, according to the NIH Panel, is a 2-week, triple therapy [see sidebar titled "Therapy Routines" at the end of this chapter]. This regimen eradicates the bacteria and reduces the risk of ulcer recurrence in 90 percent of people with duodenal ulcers. People with stomach ulcers that are not associated with NSAIDs also benefit from bacterial eradication. While triple therapy is effective, it is sometimes difficult to follow because the patient must take three different medications four times each day for 2 weeks.

In addition, the treatment commonly causes side effects such as yeast infection in women, stomach upset, nausea, vomiting, bad taste, loose or dark bowel movements, and dizziness. The 2-week, triple therapy combines two antibiotics, tetracycline (e.g., Achromycin or Sumycin) and metronidazole (e.g., Flagyl®) with bismuth subsalicylate (Pepto-Bismol®). Some doctors may add an acid-suppressing drug to relieve ulcer pain and promote ulcer healing. In some eases, doctors may substitute amoxicillin (e.g., Amoxil® or Trimox®) for tetracycline or if they expect bacterial resistance to metronidazole, other antibiotics such as clarithromycin (Biaxin®).

As an alternative to triple therapy, several 2-week, dual therapies are about 80 percent effective. Dual therapy is simpler for patients to follow and causes fewer side effects. A dual therapy might include an antibiotic, such as amoxicillin or clarithromycin, with omeprazole, a drug that stops the production of acid.

Again, an accurate diagnosis is important. Accurate diagnosis and appropriate treatment prevent people without ulcers from needless exposure to the side effects of antibiotics and should lessen the risk of bacteria developing resistance to antibiotics.

Although all of the above antibiotics are sold in the United States, the FDA has not yet approved the use of antibiotics for treatment of *H. pylori* or ulcers. Doctors may choose to prescribe antibiotics to their ulcer patients as "off label" prescriptions as they do for many conditions.

## When Is Surgery Needed?

In most eases, anti-ulcer medicines heal ulcers quickly and effectively. Eradication of *H. pylori* prevents most ulcers from recurring. However, people who do not respond to medication or who develop complications may require surgery. While surgery is usually successful in healing ulcers and preventing their recurrence and future complications, problems can sometimes result.

At present, standard open surgery is performed to treat ulcers. In the future, surgeons may use laparoscopic methods. A laparoscope is a long tube-like instrument with a camera that allows the surgeon to operate through small incisions while watching a video monitor. The common types of surgery for ulcers—vagotomy, pyloroplasty, and antrectomy—are described below:

*Vagotomy*

A vagotomy involves cutting the vagus nerve, a nerve that transmits messages from the brain to the stomach. Interrupting the messages sent through the vagus nerve reduces acid secretion. However, the surgery may also interfere with stomach emptying. The newest variation of the surgery involves cutting only parts of the nerve that control the acid-secreting cells of the stomach, thereby avoiding the parts that influence stomach emptying.

*Antrectomy*

Another surgical procedure is the antrectomy. This operation removes the lower part of the stomach (antrum), which produces a hormone that stimulates the stomach to secrete digestive juices. Sometimes a surgeon may also remove an adjacent part of the stomach that secretes pepsin and acid. A vagotomy is usually done in conjunction with an antrectomy.

*Pyloroplasty*

Pyloroplasty is another surgical procedure that may be performed along with a vagotomy. Pyloroplasty enlarges the opening into the duodenum and small intestine (pylorus), enabling contents to pass more freely from the stomach.

## What Are the Complications of Ulcers?

People with ulcers may experience serious complications if they do not get treatment. The most common problems include bleeding, perforation of the organ walls, and narrowing and obstruction of digestive tract passages.

*Bleeding*

As an ulcer eats into the muscles of the stomach or duodenal wall, blood vessels may also be damaged, which causes bleeding. If the affected blood vessels are small, the blood may slowly seep into the digestive tract. Over a long period of time, a person may become anemic and feel weak, dizzy, or tired.

If a damaged blood vessel is large, bleeding is dangerous and requires prompt medical attention. Symptoms include feeling weak and dizzy when standing, vomiting blood, or fainting. The stool may become a tarry black color from the blood.

Most bleeding ulcers can be treated endoscopically, a process in which the ulcer is located and the blood vessel is cauterized with a heating device or injected with material to stop bleeding. If endoscopic treatment is unsuccessful, surgery may be required.

*Perforation*

Sometimes an ulcer eats a hole in the wall of the stomach or duodenum. Bacteria and partially digested food can spill through the opening into the sterile abdominal cavity (peritoneum). This causes peritonitis, an inflammation of the abdominal cavity and wall. A perforated ulcer that can cause sudden, sharp, severe pain usually requires immediate hospitalization and surgery.

*Narrowing and obstruction*

Ulcers located at the end of the stomach where the duodenum is attached, can cause swelling and scarring, which can narrow or close the intestinal opening. This obstruction can prevent food from leaving the stomach and entering the small intestine. As a result, a person may vomit the contents of the stomach.

Endoscopic balloon dilation, a procedure that uses a balloon to force open a narrow passage, may be performed. If the dilation does not relieve the problem, then surgery may be necessary.

## Conclusion

Although ulcers may cause discomfort, rarely are they life threatening. With an understanding of the causes and proper treatment, most people find relief. Eradication of *H. pylori* infection is a major medical advance that can permanently cure most peptic ulcer disease.

## Additional Reading

DeCross, A. J., Peura, D. A. "Role of *H. Pylori* in Peptic Ulcer Disease." *Contemporary Gastroenterology*, 1992; 5(4): 18–28.

Fedotin, M. S. "*Helicobacter pylori* and Peptic Ulcer Disease: Reexamining the Therapeutic Approach." *Postgraduate Medicine*, 1993; 94(3): 38–45.

Gilbert, G., Chan, C. H., Thomas, E. "Peptic Ulcer Disease: How to Treat It Now." *Postgraduate Medicine*, 1991; 89(4): 91–98.

*Mayo Clinic Family Health Book*. Larson, D. E., editor. New York: William Morrow and Company, Inc., 1990. General medical guide with sections on stomach problems and ulcers.

## *The History of* Helicobacter pylori

In 1982, Australian researchers Barry Marshall and Robin Warren discovered spiral-shaped bacteria in the stomach, later named *Helicobacter pylori* (*H. pylori*). After closely studying *H. pylori*'s effect on the stomach, they proposed that the bacteria were the underlying cause of gastritis and peptic ulcers.

Marshall and Warren came to this conclusion because in their studies all patients with duodenal ulcers and 80 percent of patients with stomach ulcers had the bacteria. The 20 percent of patients with stomach ulcers who did not have *H. pylori* were those who had taken NSAIDs such as aspirin and ibuprofen, which are a common cause of stomach ulcers.

Although their findings seem conclusive, Marshall and Warren's theory was hotly debated and remained in dispute. The debate continued even after Marshall and a colleague performed an experiment in which they infected themselves with *H. pylori* and developed gastritis.

Evidence linking *H. pylori* to ulcers mounted over the next 10 years as numerous studies from around the world confirmed its presence in most people with ulcers. Moreover, researchers from the United States and Europe proved that using antibiotics to eliminate *H. pylori* healed ulcers and prevented recurrence in about 90 percent of cases.

To further investigate these findings, the National Institutes of Health (NIH) established a panel to closely review the link between *H. pylori* and peptic ulcer disease. At the February 1994 Consensus Development Conference, the panel concluded that *H. pylori* plays a significant role in the development of ulcers and that antibiotics with other medicines can cure peptic ulcer disease.

## Therapy Routines

### Typical Two-Week Triple Therapy

- Metronidazole 4 times a day
- Tetracycline (or amoxicillin) 4 times a day
- Bismuth subsalicylate 4 times a day

### Typical Two-week Dual Therapy

- Amoxicillin 2 to 4 times a day, or clarithromycin 3 times a day
- Omeprazole 2 times a day

## Points to Remember

- An ulcer is a sore or lesion that forms in the lining of the stomach or duodenum where the digestive fluids acid and pepsin are present.

- Recent research shows that most ulcers develop as a result of infection with bacteria called *Helicobacter pylori* (*H. pylori*). The bacteria produce substances that weaken the stomach's protective mucus and make the stomach more susceptible to damaging effects of acid and pepsin. *H. pylori* can also cause the stomach to produce more acid. Although acid and pepsin and lifestyle factors such as stress and smoking cigarettes play a role in ulcer formation, *H. pylori* is now considered the primary cause.

- Nonsteroidal anti-inflammatory drugs such as aspirin make the stomach vulnerable to the harmful effects of acid and pepsin, leading to an increased chance of stomach ulcers.

- Ulcers do not always cause symptoms. When they do, the most common symptom is a gnawing or burning pain in the abdomen between the breastbone and navel. Some people have nausea, vomiting, and loss of appetite and weight.

- Bleeding from an ulcer may occur in the stomach and duodenum. Symptoms may include weakness and stool that appears tarry or black. However, sometimes people are not aware they have a bleeding ulcer because blood may not be obvious in the stool.

- Ulcers are diagnosed with x-ray or endoscopy. The presence of *H. pylori* may be diagnosed with a blood test, breath test, or tissue test. Once an ulcer is diagnosed and treatment begins, the doctor will usually monitor progress.

- Doctors treat ulcers with several types of medicines aimed at reducing acid production, including $H_2$-blockers, acid pump inhibitors, and mucosal protective drugs. When treating *H. pylori*, these medications are used in combination with antibiotics.

- According to an NIH panel, the most effective treatment for *H. pylori* is a 2-week, triple therapy of metronidazole, tetracycline or amoxicillin, and bismuth subsalicylate.

- Surgery may be necessary if an ulcer recurs or fails to heal or if complications such as bleeding, perforation, or obstruction develop.

## Chapter 17

# *Peptic Ulcer Disease: Debugging the System*

Back in 1983, when Australian researchers Barry J. Marshall and J. Robin Warren first proposed that ulcers were caused by bacteria, gastroenterologists guffawed. But skepticism gave way to amazement as study after study confirmed that a particular spiral-shaped germ, originally called *Campylobacter* but later renamed *Helicobacter pylori*, thrives in the stomachs of nearly everyone with duodenal ulcers and four out of five of those with stomach ulcers.

Nine years later, a team of Texas investigators demonstrated that eradicating *H. pylori* with antibiotics protected nearly 90% of ulcer patients from subsequent attacks of their disease. That's when the world really took notice. Because this study offered unprecedented evidence that ulcers can be cured with antibiotics, the *Health Letter's* advisory board rated it as one of the ten most important medical breakthroughs of 1992. These results have since been confirmed by other researchers.

But it wasn't until early this year that the once heretical *H. pylori* hypothesis truly became part of medicine's canon. In February, the National Institutes of Health (NIH) convened a panel of medical experts to consider whether antimicrobial drugs ought to become standard therapy for people with ulcers. After scrutinizing all the evidence, the experts came down in favor of antibiotics.

The NIH consensus statement on *H. pylori* and peptic ulcer disease caught many doctors and patients by surprise. In addition to

---

This chapter is copyrighted and originally appeared in *Harvard Health Letter*, Vol. 19, No. 8 in June 1994.

raising questions about who should take antibiotics and under what circumstances, the statement also made some people wonder whether the $H_2$ blockers, antisecretory medications widely used to relieve ulcer symptoms, would become obsolete.

One of these agents, Zantac, is the largest selling prescription drug in the world and millions of people use its three competitors, Tagamet, Axid, and Pepcid.

## Rules of Thumb

The NIH panel's most important recommendation is that all patients with gastric or duodenal ulcers caused by *H. pylori* should be treated with antibiotics. But, the experts emphasized, these drugs should not be used until the physician has established the facts of the case. First, the presence of an ulcer must be confirmed by X-ray studies or direct visualization through an endoscope. Many people with healthy, intact stomach linings sometimes feel pain or discomfort that can easily be mistaken for symptoms of an ulcer. Physicians must also prove that *H. pylori* infection exists before reaching for the prescription pad. This can be most easily accomplished with a test that detects certain antibodies in blood or identifies a tell-tale enzyme in expelled breath. Alternatively, doctors can analyze a snip of stomach tissue removed during endoscopic examination.

These diagnostic guidelines benefit patients in several ways. When *H. pylori* is absent and ulcers result from the use of aspirin or other drugs, for example, it makes no sense to take unneeded antibiotics. The NIH experts also noted that the majority of people who test positive for *H. pylori* never develop ulcers but some of them suffer from belly pain, nausea, bloating, heartburn, or other gastric complaints. These symptoms should not be treated with antibiotics, the panel emphasized. Not only do these powerful drugs cause unpleasant and even dangerous side effects in some people, but they also could speed the evolution of drug resistant forms of *H. pylori* when overused. (See the *Harvard Health Letter*, April 1993.)

## Once Is Enough

Antibiotics represent a dramatic treatment advance not only because they heal ulcers, but because they prevent recurrence. Standard $H_2$ blockers do a perfectly respectable job of promoting healing, which they accomplish by reducing the secretion of gastric acid. But

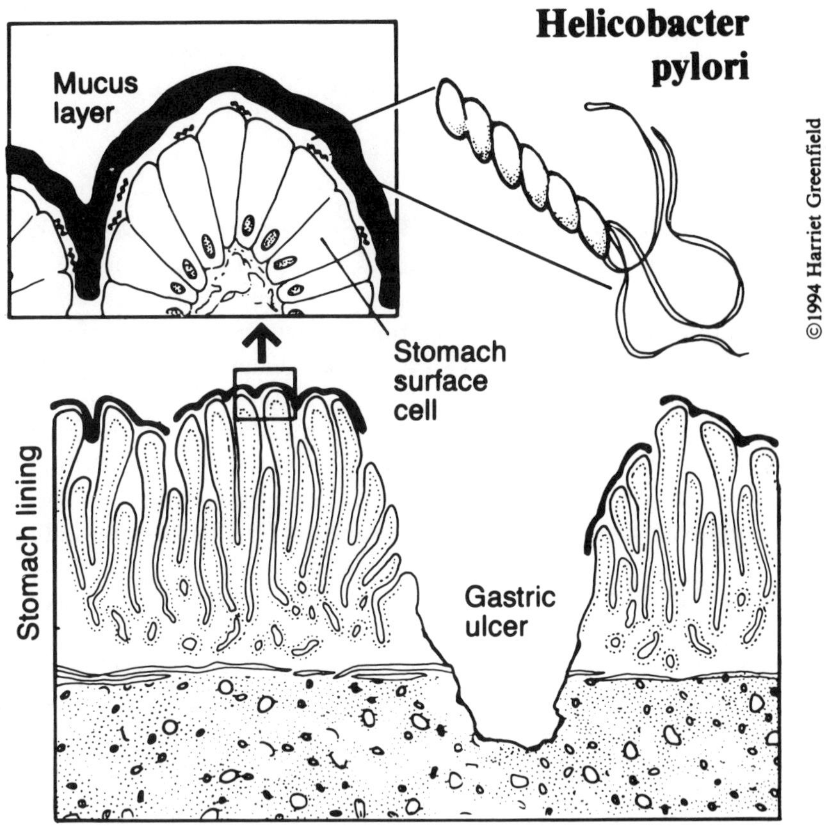

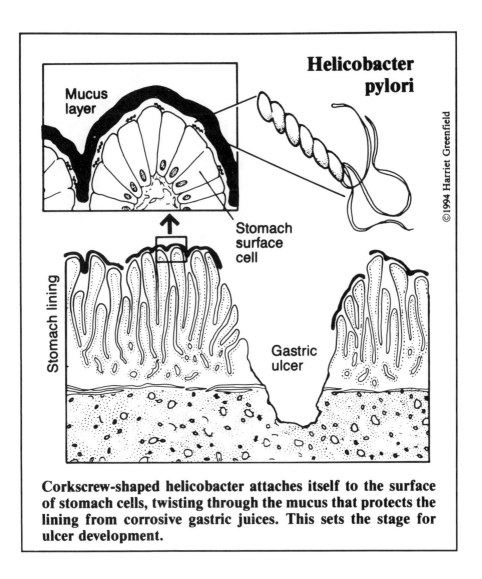

**Corkscrew-shaped helicobacter attaches itself to the surface of stomach cells, twisting through the mucus that protects the lining from corrosive gastric juices. This sets the stage for ulcer development.**

*Figure 17.1.*

85% of the time ulcers recur within a year after treatment ends. These agents have no lasting effect on any of the underlying factors that cause ulcers, such as excess acid secretion, *H. pylori* infection, emotional stress, or habitual use of tobacco and alcohol. In contrast, a proper course of antibiotic treatment can eradicate helicobacter infection and sharply reduce the risk of ever having ulcers again. In the largest study done so far. only 15% recurred after two years.

## Strategic Choices

Although the members of the NIH panel agreed that two full weeks of antibiotic therapy is almost always enough to wipe out all the *H. pylori* organisms in the stomach, they did not endorse any specific drug regimen. They advised doctors and patients to choose after weighing the effectiveness, dosing schedule, side effects, and cost of various treatment programs.

One of the best studied approaches, which combines the antibiotics tetracycline and metronidazole with bismuth subsalicylate (PeptoBismol), eradicates helicobacter about 90% of the time. Doctors sometimes substitute amoxicillin for one of the antimicrobials in this mix or use an $H_2$ blocker instead of bismuth.

Only slightly less effective is a two-drug program using amoxicillin and omeprazole (a powerful acid-blocker, sold as Prilosec), a combination that is simpler to take and associated with fewer side effects. The panel recommended that patients with bleeding ulcers, who are at greatest risk for life-threatening complications, should take maintenance doses of $H_2$ blockers after completing antibiotic therapy.

In the 1970s, $H_2$ blockers were considered wonder drugs. Although the new war on germs has diminished their role, it has not relegated them to the scrap heap. According to the NIH experts, one of these agents should be used for several weeks, overlapping with antimicrobial therapy, to promote healing of newly identified ulcers. However, the kind of long-term, low-dose antisecretory treatment that millions of people have been using to manage their ulcer disease may soon be a thing of the past. Someday it may be rare for anyone to have ulcers more than once.

*—by Stephen E. Goldfinger, M.D.*

## *Why* Helicobacter?

Most living things find the acid environment of the human stomach to be extremely inhospitable. But the spiral-shaped microbe *Helicobacter pylori* and its relatives thrive in the bellies of humans and other warm-blooded animals.

Helicobacter lives happily in the stomach because it is uniquely equipped to produce large quantities of *urease*, an enzyme that generates ammonia to neutralize the acid that quickly kills most other bacteria. Like a corkscrew, helicobacter twists itself into the viscous mucus layer that protects the stomach lining from corrosive gastric juices. Instead of penetrating stomach cells, however, it attaches itself to their surfaces. Scientists believe that it contributes to ulcers in several ways including thinning the protective mucus layer, poisoning nearby cells with ammonia or other toxins, or even increasing acid production.

Chapter 18

# *NIH Consensus Summary on* **Helicobacter Pylori** *in Peptic Ulcer Disease*

Using a combination of antibiotics to eradicate a stomach bacterium may finally offer a cure to the 25 million Americans who at some time in their lives develop peptic ulcer disease.

According to a 14-member independent panel recently convened by the National Institute of Diabetes and Digestive and Kidney Diseases and the NIH Office of Medical Applications of Research, ulcer patients who test positive for *Helicobacter pylori (H. pylori)* infection should be treated for at least two weeks with a combination of bismuth and antimicrobial drugs. Antimicrobial drugs kill microorganisms such as *H. pylori*, a bacterium said to infect 80 percent of patients with stomach ulcers. Dual and triple combinations of bismuth and antimicrobial drugs successfully cure *H. pylori* infection and reduce the rate of ulcer recurrence in up to 90 percent of ulcer patients, said the panel.

Of the several drug combinations presented during the $2^1/_2$-day conference, the panel said that triple therapies, consisting of bismuth plus the antibiotics metronidazole and tetracycline, were the most effective. In some cases, resistance to metronidazole may require a substitution of amoxicillin.

---

Originally titled *A Summary of the NIH Consensus on Helicobacter Pylori in Peptic Ulcer Disease* (February 7-9, 1994). Free single copies of the complete NIH consensus statement *Helicobacter Pylori in Peptic Ulcer Disease* may be ordered from the NIH Consensus Program Information Service, P. O. Box 2577, Kensington, MD 20891. 1-800-NIH-OMAR (1-800-644-6627).

The panel also identified several effective dual therapies, one of which combines amoxicillin with ormeprazole, a proton-pump inhibitor. Mild side effects occur with each drug combination, but they do not normally prevent patients from completing their treatment. The panel added that standard acid-suppressing drugs should be added to the antimicrobial regimen to relieve ulcer symptoms.

Until now, the traditional treatment of peptic ulcer disease involved minimizing and suppressing and secretion with drugs called $H_2$ blockers, which interfere with the release of histamine and thus reduce acid production in the stomach. The most commonly used $H_2$ blockers are ranitidine and cimetidine. Although $H_2$ blockers successfully heal ulcers, if the patient stops taking these drugs, he or she has a 50 to 80 percent chance of the ulcer recurring.

But since the 1982 isolation of *H. pylori* by Australian researchers Barry Marshall and Robin Warren, many have believed that the spiral organism plays a significant causal role in peptic ulcer disease, and there has been a growing interest in using antibiotics to treat ulcers.

Peptic ulcer disease, estimated to affect 4.5 million people each year in the United States is a chronic inflammation of the stomach lining or of the duodenum. While few people die from peptic ulcer disease, it is responsible for substantial human suffering and staggering economic costs. Every year four million people report mission approximately six days from work because of their ulcers. Now the panel believes that their recommended treatments will not only alter the way doctors treat ulcers but lower health care costs and reduce human suffering.

Research indicates that *H. pylori* infects approximately 6 in 10 people in the United States by age 60, while the infection rate in developing countries is 8 in 10 people by age 5. Although uncertainty remains about how the infection is spread, person-to-person contact appears to be a significant means of transmitting the bacteria. Whether or not *H. pylori* infection can be transmitted through contaminated food and water, and how often, requires further study.

To prevent the development of bacterial resistance to antimicrobials, the panel stressed that an accurate diagnosis should be made before a patient starts any antimicrobial treatment. The panel cited several invasive and noninvasive tests that are useful in diagnosing *H. pylori* infection.

Endoscopic biopsy and cell culture are invasive tests that provide visualization and details about the status of the gastric and duodenal lining. Sensitivity and specificity of these procedures range from 85 to 100 percent.

However, the panel said that excellent diagnostic sensitivities and specificities are also produced with noninvasive tests. These included bloodtests to measure the urease-secreting properties of *H. pylori*.

Although a number of highly accurate diagnostic tests are available, the panel said that some used only in research studies will soon be available for commercial use. Despite these diagnostic tools, the panel noted that there are no readily available, inexpensive and accurate noninvasive methods to monitor eradication of *H. pylori*. Without such tools, routine monitoring for relapse, reinfection, or treatment failure cannot be recommended.

The panel also found an association between *H. pylori* infection and gastric cancer. Considered a slow and insidious disease, the incidence of gastric cancer increases with age and occurs more frequently in blacks and Hispanics than whites. Despite the fact that gastric cancer appears to occur more frequently in some populations with higher rates of *H. pylori* infection, the panel found no conclusive evidence that treating the infection reduces cancer risk. They contend that there are factors other than *H. pylori* infection, such as geography, socioeconomic status, and ethnicity that cause the development of gastric cancer.

Finally, the experts called for future research on the mechanisms and natural history of *H. pylori* infection, whether *H. pylori* eradication prevents gastric cancer, and to analyze the comprehensive cost and impact of treating versus not treating all patients who are infected with *H. pylori*.

# Chapter 19

# *Therapeutic Endoscopy and Bleeding Ulcers*

Peptic ulcer disease is a major health problem in the United States that affects more than 4 million people each year. Bleeding is one of the most dread complications of peptic ulcer. Upper gastrointestinal (UGI) bleeding is a common cause of emergency hospitalization in the United States. It has been estimated that more than 100,000 patients with peptic ulcer disease bleed each year. Morbidity and mortality from ulcer bleeding remain significant despite major improvements in the accurate diagnosis of peptic ulcer disease and the use of $H_2$ receptor antagonist drugs and other pharmacological agents. The mortality rate from bleeding ulcers has averaged between 6 and 10 percent over the past 30 years despite advances in diagnosis and treatment.

During the past decade there has been a remarkable transition of the application of the endoscope from solely a diagnostic tool to a therapeutic modality. With the advent of this therapeutic role there has been much enthusiasm in utilizing endoscopic techniques in managing high-risk patients. A variety of approaches for endoscopic management of bleeding have evolved, and there has been continuing improvement over the past decade, resulting in considerable interest in evaluating the various treatment options for managing patients with bleeding ulcers. Unfortunately, there have been limited and conflicting clinical studies on the efficacy and safety of the various hemostatic modalities available for treating these ulcers. In an effort

---

This chapter was taken from a National Institutes of Health Consensus Development Consensus Statement (Vol. 7, No. 6, March 6–8 1989).

to define the role of these methods, the National Institute of Diabetes and Digestive and Kidney Diseases and the Office of Medical Applications of Research of the National Institutes of Health sponsored a Consensus Development Conference on Therapeutic Endoscopy and Bleeding Ulcers. The conference brought together research clinicians and other health professionals and representatives of the public on March 6–8, 1989. Following two days of presentations and discussion by the invited experts and the audience, members of a consensus panel drawn from the health care and medical communities weighed the scientific evidence in formulating a statement in response to several questions:

- Which bleeding ulcer patients are at risk for rebleeding and thus emergency surgery?
- How effective is endoscopic hemostatic therapy?
- How safe is endoscopic hemostatic therapy?
- Which bleeding patients should be treated?
- What further research is required?

It is important that certain limitations be considered when applying the findings of this conference to a particular bleeding patient. The conference was charged to address specifically the question of therapeutic endoscopy for the treatment of bleeding peptic ulcer. Other causes of UGI bleeding, including gastric and esophageal varices, diffuse erosive gastritis, and Mallory-Weiss tears were necessarily excluded from consideration. It should be noted that the conclusions reached should not be extrapolated to those diseases excluded from consideration. Moreover, a striking finding from the review of available clinical trials of therapeutic endoscopy was the selective inclusion of only a small proportion (10 to 25 percent) of the total population of patients who presented with UGI bleeding. In addition to patients with the above diagnoses, many other patients were also excluded, quite appropriately, due to hemorrhage too massive or too little to justify prudent therapeutic endoscopy.

In this conference, the need for *emergency* surgery was taken as one indicator of inadequately controlled bleeding. Although many patients treated with surgery do well, they are subjected to additional discomfort and cost and to approximately a 10-percent risk of mortality when the surgery must be performed under such emergency conditions. On the other hand, when temporary hemostasis achieved by endoscopic therapy allows resuscitation and hemodynamic control of an unstable patient, considerable benefit may be realized even if surgery must be performed ultimately. For a variety of reasons, a surgeon should be involved from the outset in the team caring for the patient with bleeding peptic ulcer.

## 1. Which Bleeding Ulcer Patients Are at Risk for Rebleeding and Thus Emergency Surgery?

### I. Clinical Features

#### A. Magnitude of Bleeding

There is consensus that a major predictor of significant persistent or recurrent bleeding is the magnitude of blood loss before initial evaluation. Clear indications of a large and clinically significant volume of blood loss are hemodynamic instability, hematemesis of grossly red material, or red stool. The hazard of hemodynamic instability underlies the importance of careful hemodynamic evaluation in order to detect significant hypovolemia before the appearance of overt shock. Another commonly used indicator of the magnitude of hemorrhage is estimation of the volume of blood lost, often quantitated as the number of units transfused or as a transfusion rate. Although there is general agreement that the volume of blood loss is important, there is substantial uncertainty about the best way to estimate it. Persistent red blood in the nasogastric aspirate correlates with an increased requirement for subsequent transfusion. Although failure of the nasogastric aspirate to clear with irrigation often is taken as an indication of rapid bleeding, this criterion may be misleading.

#### B. Host Factors

Patient-related factors also predict persistent or recurrent bleeding. The panel finds that documented coagulopathy and the onset of bleeding in a patient already hospitalized for a related or unrelated condition are predictive of recurrent bleeding. Two other factors, age and the existence of concurrent illnesses, while clearly related to mortality, bear a less clear relationship to prognosis for continued bleeding or rebleeding.

### *II. Endoscopic Features*

The first and most important endoscopic predictor of persistent or recurrent bleeding is active bleeding at the time of endoscopy, as evidenced by arterial spurting or oozing. Also of importance is the presence of a discrete protuberance within the ulcer crater, often referred to by endoscopists as a "visible vessel" or "sentinel clot." There is consensus that some pigmented protuberances (red, blue, or purple) imply a high risk of rebleeding, even when not associated with bleeding at the time of endoscopy. There is less agreement on the prognostic significance of a white or black protuberance. A white protuberance may be indicative of an older, more organized process. Although any such lesions often are referred to as "visible vessels," pathologic studies indicate that only some are true vessels. Most frequently, they represent a hemostatic plug (clot) in the underlying vessel or a false aneurysm. The prognostic implications of these distinctions remain unclear. An additional endoscopic predictor of recurrent bleeding is the presence of a clot that adheres to the ulcer base despite gentle washing (adherent clot).

Whereas the anatomic location of the ulcer often is cited as a prognostic factor, the panel members do not agree that the site is clearly predictive. Nevertheless, many endoscopists feel that deep ulcers located high on the lesser curvature of the stomach or in the posterior-inferior wall of the duodenal bulb are at greater risk for severe bleeding due to their proximity to large vessels.

Features that clearly appear to be associated with a low frequency of recurrent bleeding include a clean ulcer base or one that contains a flat pigmented spot indicative of old hemorrhage.

### *III. Value of Combined Clinical and Endoscopic Predictors*

Whereas the above clinical and endoscopic features are predictive when considered singly, they may become particularly useful as prognostic indicators when considered together.

## 2. How Effective Is Endoscopic Hemostatic Therapy?

The following consensus statements on the effectiveness of the various endoscopic hemostatic therapies are based on the limited number of studies performed. Results were reported only for the acute hospital stay; only sparse followup data are available. The level of efficacy of individual treatment modalities varies from study to study.

Some factors that may account for this variability are small sample sizes, variation in patient characteristics such as age, entry criteria, differing definitions of such terms as "visible vessel" or "rebleed," and timing of endoscopy. Nonetheless, certain conclusions can be drawn from these studies.

## *Most Promising Techniques*

### Multipolar Electrocoagulation (MPEC)

MPEC (also known as bipolar) appears to be an effective modality for achieving immediate hemostasis and preventing rebleeding in actively bleeding patients and patients with "visible vessels." The data are less clear that MPEC decreases the need for emergency surgical intervention or decreases mortality.

Further advantages of this modality are that it does not require an *en face* approach to the bleeding point, the endoscopist can control the depth of tissue injury, and the equipment is portable and easy to use.

Recommendations are evolving concerning technique in terms of probe size, power setting, pressure applied, and duration and number of pulses delivered.

### Heater Probe

In comparison with "conventional" medical therapy, the heater probe appears to achieve immediate hemostasis and to reduce rebleeding and the need for emergency surgery. The advantages of heater probe therapy are the same as for MPEC.

Early data for MPEC and heater probe suggest no delay in ulcer healing in treated patients.

## *Other Techniques*

### Neodymium-Yttrium-Aluminum-Garnet (Nd-YAG) Laser

Nd-YAG laser appears to be effective for achieving immediate hemostasis and preventing rebleeding. Studies have also shown a trend toward reducing need for emergency surgery and lowering mortality. Difficulties in using this instrument include gaining access to the bleeding lesion for an *en face* approach and training endoscopists in its use. Laser therapy is difficult to master and apply.

Furthermore, the Nd-YAG laser is costly to use in relation to other modalities. Although portability has been an obstacle in its use, new portable instruments are now available.

#### Injection Therapy

Some agents (e.g., sodium chloride, epinephrine, and ethanol) appear promising for early control of bleeding. Currently there are insufficient data to make specific recommendations concerning the proper role of this approach.

However, injection therapies warrant further study because of their technical ease of use, low cost, and promise.

### *Techniques Not Recommended*

#### Topical

There is no current evidence for efficacy of the following agents: cyanoacrylate glue, clotting factors, ferromagnetic tamponade, epinephrine lavage, and microcrystalline collagen hemostat.

#### Argon Laser

This technique appears to be effective for immediate hemostasis, but available data do not demonstrate significant reduction in rebleeding, mortality, or need for emergency surgery. This technique has been superseded by other, more effective treatment modalities.

#### Monopolar/Electrohydrothermal Coagulation

This modality appears to be effective for immediate hemostasis. However, monopolar therapy has been replaced by other techniques because of difficulty in its use due to the necessity to meet the bleeding point en face, to control the depth of injury, and to perform multiple cleanings of the probe.

## *3. How Safe Is Endoscopic Hemostatic Therapy?*

Safety may be compromised by:

- Patient characteristics: Hemodynamic instability and associated illnesses.

- Ulcer characteristics: Depth and location, especially posterior-inferior duodenal bulb and high lesser curvature of the stomach because of the proximity to large arteries.

- Method of therapy: Excessive depth of penetration of energy or injectant.

The consensus of the panel is that therapeutic endoscopy should be performed only by an endoscopist experienced and qualified in the specific therapeutic techniques. Appropriate professional organizations should develop guidelines for training and for quality assurance.

The goal of endoscopic hemostatic treatment is to stop active bleeding and prevent rebleeding while controlling depth of tissue injury and avoiding excessive necrosis, increased bleeding, and perforation. The only indication to remove an adherent clot other than by low-pressure irrigation is in the actively bleeding patient or the patient who has rebled. After clot removal, the endoscopist must be prepared to apply therapy.

The risk of precipitating bleeding with therapy is variable but has been as high as 20 percent. While this bleeding can usually be controlled by the same endoscopic hemostatic therapy, occasionally uncontrollable bleeding will require emergency surgical intervention. The risk of perforation has been approximately 1 percent and may require laparotomy should it occur.

In the patient population at high risk of rebleeding, the rate of complications of endoscopic hemostatic therapy appears to be acceptably low considering the natural history of the disease.

As the technology in this field advances, controlled observations of potential complications are needed to ensure that safety remains within acceptable limits.

## 4. Which Bleeding Ulcer Patients Should Be Treated?

Acute peptic ulcer bleeding will stop spontaneously in approximately 70 to 80 percent of patients. Therefore, there is consensus that a need exists for selectivity in applying endoscopic hemostatic therapy to bleeding ulcers. Such therapy should be directed at selected high-risk patients.

A clinical feature of high risk for rebleeding or death is rapid bleeding with substantial blood loss manifested by hemodynamic instability, ongoing transfusion requirement, red hematemesis, or red stool.

Other patient characteristics that predict a poor outcome from ulcer bleeding include age greater than 60 years and major associated diseases. Patients whose onset of bleeding occurs in the hospital or who rebleed during hospitalization are also at high risk.

Patients with high-risk clinical features are candidates for therapeutic/hemostatic endoscopy. The observations at endoscopy should then determine whether endoscopic hemostatic therapy should be carried out. There is consensus that the findings of pulsatile bleeding ("spurting") or oozing from the ulcer are indications for treatment. In addition, the finding of a pigmented protuberance ("visible vessel" or "sentinel clot") in the ulcer crater is an indication for endoscopic hemostatic therapy.

There is agreement that patients with ulcer craters that are clean with or without flat pigmented spots do not require endoscopic hemostatic treatment.

In the absence of the clinical risk factors described above, adherent clots (resisting gentle washing) without evident active bleeding should *not* be removed because of the possible risk of precipitating bleeding. In a deteriorating clinical situation, adherent clots may be removed as long as there is satisfactory endoscopic access and capability for treatment. Surgical backup should be readily available to deal with the possibility of precipitating active bleeding that cannot be controlled endoscopically, and thus the need for early surgical consultation.

Patients exsanguinating with torrential bleeding from peptic ulcer represent a special case. The panel agrees that endoscopic localization and treatment should be attempted in concert with the surgeon and without undue delay.

It should be recognized that *deep* ulcers near the left gastric artery high on the lesser curvature of the stomach and those near the to gastroduodenal artery in the posterior-inferior duodenal bulb may be at high risk for major bleeding. This emphasizes that surgical support must be available before endoscopic treatment of ulcers in these anatomic locations is undertaken.

It is important to resuscitate patients and correct coagulopathy as completely as possible before endoscopic hemostatic therapy. Uncontrollable coagulopathy appears to be a contraindication to endoscopic hemostatic therapy in the patient who is not actively bleeding. However, in the patient who is actively bleeding, endoscopic hemostatic therapy may be attempted despite uncorrectable coagulopathy with the awareness that control of hemorrhage may be temporary.

Endoscopic treatment of patients with bleeding peptic ulcers should be carried out only by individuals qualified in therapeutic endoscopy.

## *5. What Further Research Is Required?*

Despite the considerable technical advances that have been made in the past decade in endoscopic hemostatic therapy, firm conclusions regarding clinical applications are limited by a paucity of controlled trials. There is consensus that a number of important issues remain to be resolved and that high priority should be given to continuing scientific evaluation of techniques. There is a strong need to use rigorous scientific methods resolve the following issues:

- Standardize use of terminology, particularly descriptive terms such as "visible vessel" (e.g., white, blue, red, black or bare), adherent clot, persistent and recurrent bleeding.

- Quantitate rebleeding risk associated with endoscopic features such as "visible vessel," adherent clot, size, depth and location of ulcer, and timing of endoscopy.

- Quantitate rebleeding risk associated with different host factors such as aging, nonsteroidal anti-inflammatory drug use (including aspirin), and associated diseases.

- Develop a composite system using clinical and endoscopic features to predict risk of persistent or recurrent bleeding.

- Define optimal treatment regimens for individual and combined treatment modalities to maximize therapeutic effectiveness.

- Explore improved diagnostic and therapeutic technology through collaboration with bioengineers.

Clinical effectiveness and safety of endoscopic hemostatic therapies would be best assessed by multicenter, randomized controlled trials. Ulcer patients at high risk but without active bleeding at endoscopy should be entered into studies comparing endoscopic therapies with medical therapies. There is a lack of consensus regarding the need for a medical therapy control group of patients with active bleeding at endoscopy.

## Conclusions and Recommendations

- In the United States, more than 100,000 patients a year bleed from peptic ulcers.
- Despite advances in diagnosis and treatment, the mortality rate from bleeding ulcers has remained largely unchanged, averaging between 6 and 10 percent over the past 30 years.
- Bleeding from peptic ulcers will stop spontaneously in 70 to 80 percent of patients.
- A surgeon should be involved from the outset in the team caring for the patient with a bleeding peptic ulcer.
- Patients at high risk for persistent or recurrent bleeding are those with a large initial blood loss and active bleeding or a pigmented protuberance ("visible vessel") at endoscopy.
- Patients at low risk for subsequent bleeding are those with a clean ulcer base or one that contains a flat pigmented spot at endoscopy.
- Heater probe and multipolar electrocoagulation (also known as bipolar) are the most promising modalities for endoscopic hemostatic therapy.
- In the hands of the qualified therapeutic endoscopist, the rate of complications of endoscopic hemostatic therapy is acceptably low considering the natural history of bleeding peptic ulcers.
- Endoscopic hemostatic therapy should be used only in patients who are at high risk for persistent or recurrent bleeding and death.
- Clinical efficacy and safety of endoscopic hemostatic therapy should be assessed by multicenter, randomized controlled trials.

*—by Michael J. Bernstein,*
*Director of Communications,*
*Office of Medical Applications of Research,*
*and James N. Fordham,*
*Writer / Editor,*
*National Institute of Diabetes and*
*Digestive and Kidney Diseases,*
*National Institutes of Health,*
*Bethesda, Maryland.*

The conference was sponsored by:

National Institute of Diabetes and Digestive and Kidney Diseases
Phillip Gorden, M.D.
Director

NIH Office of Medical Applications of Research
John H. Ferguson, M.D.
Director

NIH Consensus Development Conferences are convened to evaluate available scientific information and resolve safety and efficacy issues related to a biomedical technology. The resultant NIH Consensus Statements are intended to advance understanding of the technology or issue in question and to be useful to health professionals and the public.

*NIH Consensus Statements are prepared by a nonadvocate, nonfederal panel of experts, based on: (1) presentations by investigators working in areas relevant to the consensus question during a 1½ day public session; (2) questions and statements from conference attendees during open discussion periods that are part of the public session; and (3) closed deliberations by the panel during the remainder of the second day and morning of the third. This statement is an independent report of the panel and is not a policy statement of the NIH or the Federal Government. Copies of this statement and bibliographies prepared by the National Library of Medicine are available from the Office of Medical Applications of Research, National Institutes of Health, Building 1, Room 260, Bethesda, MD 20892.*

## Chapter 20

# *Surprise Cause of Gastritis Revolutionizes Ulcer Treatment*

Mention "ulcer" and most people envision a stressed-out, workaholic, junk-food-gobbling worrywart. Since the turn of the century, ulcers have been equated with stress and poor diet. But that image may be substantially incorrect. Now, the medical community is beginning to look at painful ulcers in a new light—as an easily treatable bacterial infection. The name of the bug—*Helicobacter pylori*.

For many of the 4 million ulcer sufferers in the United States, the new view of ulcers may mean a course of antibiotics. This treatment may reduce recurrence to below the 10 to 15 percent a year for current, non-antibiotic drug therapies. In ulcer sufferers who receive no treatment, recurrence is up to 80 percent.

"Now there is the possibility of curing the condition, which was unthought of before," says Hugo Gallo-Torres, M.D., medical officer in the Food and Drug Administration's division of gastrointestinal and coagulation drug products.

The agency is considering particular combinations of drugs for ulcer treatment, following conclusions of a consensus development conference convened by the National Institutes of Health in February 1994. The conference gathered experts to review data accumulating since 1983 implicating bacteria in causing ulcers. The drugs under consideration aren't new, but their use to treat ulcers is.

---

Originally appeared in *FDA Consumer Magazine*, December 1994.

## Anatomy of an Ulcer

Sufferers describe an ulcer as a burning, cramping, gnawing, or aching in the abdomen that comes in waves, for three to four days at a time, but may subside completely for weeks or months. Pain is worst before meals and at bedtime, when the stomach is usually empty. The ulcer itself is an open sore in the lining of the stomach (gastric ulcer) or in the upper part of the small intestine, or duodenum (duodenal ulcer). Both types are also called peptic ulcers.

The stomach is the most acidic part of the body, setting the stage both for ulcer development and infection. Three types of cells pump out the ingredients of gastric juice: mucous-secreting cells, chief cells that release digestive enzymes, and parietal cells that produce hydrochloric acid. The mucous-secreting cells also produce histamine, which stimulates the parietal cells to release acid. The stomach needs the acid environment for the digestive enzyme pepsin to break down proteins in foods.

Acidity is measured using the pH scale. A neutral pH is neither acid nor base—it has a value of 7; acids are less than 7, and bases (also called alkaline substances) are greater than 7. Many body fluids, including blood, tears, pancreatic juice, and bile, are in the 7 to 8 pH range. Gastric juice, in contrast, has a pH of 1.6 to 1.8. That's more acidic than lemon juice, cola drinks, and coffee. The environment in the small intestine is far less acidic than in the stomach, but because it receives the acidic mixture of semi-digested food from the stomach, it is prone to ulceration too.

The stomach's innermost lining, the mucosa, protects it from digesting itself. The mucosa consists of lining cells, connective tissue, and muscle. An ulcer hurts when it penetrates the mucosa into the underlying submucosa, which is rich in nerves and blood vessels.

A vat of churning acidic goop may not seem a hospitable place for a microbe, but the type that causes ulcers thrives in the low pH environment. "They have outgrowths called flagella that allow them to penetrate the mucus layer of the stomach, where the pH is more tolerable. "Eradicating these bacteria is not simple," says Gallo-Torres. The antibiotic drug must be able to kill the bacteria, yet also resist breakdown in the acidic surroundings.

Researchers aren't certain how people acquire the bacteria. However, person-to-person transmission is believed to be the most likely route in developed countries. In developing countries, fecal-oral transmission may play a more important role, similar to the way a person contracts cholera and hepatitis A.

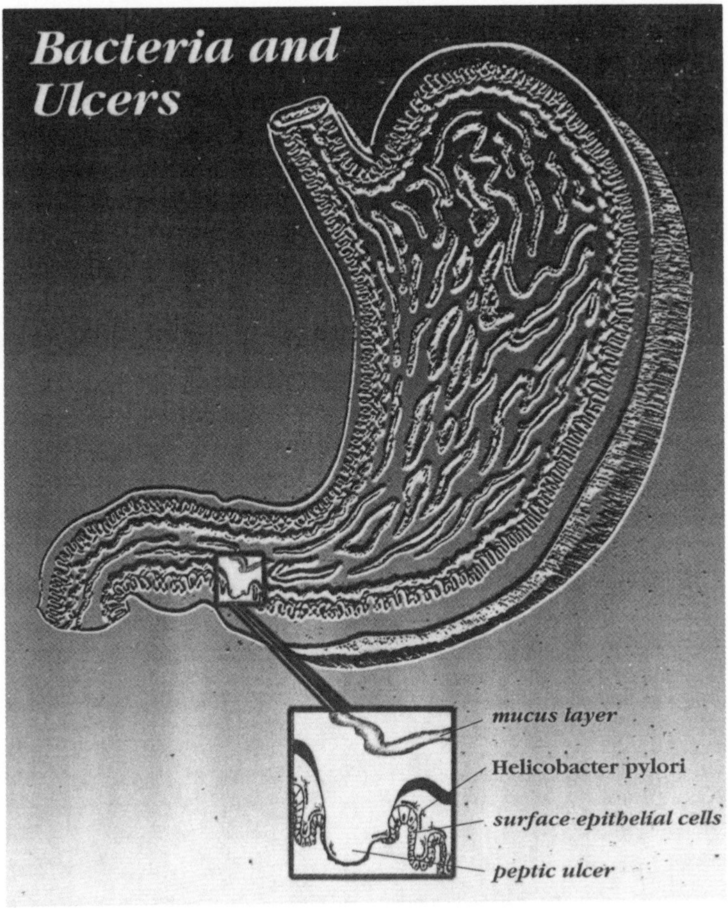


***Figure 20.1.*** *Spiral-shaped* Helicobacter pylori *bacteria attach to the surface epithelial cells of the stomach lining after eating a hole in the mucus layer that normally protects the lining from gastric juice. Gastritis results and a peptic ulcer may develop.*

Early in the 20th century, the prescription for an ulcer was bed rest and a bland diet, in a hospital if the patient could afford it. Antacids were added to the treatment regimen when researchers learned that ulcer patients produce excess stomach acid. By 1971, the control site of acid secretion was identified—histamine ($H_2$) receptors on the parietal cells.

When histamine binds such receptors, acid output increases. Four approved ulcer drugs—Zantac (ranitidine), Tagamet (cimetidine), Pepcid (famotidine), and Axid (nizatidine)—block $H_2$ receptors, thwarting the signal to secrete acid. A second type of ulcer drug, called an acid- or proton-pump inhibitor, works at a different point in digestion, blocking parietal cells from releasing acid. Prilosec (omeprazole) is the only acid-pump inhibitor approved in the United States at this time.

The problem with existing drugs is that they only temporarily improve symptoms; the ulcer is likely to return. If bacteria causing some ulcers are eradicated, however, the likelihood of ulcer recurrence is much less because the problem is attacked at its source. But acceptance of the role of bacteria in the production of peptic ulcer disease has been slow.

## Discovering the Infection Connection

In 1982, two young Australian physicians, Barry J. Marshall and J. Robin Warren, isolated bacteria from patients with ulcers or gastritis (stomach inflammation). In a paper published in the medical journal *Lancet* in early 1983, they proposed that a spiral-shaped bacterium, later named *Helicobacter pylori*, causes gastritis and possibly ulcers. But few physicians accepted their work, so entrenched was the idea that ulcers stem from stress. So Marshall and Warren took drastic measures to prove their point—they swallowed some of the bacteria. And their digestive tracts soon became inflamed.

But most of the medical community felt this was not sufficient proof to definitively implicate the bacteria in causing ulcers. A medical dictionary published in 1986, for example, lists the causes of ulcers in order of importance as high acid, irritation, decreased blood supply to the digestive tract, decreased mucus, and last, with a question mark, infection.

"We had treated ulcers with anti-secretory compounds for so many years, it was hard to accept that a germ, a bacterium, would produce a disease like that. It took a while. Even academicians were not convinced. Gradually other people found the same thing," says Gallo-Torres.

The accumulating evidence became the basis of the February 1994 consensus development conference, which concluded: "Ulcer patients with *Helicobacter pylori* infection require treatment with anti-microbial agents in addition to anti-secretory drugs."

In a nutshell, the evidence for the link between bacteria and ulcers is that:

- All patients examined who are infected with the bacteria have evidence at the tissue level of gastritis (inflammation), but most are asymptomatic.
- Clearing up the infection cures the gastric inflammation.
- Giving the bacteria to laboratory animals (and Warren and Marshall) causes gastritis.

However, even though nearly all people who are infected develop gastritis, not all develop ulcers. This suggests that other factors—such as heredity, diet, stress, and other environmental influences—may be important for the development of peptic ulcers. According to the consensus development report, "the strongest evidence for the pathogenic role of *H. pylori* in peptic ulcer disease is the marked decrease in recurrence rate of ulcers following the eradication of infection."

How common are bacterial ulcers? The consensus report estimates that "almost all" duodenal ulcers are attributable to *H. pylori*, as are about 80 percent of gastric ulcers, making the microbes a very major cause. A very small percentage of ulcer sufferers develop ulcers from using aspirin or a nonsteroidal anti-inflammatory drug (NSAID) such as Voltaren (diclofenac), Feldene (piroxicam), or Ansaid (flurbiprofen). Ibuprofen, also an NSAID, is less likely to cause gastric inflammation.

## Diagnosis

For ulcer patients, diagnosis and treatment are changing.

Several different tests detect *H. pylori*. "You can biopsy [take tissue samples of] gastric and duodenal mucosa, then culture bacteria and identify them. But this approach is not very sensitive because it depends upon where you biopsy," says Gallo-Torres.

To sample stomach or intestinal tissue, a physician snakes a lighted tube called an endoscope down through the throat. Less invasive techniques are available, too. Blood tests can detect IgG antibodies to

*H. pylori* in a person's blood, representing the immune system's response to the microbe. These tests are cleared for marketing by FDA.

Other diagnostic tests in development, but not yet evaluated by FDA, are based on the ability of *H. pylori* to break down urea, human metabolic waste, with an enzyme called urease, which humans do not produce. Elevated levels of breakdown products of urea, detected in a person's breath after drinking chemically labeled urea, indicate *H. pylori* infection.

## Treatment

Quite a few helpful drugs are already on the market, though they are not approved for treating ulcers. FDA's role now is to wade through studies, old and new, to identify the best combinations of drugs, a process that was under way when this issue of *FDA Consumer* went to press. FDA is also considering new drugs to treat bacterial ulcers.

"We would really like to inform physicians quickly and also evaluate the data. There are many regimens proposed," says Gallo-Torres.

The consensus development conference examined several treatment plans. Its report said that there had been extensive studies of bismuth subsalicylate (better known as Pepto Bismol), an antiprotozoan drug, Flagyl (metronidazole), and either the antibiotic tetracycline (giving an overall 90 percent cure rate) or amoxicillin (with an overall 80 percent cure rate).

According to the consensus development report, there had been one study of another regimen, consisting of amoxicillin, metronidazole and ranitidine, that showed a 90 percent effective rate. However, all of these approaches require a patient to take several different pills several times a day. The committee reported that a two-drug alternative, consisting of amoxicillin, taken four times a day, and Prilosec (omeprazole), taken twice a day, offers 80 percent effectiveness. However, at press time FDA had not verified these regimens.

Clearly, doctors will have many choices. But at the time of the conference, only 1 to 2 percent of U.S. physicians were treating an ulcer as they would a bacterial infection, according to the conference report.

Concluded conference member Daniel K. Podolsky, M.D., of Massachusetts General Hospital, "These recommendations represent a sea change in how we approach this problem. From this time forward, I would consider use of these drugs to be essential."

As data confirming the bacteria-ulcer link continue to pour in, medical researchers are already asking questions that will form the basis of future studies: What factors cause bacterial gastritis to develop into an ulcer? Do children have bacterial ulcers? Can the new treatments prevent complications, such as bleeding ulcers? Does *H. pylori* cause stomach cancer, and, if so, can we prevent it?

Meanwhile, the future of current ulcer sufferers looks brighter than ever. Says consensus team member Ann L. B. Williams, M.D., of George Washington University Medical College, "We now have an opportunity to cure a disease that previously we had only been able to suppress or control."

## Can the Ulcer Bacterium Also Cause Cancer?

It's been known for several years that people with a form of stomach cancer called gastric carcinoma are very often infected with *H. pylori*, and there is evidence that the infection precedes the cancer. More recently, researchers linked the microbe to a second type of stomach cancer, called primary gastric lymphoma.

This second type of malignancy affects lymphoid tissue-antibody-producing cells in the stomach. However, such cells are not normally present in the stomach unless there is an infection.

In the May 5, 1994, issue of *The New England Journal of Medicine*, a multi-center team led by Julie Parsonnet, M.D., of Stanford University, reported that people with gastric lymphoma also have *H. pylori* infection, and that the infection precedes the cancer. In an accompanying editorial, Peter G. Isaacson, D.M., of University College London Medical School, suggests that the bacterial infection initiates a chain reaction leading to cancer. He suggests that first infection causes chronic gastritis; then, the inflammation causes stomach lining tissue to overgrow; and, ultimately, excess growth may blossom into cancer, given some as-yet unidentified environmental trigger or genetic susceptibility.

But, so far, the link between *H. pylori* and cancer is far more tenuous than that between the bacteria and gastritis or ulcers. Fewer than 1 percent of people infected with the microbe develop cancer, and some populations in which many people are infected have very low stomach cancer rates. These facts, researchers say, suggest that several factors are at play. Still, it will be interesting to see if antibiotic/anti-secretory treatment can reduce incidence of these already rare cancers.

The consensus development conference convened to study *H. pylori* in February 1994 concluded, "if there is any causal relationship between *H. pylori* infection and gastric cancer, clearly other facts are also important." They recommend further study into whether eradicating the infection can prevent cancer.

*—By Ricki Lewis, a geneticist and college biology textbook writer.*

# Part Four

# Intestinal and Anorectal Disorders

Chapter 21

# *Diverticulosis and Diverticulitis*

Diverticulosis is a condition in which outpouchings form in the walls of the intestines. These pouches, known as diverticula, are about the size of large peas. They form in weakened areas of the bowels, most often in the lower part of the colon (large bowel). (See Figure 21.1.)

***Figure 21.1.***

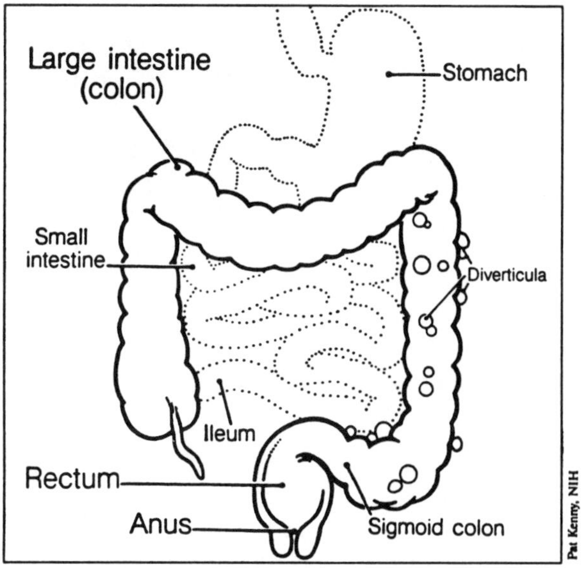


NIH Pub. 92–1163. This chapter was originally published as a Diverticulosis and Diverticulitis Fact Sheet, by the DD Clearinghouse, National Institutes of Health.

## What Are the Symptoms of Diverticulosis?

Most people with diverticula do not have any symptoms from them. They may never know they have the condition. Some people feel tenderness over the affected area or muscle spasms in the abdomen. Pain may be felt on the lower left side of the abdomen or, less often, in the middle or on the right side.

Although the diverticula themselves do not cause symptoms, complications such as bleeding and infection may occur. Bleeding is an uncommon symptom and is usually not severe. Sometimes the pouches become infected and inflamed, a more serious condition known as diverticulitis. (See Figure 21.2.) When inflammation is present, there may be fever and an increased white blood cell count, as well as acute abdominal pain. Diverticulitis also may result in large abscesses (infected areas of pus), bowel blockage, or breaks and leaks through the bowel wall.

## How Are These Disorders Diagnosed?

Often diverticulosis is unsuspected and is discovered by an x-ray or intestinal examination done for an unrelated reason. The doctor may see the diverticula through a flexible tube (colonoscope) that is inserted through the anus. Through this scope, the diverticula may be seen as dark passages leading out of the normal colon wall. The doctor also may do a barium enema, an x-ray that reveals the outpouchings in the walls of the colon.

If rectal bleeding occurs, the doctor may take a special x-ray (angiography). In this procedure, dye is injected into an artery that goes to the colon, so that the site of the bleeding problem can be located. Diverticulitis may be diagnosed when a patient has pain and tenderness in the lower abdomen with disturbed bowel function and fever.

## How Common Are These Disorders?

Diverticulosis is very common, especially in older people. Studies show that about 10 percent of people over the age of 40 and nearly half of people over age 60 have diverticulosis. But among those who are found to have diverticula, only about 20 percent develop diverticulitis, and of those, only a small number have very serious or life-threatening complications.

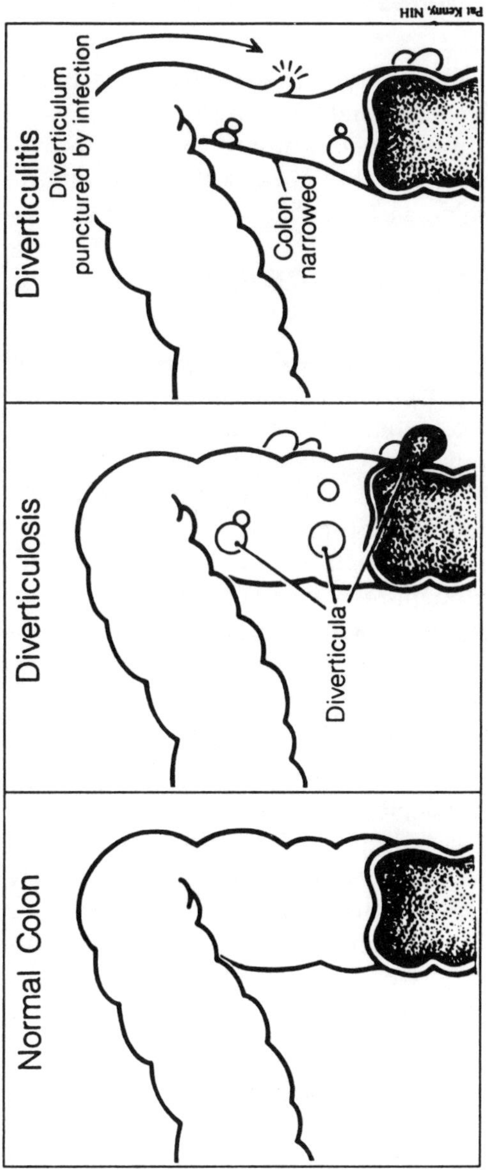

Normal Colon
Diverticulosis
Diverticula
Diverticulitis
Diverticulum punctured by infection
Colon narrowed
Pat Kenny, NIH


*Figure 21.2.*

## What Causes Diverticula to Form?

No one knows for sure why the pouches form. Scientists think they may be caused by increased pressure inside the colon due to muscle spasms or straining. The sacs might form when increased pressure acts on soft spots along the bowel wall, especially if the person has constipation problems or uses laxatives too often.

## How Serious Are These Disorders?

For most people, diverticulosis is not a problem. Diverticulitis, on the other hand, is a problem, sometimes a serious one. (See Figure 21.2.) For instance, when one of the sacs (a diverticulum) becomes infected and inflamed, bacteria enter small tears in the surface of the bowel. This leads to small abscesses. Such an infection may remain localized and go away within a few days. In rare cases, the infection spreads and breaks through the wall of the colon causing peritonitis (infection of the abdominal cavity) or abscesses in the abdomen. Such infections are very serious and can lead to death unless treated without delay.

## What Are the Treatments?

If you have diverticulosis with no symptoms, no treatment is needed. Some doctors advise eating a high-fiber diet and avoiding certain foods. Laxatives and enemas should not be used regularly. Patients with diverticulitis may be hospitalized and treated with bed rest, pain relievers, antibiotics, fluids given by vein, and careful monitoring.

## Is Surgery Ever Necessary?

The majority of patients will recover from diverticulitis without surgery. Sometimes patients need surgery to drain an abscess that has resulted from a ruptured diverticulum and to remove that portion of the colon. Surgery is reserved for patients with very severe or multiple attacks. In those cases, the involved segment of colon can be removed and the colon rejoined.

In some cases, the two ends of the colon cannot be rejoined right away, so more than one operation is needed. For instance, an operation may be performed to drain an abscess and remove diseased colon and a second operation done to rejoin the colon. In this case, the surgeon must connect the colon to a surgically created hole on the body's surface (colostomy) until a second operation can be done to reconnect the colon.

The delay between operations may be only a few weeks, or it might be several months if the patient needs time to overcome infection and build up strength. In rare cases, three operations are needed: the first to drain an abscess, the second to remove part of the colon, and the third to rejoin the bowel.

## What About Diet?

If you have diverticulosis with no symptoms, you don't need treatment, but it is a good idea to watch your diet. The diet some doctors recommend is the same kind that is healthy for most people—eat more foods high in fiber. (See *Diet, Nutrition & Cancer Prevention: The Good News* in the additional readings section.) A fiber-rich diet helps prevent constipation and promotes a healthy digestive tract. Fiber-rich foods include whole-grain cereals and breads, fruits, and vegetables. A fiber-rich diet is also thought to help prevent diverticula from forming.

Remember, diverticula usually cause no problems at all, so a diagnosis of diverticulosis should not be a serious concern.

## Additional Readings

*Diet, Nutrition & Cancer Prevention: The Good News* (NIH Publication No. 87-2878). Pamphlet available from the Cancer Information Service, Office of Cancer Communications, National Cancer Institute, 9000 Rockville Pike, Bethesda, MD 20892. 1-800-4-CANCER. Discusses high-fiber diet and fiber-rich foods.

*Diverticulitis and Diverticulosis.* Fact sheets available from the National Organization for Rare Disorders, Inc., P.O. Box 8923, New Fairfield, CT 06812-1783. (203) 746-6518.

Ertan A. Colonic diverticulitis: recognizing and managing its presentations and complications. *Postgraduate Medicine* 1990; 88(3): 67–72, 77. This article for primary care physicians discusses how to recognize, evaluate, and manage diverticulitis.

Larson DE, Editor-in-chief. *Mayo Clinic Family Health Book*. New York: William Morrow and Company, Inc., 1990. General medical guide with section on diverticular disease. Available in libraries and bookstores.

Weck E. New hope for those with diverticular disease. *FDA Consumer* 1987; 21(6):23–5. Article reprint available from the Food and Drug Administration, 5600 Fishers Lane, Rockville, MD 20857 or in libraries.

## Chapter 22

# *Dietary Changes that Help Prevent Diverticular Disease*

As the U.S. population grows older, experts have warned, Americans can expect to suffer from an increasing number of health problems. In recent years, however, attention has turned to the possibility that most Americans—by changing their lifestyles—may be able to avoid or control many of the diseases traditionally associated with aging, if they act in time.

One condition associated with aging for which new hope has emerged in recent years is diverticular disease, [that is, the] inflammation or infection of the large intestine, or colon. Diverticular disease rarely touches people under 40. But more than half of Americans have it by the time they reach 60.

Most people with a milder form of diverticular disease (diverticulosis) aren't aware they have it because they experience no symptoms. However, when it progresses to diverticulitis, they may suffer a variety of symptoms, including severe pain. Diverticulitis may lead to dangerous bowel complications requiring hospitalization and even major surgery. Though the disease itself is rarely fatal, complications from diverticulitis can cause death.

Diverticular disease consists of small sacs of grape-like protrusions formed when the lining of the intestine is forced out through the gut's muscular wall. The lesions may occur anywhere in the gut, but are found mostly in the colon. Doctors call them diverticula or a diverticulum when there is only one. (It's from the Latin verb *divertere*,

---

This chapter originally appeared as "New Hope for Those with Diverticular Disease" in *FDA Consumer* magazine, July/August 1987.

which means to turn aside.) These small, self-contained hernias of the colon wall vary in size from a fraction of an inch to slightly over an inch in diameter.

The small hernias in the gastrointestinal tract that give rise to diverticula usually occur in the last segment, called the sigmoid (for S-shaped), or descending, colon. So, to understand how diverticula develop, it's helpful to see how the large intestine functions.

The colon, [which is] five to seven feet long and three to four inches in diameter, is composed, in part, of two sets of muscles. One set runs lengthwise in three roughly parallel lines. The other encircles the colon in parallel rings, giving the organ a bumpy appearance like that of a long balloon ringed by strings that partially restrict its cross-section every inch or so.

The colon receives watery, undigested material from the small intestine. Acting in concert, the two sets of muscles push this residue from one end to the other in wave-like, squeezing motions. In the process, the colon wall may contract and expand up to 10 times a minute. As the undigested material moves through the colon, some vitamins, water and minerals are absorbed into the bloodstream. Finally, bacteria break down the residue before it is expelled through the rectum.

In diverticulosis, the colon contracts and its walls tend to thicken. This is particularly true of the sigmoid, the narrowest and most muscular section. The normally pillow-like external convolutions may take on a corrugated appearance instead. This process of constriction occurs as the sigmoid exerts more pressure on its contents. This added pressure is probably one of the causes of diverticula, although researchers are far from certain about how diverticulosis begins.

Weak spots often form in the intestinal wall, particularly along the corrugated ridges of the colon. At these weak spots, diverticula made up of mucous membrane and connective tissue may balloon through the muscle wall like bubble gum from the mouth of a child. They usually occur where arterioles (small arteries) enter the colon through small gaps in the muscle wall. Occasionally these arterioles balloon out with the diverticula.

According to one estimate, of the millions who harbor diverticula, only one in five will develop symptoms or become sick. Those with symptoms may complain of occasional nausea, constipation, gas, bloating and, sometimes, pain. (These same symptoms can arise from other diseases, such as irritable bowel syndrome, gastric ulcer, hiatal hernia, and liver disease.)

Physicians have two ways to diagnose diverticular disease: the diverticula can be seen on a barium enema X-ray of the lower digestive tract, and the tiny telltale hernias inside the colon wall often can be detected by examination with an endoscope (a flexible fiber device for seeing inside hollow organs of the body).

Physicians use such diagnostic procedures to follow up many gastrointestinal complaints. For example, sigmoidoscopy, an endoscopic examination of the sigmoid colon, is often part of routine physical checkups, particularly in middle-aged men, who tend to suffer a higher incidence of colon cancer. So diverticula may be discovered during routine physical examinations or as physicians diagnose other problems of the digestive tract.

When diverticula become inflamed, diverticulosis turns into diverticulitis. The likelihood of developing this inflammatory complication rises if diverticula are numerous or widely distributed in the colon, if they appear at an early age, or if they have been present 10 years or longer.

Inflamed diverticula may lead to several complications. The inflammation may give rise to an abscess when fecal matter, which occasionally lodges in diverticula, leaks out and contaminates the exterior surface of the colon; the inflamed tissue may adhere to nearby pelvic organs such as the bladder or vagina; a fistula, or hollowing, may develop between the colon and the organ stuck to the diverticula, allowing dangerous wastes to pass between them; a hole may open in a diverticulum and cause fecal matter or pus from an abscess to flow more freely into the pelvic or abdominal cavity, causing peritonitis, a dangerous inflammation of the abdominal cavity's lining; or tiny blood vessels that often form part of the diverticula may bleed.

Patients with diverticulitis may have pain, at times severe, and local tenderness near the groin in the lower left or, occasionally, the lower right abdominal quadrant. Some patients may complain of pain even when the disease is not inflammatory. Other symptoms may include pain when urinating; constipation, often interrupted by diarrhea or other changes in bowel movements; fever; and rectal bleeding.

Doctors advise patients with diverticular disease to stay away from harsh laxatives and avoid straining during bowel movements in order to lessen discomfort.

Diverticulitis often clears up spontaneously. When treatment is necessary it depends on the nature and degree of inflammation. For severe and persistent cases, bed rest or hospitalization may be prescribed. In an acute phase of diverticular disease, the first objective may be to rest the colon. So a physician may prescribe a bland diet or even intravenous feeding until flare-ups subside. Antibiotics and pain-killing drugs may be indicated in some cases. However, physicians must be careful to differentiate cases of painful diverticulosis from diverticulitis because antibiotics are not prescribed for the former, which is not inflammatory or infected.

Although medical science lacks experimental evidence in humans to demonstrate exactly how diverticula arise, animal studies and epidemiological evidence support the view that dietary fiber plays a role. Before the turn of the century, diverticular disease was virtually unknown in the United States. But since then the number of cases has risen in Western countries, particularly the United States, England and Australia. Epidemiologists (doctors who study the causes and control of diseases in populations) note that the increased incidence of diverticular disease has paralleled the introduction of highly refined foods starting early in the 20th century. Some have associated the rise with the introduction, in the 19th century, of steel flour mills, which produce pulverized flour low in fiber.

Other epidemiologists have observed that diverticular disease is virtually unknown among rural Asian and African peoples who subsist largely on a high-fiber vegetable diet. Comparing the incidence of the disease in the developed countries and the Third World, some researchers, such as Dr. D. P. Burkitt—who spent many years studying nutrition and disease in Africa—have concluded that dietary fiber does play a key role in preventing diverticular disease.

After Dr. Burkitt and others published their epidemiological evidence in the *American Journal of Digestive Diseases* in 1971, physicians began to advise patients with diverticular disease to add fiber to their diets.

A study of 100 hospitalized patients with diverticular disease, published in the *British Journal of Surgery* in February 1980, showed that by adding fiber to their diets, over 90 percent of the patients remained symptom-free for five to seven years after release from the hospital. Older studies done before dietary fiber was used reported that only 38 percent to 64 percent of such discharged patients remained symptom free. So, although dietary fiber is not a cure, it appears that it can reduce or eliminate symptoms.

The precise role of fiber in preventing diverticular disease or controlling its symptoms is not yet known. However, dietary fiber increases the volume of the stool. The bulkier the stool, the faster it moves through the intestine. Stools high in fiber also retain moisture. This keeps them soft and bulky, thereby stimulating healthy colon function. Stools low in fiber, on the other hand, tend to lack water, leaving them compact and hard. The colon responds by exerting greater pressure to move the residue, giving rise to constipation and then diverticula.

How can you be sure that you are getting enough dietary fiber?

Foods rich in dietary fiber include breads, cereals and other products made from whole grains; brown rice; raw fruit (including edible skin and pulp) such as apples, peaches, berries, and citrus fruits; cabbage, broccoli, spinach and other leafy green vegetables, carrots, celery, most varieties of beans, squash, asparagus and string beans.

One substance that has proven to be most effective in retaining the bulk and moisture of stool in the colon is wheat bran. Wheat bran is readily available either alone or as an ingredient in products such as breakfast cereals or muffins.

*—By Egon Weck*

Egon Weck is a free-lance writer who has written extensively on health and medical issues.

## *One Patient's Bout with Diverticulitis*

Dr. William R. Stern, chairman of the Department of Gastroenterology at Shady Grove Adventist Hospital in Rockville, MD, treats many patients with diverticular disease. He first saw a 61-year-old male diverticular patient (we'll call him Gus) in 1985 when Gus came in with stomach pains. In Dr. Stern's office, Gus complained that he had stomach cramps and discomfort in his rectum.

Gus was diagnosed as having diverticulosis, and Dr. Stern put him on a high-fiber diet. "For about 18 months, from followup visits, we felt that Gus's problem was under control," Dr. Stern notes. "By last December, however, he complained of more severe rectal discomfort. Though there was no fever or bleeding, we brought him into the hospital because he was so uncomfortable and somewhat dehydrated."

In the hospital, lab tests and studies showed that Gus had a mild case of diverticulitis, meaning the diverticula had become inflamed or infected. He was given antibiotics to clear up the infection and put on a low-fiber diet to prevent further irritation of the inflamed areas. (During certain acute phases of diverticulitis, it's best to avoid fiber until symptoms subside.) He was released after four days.

Gus seemed to be doing well at home for about a week. But then he began feeling more uncomfortable. This time the discomfort was accompanied by fever and shaking chills.

Back in the hospital, tests showed that there was an abscess, or infection, on the outside of the diverticula. Dr. Stern began intravenous feeding and administered more antibiotics. “Once the infection is under control,” explains Dr. Stern, “he’ll need to have surgery to remove about a one-foot section of his colon which includes the inflammation and the abscess.”

In cases where the infection that accompanies diverticulitis can’t be brought under control with antibiotics, surgeons are forced to go in more promptly. In such cases they perform two operations: first a colostomy to bring the abscessed part of the colon out to the abdominal wall and drain the area of the abscess. Then, once the infection subsides, the colon is reconnected in a second operation.

In rare cases, three operations may be necessary: the first to circumvent the infection with a colostomy, the second to resect—or cut out—the diseased part of the colon, and the third to reconnect the two ends of the colon.

“Such complications are unusual,” observes Dr. Stern. “We can usually control acute cases of diverticulitis with antibiotics and low-residue diets until the inflammation resolves.”

Four months after surgery, Gus is doing well. According to Dr. Stern, “Gus has no pain, fever, or pressure in the rectum. And, although diverticula are present in other areas of Gus’s colon, the probability that he will require more surgery is low, because inflammation is most common in the sigmoid, which is the section that has been removed.”

## Chapter 23

# *Crohn's Disease*

Inflammatory bowel disease (IBD) is a group of chronic disorders that cause inflammation or ulceration in the small and large intestines. Most often IBD is classified as ulcerative colitis or Crohn's disease but may be referred to as colitis, enteritis, ileitis, and proctitis.

Ulcerative colitis causes ulceration and inflammation of the inner lining of the colon and rectum, while Crohn's disease is an inflammation that extends into the deeper layers of the intestinal wall.

Ulcerative colitis and Crohn's disease cause similar symptoms that often resemble other conditions such as irritable bowel syndrome (spastic colitis). The correct diagnosis may take some time.

Crohn's disease usually involves the small intestine, most often the lower part (the ileum). In some cases, both the small and large intestine (colon or bowel) are affected. In other cases, only the colon is involved. Sometimes, inflammation also may affect the mouth, esophagus, stomach, duodenum, appendix, or anus. Crohn's disease is a chronic condition and may recur at various times over a lifetime. Some people have long periods of remission, sometimes for years, when they are free of symptoms. There is no way to predict when a remission may occur or when symptoms will return.

## *What Are the Symptoms?*

The most common symptoms of Crohn's disease are abdominal pain, often in the lower right area, and diarrhea. There also may be

---

NIH Pub. No. 95–3410.

rectal bleeding, weight loss, and fever. Bleeding may be serious and persistent, leading to anemia (low red blood cell count). Children may suffer delayed development and stunted growth.

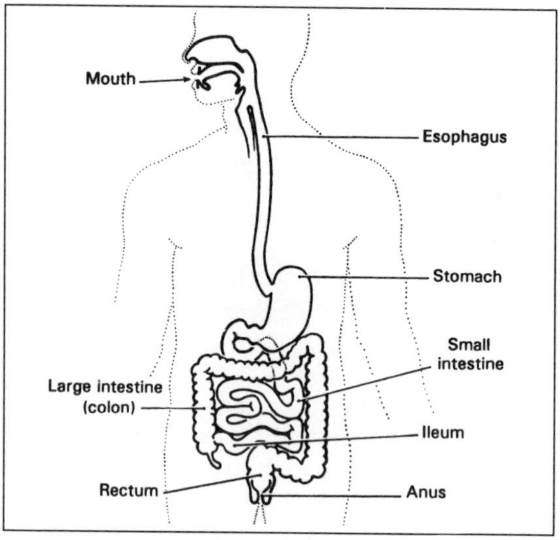


*Figure 23.1.*

## What Causes Crohn's Disease and Who Gets It?

There are many theories about what causes Crohn's disease, but none has been proven. One theory is that some agent, perhaps a virus or a bacterium, affects the body's immune system to trigger an inflammatory reaction in the intestinal wall. Although there is a lot of evidence that patients with this disease have abnormalities of the immune system, doctors do not know whether the immune problems are a cause or a result of the disease. Doctors believe, however, that there is little proof that Crohn's disease is caused by emotional distress or by an unhappy childhood.

Crohn's disease affects males and females equally and appears to run in some families. About 20 percent of people with Crohn's disease have a blood relative with some form of inflammatory bowel disease, most often a brother or sister and sometimes a parent or child.

## [How Does Crohn's Disease Affect Pregnancy?

Research has shown that the course of pregnancy and delivery is usually not impaired in women with Crohn's disease. Even so, it is a good idea for women with Crohn's disease to discuss the matter with their doctors before pregnancy.

## How Does Crohn's Disease Affect Children?

Women with Crohn's disease who are considering having children can be comforted to know that the vast majority of such pregnancies will result in normal children. Children who do get the disease are sometimes more severely affected than adults, with slowed growth and delayed sexual development in some cases.]

## How Is Crohn's Disease Diagnosed?

If you have experienced chronic abdominal pain, diarrhea, fever, weight loss, and anemia, the doctor will examine you for signs of Crohn's disease. The doctor will take a history and give you a thorough physical exam. This exam will include blood tests to find out if you are anemic as a result of blood loss, or if there is an increased number of white blood cells, suggesting an inflammatory process in your body. Examination of a stool sample can tell the doctor if there is blood loss, or if an infection by a parasite or bacteria is causing the symptoms.

The doctor may look inside your rectum and colon through a flexible tube (endoscope) that is inserted through the anus. During the exam, the doctor may take a sample of tissue (biopsy) from the lining of the colon to look at under the microscope.

Later, you also may receive x-ray examinations of the digestive tract to determine the nature and extent of disease. These exams may include an upper gastrointestinal (GI) series, a small intestinal study, and a barium enema intestinal x-ray. These procedures are done by putting the barium, a chalky solution, into the upper or lower intestines. The barium shows up white on x-ray film, revealing inflammation or ulceration and other abnormalities in the intestine.

If you have Crohn's disease, you may need medical care for a long time. Your doctor also will want to test you regularly to check on your condition.

## What Is the Treatment?

Several drugs are helpful in controlling Crohn's disease, but at this time there is no cure. The usual goals of therapy are to correct nutritional deficiencies; to control inflammation; and to relieve abdominal pain, diarrhea, and rectal bleeding.

Abdominal cramps and diarrhea may be helped by drugs. The drug sulfasalazine often lessens the inflammation, especially in the colon. This drug can be used for as long as needed, and it can be used along with other drugs. Side effects such as nausea, vomiting, weight loss, heartburn, diarrhea, and headache occur in a small percentage of cases. Patients who do not do well on sulfasalazine often do very well on related drugs known as mesalamine or 5-ASA agents. More serious cases may require steroid drugs, antibiotics, or drugs that affect the body's immune system such as azathioprine or 6-mercaptopurine (6-MP).

## Can Diet Control Crohn's Disease?

No special diet has been proven effective for preventing or treating this disease. Some people find their symptoms are made worse by milk, alcohol, hot spices, or fiber. But there are no hard and fast rules for most people. Follow a good nutritious diet and try to avoid any foods that seem to make your symptoms worse. Large doses of vitamins are useless and may even cause harmful side effects.

Your doctor may recommend nutritional supplements, especially for children with growth retardation. Special high-calorie liquid formulas are sometimes used for this purpose. A small number of patients may need periods of feeding by vein. This can help patients who temporarily need extra nutrition, those whose bowels need to rest, or those whose bowels cannot absorb enough nourishment from food taken by mouth.

## What Are the Complications of Crohn's Disease?

The most common complication is blockage (obstruction) of the intestine. Blockage occurs because the disease tends to thicken the bowel wall with swelling and fibrous scar tissue, narrowing the passage. Crohn's disease also may cause deep ulcer tracts that burrow all the way through the bowel wall into surrounding tissues, into adjacent segments of intestine, into other nearby organs such as the urinary bladder or vagina, or into the skin. These tunnels are called fistulas. They are a common complication and often are associated with pockets of infection or abscesses (infected areas of pus). The areas around the anus and rectum often are involved. Sometimes fistulas can be treated with medicine, but in many cases they must be treated surgically.

Crohn's disease also can lead to complications that affect other parts of the body. These systemic complications include various forms of arthritis, skin problems, inflammation in the eyes or mouth, kidney stones, gallstones, or other diseases of the liver and biliary system. Some of these problems respond to the same treatment as the bowel symptoms, but others must be treated separately.

## Is Surgery Often Necessary?

Crohn's disease can be helped by surgery, but it cannot be cured by surgery. The inflammation tends to return in areas of the intestine next to the area that has been removed. Many Crohn's disease patients require surgery, either to relieve chronic symptoms of active disease that does not respond to medical therapy or to correct complications such as intestinal blockage, perforation, abscess, or bleeding. Drainage of abscesses or resection (removal of a section of bowel) due to blockage are common surgical procedures.

Sometimes the diseased section of bowel is removed. In this operation, the bowel is cut above and below the diseased area and reconnected. Infrequently some people must have their colons removed (colectomy) and an ileostomy created.

In an ileostomy, a small opening is made in the front of the abdominal wall, and the tip of the lower small intestine (ileum) is brought to the skin's surface. This opening, called a stoma, is about the size of a quarter or a 50-cent piece. It usually is located in the right lower corner of the abdomen in the area of the beltline. A bag is worn over the opening to collect waste, and the patient empties the bag periodically. The majority of patients go on to live normal, active lives with an ostomy.

The fact that Crohn's disease often recurs after surgery makes it very important for the patient and doctor to consider carefully the benefits and risks of surgery compared with other treatments. Remember, most people with this disease continue to lead useful and productive lives. Between periods of disease activity, patients may feel quite well and be free of symptoms. Even though there may be long-term needs for medicine and even periods of hospitalization, most patients are able to hold productive jobs, marry, raise families, and function successfully at home and in society.

## Additional Readings

*Bleeding in the Digestive Tract* and *Ulcerative Colitis*. National Digestive Diseases Information Clearinghouse, 2 Information Way, Bethesda, MD 20892-3570; (301) 654-3810. General patient information fact sheets.

Brandt, LJ, Steiner-Grossman, P, eds. *Treating IBD: A Patient's Guide to the Medical and Surgical Management of Inflammatory Bowel Disease*. New York: Raven Press, 1989. General guide for patients with sections on treatment and descriptions and drawings of surgical procedures. Available from the Crohn's & Colitis Foundation of America.

Hanauer, SB, Peppercorn, MD, Present, DH. "Current Concepts, New Therapies in IBD." *Patient Care*, 1992; 26(13): 79–102. General review article for health care professionals.

Steiner-Grossman, P, Banks PA, Present, DH, eds. *The New People Not Patients: A Source Book for Living with IBD*. Dubuque, Iowa: Kendall/Hunt Publishing Company, 1992. Book for patients with sections on diagnostic tests, medications, nutrition, coping with employment and health insurance problems, and IBD in children and teenagers, older adults, and during pregnancy. Available from the Crohn's & Colitis Foundation of America.

## Additional Resources

Crohn's & Colitis Foundation of America, Inc.
386 Park Avenue South, 17th Floor
New York, NY 10016–8804
(800) 932-2423 or (212) 685-3440

Pediatric Crohn's & Colitis Association, Inc.
PO. Box 188
Newton, MA 02168
(617) 244-6678

Reach Out for Youth with Ileitis and Colitis, Inc.
15 Chemung Place
Jericho, NY 11753
(516) 822-8010

United Ostomy Association
36 Executive Park, Suite 120
Irvine, CA 92714
(800) 826-0826 or (714) 660-8624

# Chapter 24

# *Ulcerative Colitis*

Inflammatory bowel disease (IBD) is a group of chronic disorders that cause inflammation or ulceration in the small and large intestines. Most often IBD is classified as ulcerative colitis or Crohn's disease but may be referred to as colitis, enteritis, ileitis, and proctitis.

Ulcerative colitis causes ulceration and inflammation of the inner lining of the colon and rectum, while Crohn's disease is an inflammation that extends into the deeper layers of the intestinal wall. Crohn's disease also may affect other parts of the digestive tract, including the mouth, esophagus, stomach, and small intestine.

Ulcerative colitis and Crohn's disease cause similar symptoms that often resemble other conditions, such as irritable bowel syndrome (spastic colitis). The correct diagnosis may take some time.

In ulcerative colitis, the inner lining of the large intestine (colon or bowel) and rectum becomes inflamed. The inflammation usually begins in the rectum and lower (sigmoid) intestine and spreads upward to the entire colon. Ulcerative colitis rarely affects the small intestine except for the lower section, the ileum. The inflammation causes the colon to empty frequently, resulting in diarrhea. As cells on the surface of the lining of the colon die and slough off, ulcers (tiny open sores) form, causing pus, mucus, and bleeding.

An estimated 250,000 Americans have ulcerative colitis. It occurs most often in young people ages 15 to 40, although children and older people sometimes develop the disease. Ulcerative colitis affects males and females equally and appears to run in some families.

---

NIH Pub. 95-1597.

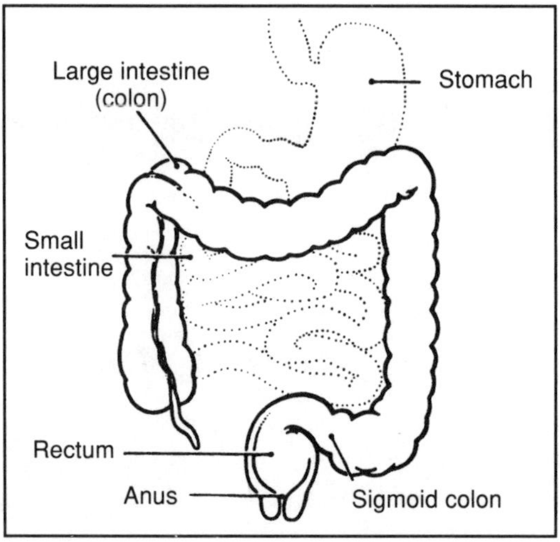


*Figure 24.1.*

## What Are the Symptoms of Ulcerative Colitis?

The most common symptoms of ulcerative colitis are abdominal pain and bloody diarrhea. Patients also may suffer fatigue, weight loss, loss of appetite, rectal bleeding, and loss of body fluids and nutrients. Severe bleeding can lead to anemia. Sometimes patients also have skin lesions, joint pain, inflammation of the eyes, or liver disorders. No one knows for sure why problems outside the bowel are linked with colitis. Scientists think these complications may occur when the immune system triggers inflammation in other parts of the body. These disorders are usually mild and go away when the colitis is treated.

## What Causes Ulcerative Colitis?

The cause of ulcerative colitis is not known, and currently there is no cure, except through surgical removal of the colon. Many theories about what causes ulcerative colitis exist, but none has been proven. The current leading theory suggests that some agent, possibly a virus or an atypical bacterium, interacts with the body's immune system to trigger an inflammatory reaction in the intestinal wall.

Although much scientific evidence shows that people with ulcerative colitis have abnormalities of the immune system, doctors do not know whether these abnormalities are a cause or result of the disease. Doctors believe, however, that there is little proof that ulcerative colitis is caused by emotional distress or sensitivity to certain foods or food products or is the result of an unhappy childhood.

## How Is Ulcerative Colitis Diagnosed?

If you have symptoms that suggest ulcerative colitis, the doctor will look inside your rectum and colon through a flexible tube (endoscope) inserted through the anus. During the exam, the doctor may take a sample of tissue (biopsy) from the lining of the colon to view under the microscope. You also may receive a barium enema x-ray of the colon to determine the nature and extent of disease. This procedure involves putting a chalky solution (barium) into the colon. The barium shows up white on x-ray film, revealing growths and other abnormalities in the colon.

The doctor will give you a thorough physical exam, including blood tests to see if you are anemic (as a result of blood loss), or if your white blood cell count is elevated (a sign of inflammation). Examination of a stool sample can tell the doctor if an infection, such as by amoebae or bacteria, is causing the symptoms.

If you have ulcerative colitis, you may need medical care for some time. Your doctor also will want to see you regularly to check on the condition.

## How Serious Is This Disease?

About half of patients have only mild symptoms. Others suffer frequent fever, bloody diarrhea, nausea, and severe abdominal cramps. Only in rare cases, when complications occur, is the disease fatal. There may be remissions (periods when the symptoms go away) that last for months or even years. However, most patients' symptoms eventually return. This changing pattern of the disease can make it hard for the doctor to tell when treatment has helped.

## What Is the Treatment?

While no special diet for ulcerative colitis is given, patients may be able to control mild symptoms simply by avoiding foods that seem to upset their intestine. In some cases, the doctor may advise avoiding highly seasoned foods or milk sugar (lactose) for a while. When treatment is necessary, it must be tailored for each case, since what may help one patient may not help another. The patient also should be given needed emotional and psychological support.

Patients with either mild or severe colitis are usually treated with the drug sulfasalazine. This drug can be used for as long as needed, and it can be used along with other drugs. Side effects such as nausea, vomiting, weight loss, heartburn, diarrhea, and headache occur in a small percentage of cases. Patients who do not do well on sulfasalazine often do very well on related drugs known as 5-ASA agents.

In some cases, patients with severe disease, or those who cannot take sulfasalazine-type drugs, are given adrenal steroids (drugs that help control inflammation and affect the immune system) such as prednisone or hydrocortisone. All of these drugs can be used in oral, enema, or suppository forms. Other drugs may be given to relax the patient or to relieve pain, diarrhea, or infection.

Patients with ulcerative colitis occasionally have symptoms severe enough to require hospitalization. In these cases, the doctor will try to correct malnutrition and to stop diarrhea and loss of blood, fluids, and mineral salts. To accomplish this, the patient may need a special diet, feeding through a vein, medications, or, sometimes, surgery.

The risk of colon cancer is greater than normal in patients with widespread ulcerative colitis. The risk may be as high as 32 times the normal rate in patients whose entire colon is involved, especially if the colitis exists for many years. However, if only the rectum and lower colon are involved, the risk of cancer is not higher than normal.

Sometimes precancerous changes occur in the cells lining the colon. These changes in the cells are called "dysplasia." If the doctor finds evidence of dysplasia through endoscopic exam and biopsy, it means the patient is more likely to develop cancer. Patients with dysplasia, or whose colitis affects the entire colon, should receive regular followup exams, which may involve colonoscopy (examination of the entire colon using a flexible endoscope) and biopsies.

About 20 to 25 percent of ulcerative colitis patients eventually require surgery for removal of the colon because of massive bleeding, chronic debilitating illness, perforation of the colon, or risk of cancer. Sometimes the doctor will recommend removing the colon when medical treatment fails or the side effects of steroids or other drugs threaten the patient's health. Patients have several surgical options, each of which has advantages and disadvantages. The surgeon and patient must decide on the best individual option.

The most common surgery is the proctocolectomy, the removal of the entire colon and rectum, with ileostomy, creation of a small opening in the abdominal wall where the tip of the lower small intestine, the ileum, is brought to the skin's surface to allow drainage of waste. The opening (stoma) is about the size of a quarter and is usually located in the right lower corner of the abdomen in the area of the beltline. A pouch is worn over the opening to collect waste and the patient empties the pouch periodically.

The proctocolectomy with continent ileostomy is an alternative to the standard ileostomy. In this operation, the surgeon creates a pouch out of the ileum inside the wall of the lower abdomen. The patient is able to empty the pouch by inserting a tube through a small leak-proof opening in his or her side. Creation of this natural valve eliminates the need for an external appliance. However, the patient must wear an external pouch for the first few months after the operation.

Sometimes an operation that avoids the use of a pouch can be performed. In the ileoanal anastomosis ("pullthrough operation"), the diseased portion of the colon is removed and the outer muscles of the rectum are preserved. The surgeon attaches the ileum inside the rectum, forming a pouch, or reservoir, that holds the waste.

This allows the patient to pass stool through the anus in a normal manner, although the bowel movements may be more frequent and watery than usual.

The decision about which surgery to have is made according to each patient's needs, expectations, and lifestyle. If you are ever faced with this decision, remember that getting as much information as possible is important. Talk to your doctor, to nurses who work with patients who have had colon surgery (enterostomal therapists), and to other patients. In addition, read pamphlets and books, such as those available from the Crohn's & Colitis Foundation of America, before you decide.

Most people with ulcerative colitis will never need to have surgery. If surgery ever does become necessary, however, you may find comfort in knowing that after the surgery, the colitis is cured and most people go on to live normal, active lives.

## *Additional Readings*

*Bleeding in the Digestive Tract and Crohn's Disease*. National Digestive Diseases Information Clearinghouse, 1992. 2 Information Way, Bethesda, MD 20892-3570; (301) 654-3810. General patient information fact sheets.

Brandt LJ, Steiner-Grossman F eds. *Treating IBD: A Patient's Guide to the Medical and Surgical Management of Inflammatory Bowel Disease*. New York: Raven Press, 1989. This book, produced by the Crohn's & Colitis Foundation of America, addresses many aspects of treatment and living with inflammatory bowel disease.

Hanaver SB, Peppercorn MD, Present DH. Current concepts, new therapies in IBD. *Patient Care*, 1992; 26 (13): 79–102. General review article for health care professionals.

Steiner-Grossman P, Banks PA, Present DH, eds. *The New People Not Patients: A Source Book for Living with IBD*. Dubuque, Iowa: Kendall/Hunt Publishing Company, 1992. This book for patients includes sections on diagnostic tests, medications, nutrition, coping with employment and health insurance problems, and IBD in children and teenagers, older adults, and during pregnancy. Available from the Crohn's & Colitis Foundation of America.

## Resources

Crohn's & Colitis Foundation of America, Inc.
386 Park Avenue South, 17th floor
New York, NY 10016-8804
(800) 932-2423 or (212) 685-3440

The Greater New York Pull-thru Network
62 Edgewood Avenue
Wyckoff, NJ 07481
(201) 891-5977

Pediatric Crohn's & Colitis Association, Inc.
Box 188
Newton, MA 02168
(617) 244-6678

Reach Out for Youth with Ileitis and Colitis, Inc.
15 Chemung Place
Jericho, NY 11753
(516) 822-8010

United Ostomy Association
36 Executive Park, Suite 120
Irvine, CA 92714
(800) 826-0826 or (714) 660-8624

Chapter 25

# Living with Inflammatory Bowel Disease

Both ulcerative colitis and Crohn's disease are caused by inflammation of the small or large bowel. Because they are similar, these two conditions are often referred to as inflammatory bowel disease (IBD). Inflammation is a natural process that helps the body get rid of dangerous materials. But if inflammation gets out of control, as it does with IBD, arthritis, and other conditions, it can cause damage and pain.

## What Happens If You Have IBD

Abdominal pain, cramps, and diarrhea are common symptoms. But some people may also experience bleeding from the rectum, tenderness of the abdomen, and awakening at night because of diarrhea. Other symptoms are fever, weight loss, and constipation. Children with IBD may not grow and develop as they should. Arthritis, skin rashes, and inflamed eyes may also occur. Many of these symptoms come and go, as the disease flares up or tapers off.

Unfortunately, IBD affects many people when they are young and stays with them throughout their lives. Patients generally need to take drugs for years. Some patients may need surgery later when the disease becomes worse and severely affects bowel function.

The good news is that IBD can be successfully treated, and most patients can carry on normal lives and live as long as anyone else.

---

This chapter was originally published in *Patient Care*, August 15, 1992. Reprinted with permission.

Today a number of helpful drugs are available, and several operations have been perfected to give relief to IBD victims—and sometimes cure them.

## When You See a Doctor

Your doctor will ask about past illnesses you have had and whether anyone in your family has had IBD. He or she will probably take a blood sample and also ask you to bring in a stool sample to check for blood cells. The doctor may also examine your large bowel through a tube inserted in the rectum or take X-rays of your intestines.

Your doctor will probably give you medication to reduce the inflammation in your bowels. If one drug doesn't help, another one may work better or not have unpleasant side effects. Even after the pain and other symptoms let up, it is important to keep on taking the medicine to avoid a flare-up of the symptoms. Many medications can be taken by mouth, but the doctor may ask you to use an enema or a suppository.

## Changing Your Diet May Help

Another way to relieve symptoms is to make changes in your diet. If you have diarrhea, your doctor may ask you to avoid foods containing roughage, such as fruits and vegetables. But if you are constipated, he may tell you to add roughage to your diet. Spicy foods, fatty foods, and beverages containing caffeine may be forbidden. You will probably learn by trial and error which foods agree with you. You should understand, however, that foods of one kind or another do not cause IBD: They only make the symptoms better or worse. If you are not getting enough nourishment with your diet to keep healthy and active, a doctor may suggest vitamins or concentrated food supplements in liquid form.

## If Surgery Is Needed for IBD

Sometimes, in both ulcerative colitis and Crohn's disease, the symptoms and damage to the intestines get gradually worse, especially after a few years. Then your doctor may recommend surgery so that you can feel and function better. In some cases, a surgeon can remove diseased parts of the small or large intestine and sew the healthy sections together. In other cases, the surgeon will have to make a hole in the abdominal wall (ostomy) so that the end of the remaining intestine can be attached. Waste matter then passes through the hole and into a bag on the outside of the person's body. Today surgeons are sometimes able to perform an operation that avoids the hole and bag and allows bowel movements through the rectum. The kind of operation recommended depends on which parts of the intestines are diseased and how serious the condition is. Most patients find that their lives improve considerably after surgery, although a few may require surgery again later on.

## If You Need Help with Problems

In some cases, patients become discouraged with the symptoms they must live with for the rest of their lives. They may find that it helps to talk to other people with the same problems.

A nationwide support organization has been set up and may be able to refer you to a local support group where you can obtain information and discuss your problems. Contact the Crohn's & Colitis Foundation of America, Inc.. 444 Park Ave. S, 11th Floor, New York. N.Y. 10016-7374; (212) 685-3440 or (800) 343-3637. Patients who must wear an ostomy bag can get help from the United Ostomy Association, 36 Executive Park, Suite 120, Irvine, Calif. 92714; (714) 660-8624.

## You Can Live with IBD!

People with IBD can generally lead normal lives, holding jobs, marrying, having children, and engaging in almost every kind of activity. In fact, patients can freely choose their mates, and women should not worry about pregnancy or nursing. Doctors can switch drugs for their female patients if any of the commonly used drugs might be harmful during pregnancy.

## Chapter 26

# *FDA Consumer: Living with Inflammatory Bowel Disease*

Inflammatory bowel disease (IBD), the collective term for Crohn's disease and ulcerative colitis, spells tough times for the 1 million to 2 million Americans wrestling lifelong with its fever, cramps, weight loss, and persistent diarrhea. Crohn's occurs mainly in the ileum (the lowest part of the small intestine) and colon (the large intestine). Ulcerative colitis is limited to the colon.

Symptoms lessen or disappear during remissions, but the disease lurks doggedly within until, unpredictably, its threat to health begins anew. The IBD specter can so hover over career, sex life, social plans, and even shopping that feelings of isolation and discouragement may force social withdrawal. As one patient put it, "My life revolves around the bathroom."

No one knows the cause of IBD. No drug offers a cure. But the outlook for IBD patients is far from hopeless:

- Many IBD patients have relatively mild symptoms.
- Even severe disease can usually be managed.
- Drug treatment helps induce and maintain remission, which can last for years.
- The Food and Drug Administration recently approved a new IBD drug. Others are undergoing clinical testing.

---

This article originally appeared in *FDA Consumer*, April 1988.

- As a last resort, the colon can be removed and stool passed some other way, usually through an artificial opening called a stoma.

Actually, with proper treatment and personal determination, most people with IBD (including those with stomas) can engage in athletics, build successful careers, enjoy sex, and otherwise participate in life in nearly any way they wish. Further, normal deliveries and healthy babies are as likely in women with IBD—except during severe, active Crohn's—as in healthy women.

And yet, "people are suffering needlessly because of ignorance," said Pearl Lewis recently in the *Baltimore Jewish Times*. Lewis is patient advocacy and government relations director of the National Foundation for Ileitis (another name for Crohn's disease) and Colitis, Inc. Indeed, a recent survey sponsored by grants to the Coalition of Digestive Disease Organizations showed that Americans are "largely uninformed and misinformed" about all digestive diseases, including IBD. More than half the people interviewed mistakenly believed, for instance, that IBD is caused by emotional stress. Most medical experts disagree.

So, what *are* the facts concerning ulcerative colitis and Crohn's disease?

Foremost, the two conditions are more alike than different. Anyone can develop IBD, but some factors add to a person's risk. Jews are the most susceptible, blacks and Orientals the least. Those aged 12 to 40 constitute the highest risk group, with 10 percent of patients under 18. Twenty percent to 25 percent of IBD patients have one or more relatives with colitis or Crohn's. Both diseases occur in both sexes with about the same frequency. Both are reported mainly in developed countries.

In addition to the characteristic fever, cramps, weight loss, and persistent—often bloody—diarrhea, IBD may cause so-called "systemic" problems such as arthritis and eye and skin inflammation. In children, growth and sexual development may be retarded, possibly from too little food intake because the child feels ill so much of the time.

## Inflammatory Response

But the most important similarity shared by ulcerative colitis and Crohn's disease is bowel inflammation, hence the term "inflammatory bowel disease." Inflammation is the normal response of the immune system to protect the body from outside offenders such as bacteria. Several kinds of inflammatory cells move to the attacked area, fight the invaders, and release chemicals to attract more cells.

While scientists don't know the exact cause of IBD's chronic inflammation, they have a number of theories. Some think that an unknown infectious or toxic substance triggers the initial immune response and that the inflammation is then perpetuated, or made chronic, as irritating substances (such as chemicals in the cell walls of bacteria) leak repeatedly through the ulcerated intestinal wall. Others suspect the inflammatory response is actually against the patient's own cells as if they were invaders, a condition called autoimmunity.

However this abnormal cycle begins, harmful changes to the intestinal lining or wall occur, creating a break in the body's protection there. The body responds with inflammation. Blood flow increases to the area, making it red, painful and swollen.

At the microscopic level, damage includes depletion of the intestine's "goblet" cells in ulcerative colitis; in Crohn's, certain blood cells cluster together in "granulomas." Open sores called ulcers may form. Bloody fluid may leak. Segments of the intestine may become so narrowed from scarring and swelling of the wall that body wastes can't pass. Ulcers may penetrate so deeply that they perforate the intestine, causing infection or fistulas—deep ulcer channels tunneled between bowel segments or between the bowel and the skin surface or another organ, such as the bladder.

The links that bind ulcerative colitis and Crohn's together under the IBD umbrella are strong. But the differences that separate them are significant, too.

## *Ulcerative Colitis*

Ulcerative colitis is limited to the inner mucous membranes lining the colon, with inflammation nearly always beginning at the rectum and spreading backwards through the colon in a continuous fashion. The lining becomes fragile and filled with blood and, so, bleeds easily. A frequent, urgent need to move the bowels may interrupt sleep, meals, and other activities. When inflammation involves the entire colon, there may be fever, muscle aches, heavy sweating, and poor appetite. Symptoms are milder in the 25 percent of cases that affect only the rectum and left colon, [a condition] known as "left-sided" colitis.

Most patients never face the complications of ulcerative colitis. But for those who do, rapid, deep growth of ulcers can cause severe rectal bleeding, acute colon dilation (toxic megacolon), and leakage of the colon's contents into the sterile abdominal cavity to cause peritonitis. Long-term, "smoldering" ulcerative colitis (usually involving most of the colon for 10 years or more) may increase a person's risk of developing colon and rectal cancers.

Not to be confused with ulcerative colitis is irritable bowel syndrome, or IBS, a disorder of the colon's contractions sometimes also called spastic colon or mucous colitis. IBS ranks close to the common cold as the number one health-related reason for time off from work. The major symptoms are abdominal pain and diarrhea or constipation or alternating bouts of both. Contrary to what some may think, IBS does not cause inflammation, has no relationship to ulcerative colitis, and hasn't been shown to lead to serious illnesses such as IBD or cancer. A person can have IBD and IBS at the same time.

## Crohn's Disease

Unlike ulcerative colitis, Crohn's disease (named for Burrill Crohn, M . D., who described it in a paper in 1932) causes inflammation that affects all layers of the intestinal wall and occurs in patches, skipping portions of the intestine. Crohn's is most commonly found in the ileum or in the ileum and upper colon; [hence] its other names: regional ileitis and regional enteritis. When [the condition affects] the colon only, it is called Crohn's colitis. Infrequently, Crohn's may occur in [any other part] of the digestive tract from the mouth to the anus.

Patients usually have abdominal pain and diarrhea. Rectal bleeding is less likely in Crohn's than in ulcerative colitis because Crohn's often spares the rectum. Still, first signs often show up at the anus: hemorrhoids, unhealing cracks, and fistulas. Some people develop kidney stones, urinary tract obstructions, or fistulas into the bladder or vagina [that are] marked by pain or difficulty in urinating or by passing blood, gas or feces with the urine or through the vagina. Eventually, the person runs a fever, loses weight, and feels weak. Onset tends to be gradual, so Crohn's may be unnoticed for years.

## Diagnosis

Diagnosing IBD can be a difficult, lengthy task. Typically, ulcerative colitis shows up as watery bowel movements and abdominal cramping that lead the person to suspect an intestinal "bug." But as days go by and diarrhea continues, especially if there's bleeding, the need for medical help becomes clear. Diagnosis can be complicated, however, because a number of intestinal diseases mimic ulcerative colitis.

When a patient reports persistent abdominal pain, fever, diarrhea, weight loss, and anemia, the doctor will likely consider Crohn's as a possible cause. But when Crohn's presents only subtle symptoms—say, a general feeling of fatigue and aching joints—detection may be impeded. Such patients may suffer for years without help. They may even believe their feeling ill is "all in the head."

People who think their symptoms might be caused by IBD should point this out to their doctor, who may suggest seeing a gastroenterologist, a physician who specializes in diseases of the gastrointestinal tract.

Generally, a diagnosis can be established with a complete medical history, physical examination, and laboratory analysis of stool, blood and urine samples. A biopsy of intestinal tissue and radiological tests, such as X-rays, also may be needed.

In the physical examination, the doctor will probably use an endoscope, a lighted tubular instrument inserted into a body opening such as the anus or mouth for viewing internal organs. (The FDA's Center for Devices and Radiological Health regulates such instruments as medical devices.) An endoscope inserted into the mouth can be passed down the throat and through the stomach to show the upper few inches of the small intestine. Inserted into the anus, an endoscope can display tissue inside the rectum, the sigmoid colon (the colon's lower 10 to 12 inches), or, in fact, the entire length of the colon, since the flexible fiberoptic colonoscope bends with the intestine. Such procedures may seem threatening, but apprehension is likely the worst part. "I'm so relaxed when the doctor is looking at my colon that I really don't feel much," said a teenager in *Living with IBD*, by George Ferry, M.D., and L. Kay Bartholomew, M.P.H. (See also "A Physician's Spyglass for Looking Inward" in the December 1982–January 1983 *FDA Consumer*.)

## Drug Treatment

While no drug can cure IBD, several have been approved by FDA's Center for Drug Evaluation and Research as safe and effective treatment. These therapies can suppress inflammation, promote tissue healing, and relieve symptoms for most people. The remission that occurs doesn't necessarily mean that all inflammation is gone or that healing is complete, but the person does enjoy a period of comfort. Treatment may or may not be needed for remission to continue.

The corticosteroids prednisone and prednisolone are for use during critical periods of Crohn's disease and ulcerative colitis. Bothersome side effects include headache, puffy rounding of the face, fluid retention, and increased sweating. The drugs may produce such serious effects as osteoporosis (thinning of the bones), high blood pressure, activation of latent diabetes mellitus, cataracts, glaucoma, impaired resistance to infection, mood swings, potassium loss, and suppressed growth in youngsters. Corticosteroids are very potent drugs, to be used with care and delicacy. Patients should follow instructions exactly. The drug labeling cautions that the lowest possible dose should be used, that dosage reduction must be gradual, and that anyone with a systemic fungal infection should not take the drugs. The labeling also gives special guidance on vaccination during therapy and on use of the drugs with tuberculosis patients.

Sulfasalazine is used [in several ways] to treat ulcerative colitis: as the principal drug in mild to moderate disease, as additional therapy in severe cases, and in extending remission. Patients can have flare-ups while taking sulfasalazine, but the risk is much lower than without it. Some people are allergic to the drug. If an allergic reaction is suspected—symptoms can include breathing difficulty, swelling around the eye, hives, or rash—the person should call the doctor right away or, if the doctor is unavailable, [he or she should go to] a hospital emergency room.

The most common side effects [of sulfasalazine] are headache, nausea, vomiting, loss of appetite, and reduced fertility (apparently reversible) in men. Starting with small doses may help prevent those effects and may help hypersensitive people to tolerate the drug. Other effects include impaired folic acid absorption, orange-yellow discoloring of the urine, hearing loss, insomnia, abdominal pain, and increased sensitivity to sunlight. Rare, serious adverse effects include bone marrow toxicity and inflammation of the liver; regular blood and urine tests are vital to alert the doctor if such effects include bone marrow toxicity and inflammation of the liver; regular blood and urine tests are vital to alert the doctor if such occur.

In December 1987, FDA approved an enema form of mesalamine (trade name Rowasa), also known as 5-aminosalicylic acid (5-ASA), for mild to moderate ulcerative colitis extending from the anus no further than the left side of the colon. This drug could mean improved treatment for patients with left-sided colitis. In one small clinical trial, there were no reports of infertility in men. Some of the patients who were hypersensitive to sulfasalazine were able to take these enemas without an allergic reaction. Mesalamine does contain a sulfite, so it shouldn't be used by anyone known to be sensitive to sulfites—a sensitivity most frequently reported among people with asthma. The primary symptom in sulfite allergy is breathing difficulty. If an allergic reaction is suspected, the patient should call the doctor right away.

Mesalamine may cause an acute intolerance syndrome, with cramping, abdominal pain, bloody diarrhea, and sometimes fever, headache and a rash. If this syndrome appears, the person should call the doctor about withdrawal from the drug. Other side effects include nausea, leg and joint pain, dizziness, and mild hair loss. Kidney damage was noted during animal testing, but not in human studies. Nevertheless, the possibility of this toxicity should be kept in mind, and anyone with existing kidney disease should be monitored carefully while on mesalamine.

Another drug that may be used during a severe flare-up of IBD is adrenocorticotropic hormone (ACTH), which stimulates the release of the body's own type of corticosteroid.

Drugs to relieve diarrhea include diphenoxylate and loperamide. Iron and folic acid may be given to prevent or treat anemia, which may result from bleeding and impaired intestinal absorption of those nutrients. Other dietary supplements may be needed, too.

A woman who is breast-feeding or who thinks she is pregnant or is planning a pregnancy should tell the doctor before taking any medication. During drug therapy, a person should follow instructions exactly, know what side effects are possible and what to do if any occur, and have regular checkups.

## *Alternative Feeding*

It's important to maintain proper nutrition by eating sufficient calories, protein, and other nutrients supplied by a balanced diet. Foods that are particularly irritating to the bowels vary from person to person, however, so there is no one diet that is well-tolerated and nutritious for everyone.

Sometimes, poor appetite, weight loss, or continued vomiting or diarrhea can lead to malnutrition. Even dietary supplements may not relieve this. The doctor may advise some type of alternative feeding.

This may be done at home, but often a hospital stay is required. In the "elemental diet," a solution of essential nutrients is pumped through a thin, flexible, plastic tube passed into the nose to the stomach or through a rubber tube inserted through the skin into the abdomen to the stomach. If the digestive system needs complete rest to heal, "total parental nutrition" may be needed. All life-sustaining nutrients are then given through a tube into a large vein near the shoulder.

## Surgery

Surgery is needed by less than half the people with ulcerative colitis, but by two-thirds of Crohn's patients—some 40 percent of whom may require it again. The most common operations are to remove fistulas, blockages and tissue that stubbornly resist long-term medication. While not cures, these operations offer a fresh start.

In severe uncontrolled disease, there is the possibility a person may need the rectum or colon surgically removed. When that's the case, the surgeon may perform an operation called an ostomy to create an artificial passage for eliminating stool. About 83,000 such operations were performed in the United States in 1986, according to the National Center for Health Statistics. An ostomy is six times more likely with ulcerative colitis than with Crohn's, but IBD accounts for only about 18 percent of all ostomies. Removal of the colon cures ulcerative colitis, but not Crohn's, which can recur in some other part of the digestive tract.

In a colostomy operation, an opening (stoma) is created through the abdomen into the colon. An ileostomy procedure creates an opening into the ileum. Wastes are then diverted into a pouch attached outside the skin with adhesive. The pouch is periodically emptied. Today's ostomy pouches can't be seen under even tight jeans.

Certain patients with ulcerative colitis have alternatives to the standard ileostomy. The continent ileostomy, for instance, involves constructing a pouch inside the body from a segment of small intestine. Drainage is via a small tube inserted periodically through a stoma in the lower abdomen. Another procedure, called ileoanal anastomosis (with reservoir), or pull-through operation, allows normal evacuation. The rectum is retained, but the innermost mucosal layer is stripped off. A pouch is made from a portion of the ileum, which is then brought down through a rectal cuff and stitched just above the anus so that the patient passes stool normally through the anus.

Local chapters of groups like the United Ostomy Association, Inc., encourage the 1.5 million people who have had ostomy surgery to lead full lives and have positive feelings about themselves.

## Research

Though the cause and medical cure for ulcerative colitis and Crohn's disease remain elusive, millions of dollars are going into IBD research. The National Foundation for Ileitis and Colitis alone spent $3.7 million over the past three years.

For half a century now, scientists have been trying to identify an infectious agent as the cause of IBD. Pointing to the idea that bacteria are somehow involved is the recent identification of a new species of Mycobacterium in the intestines of some Crohn's disease patients.

Other research centers on various findings about the immune system, the role nutrition plays in healing, the possibility that genes may predispose a person to IBD, and the perfection of surgical procedures. Scientists also are investigating the use of the antibacterial drug metronidazole as an alternative treatment for Crohn's and the use . . . of such drugs as azathioprine and 6-mercaptopurine [as additional therapies] to suppress the immune system. A number of oral 5-ASA drugs are undergoing clinical testing for safety and effectiveness.

## Living with IBD

The keys to living successfully with ulcerative colitis or Crohn's disease, the two forms of inflammatory bowel disease (IBD), are [lifelong] proper treatment and personal commitment. Triumphs over these serious diseases abound, as in the following examples from *People . . . Not Patients*, published by the National Foundation for Ileitis and Colitis, Inc. (NFIC).

Despite developing Crohn's at a young age, Peter Nielsen earned, by age 23, the greatest number of titles ever in the sport of body building, including "Mr. International Universe."

Rolf Benirschke had his colon and rectum removed because of ulcerative colitis in 1982, yet rebuilt his strength to resume a physically vigorous life. As a place kicker for the San Diego Chargers, he was named National Football League Man of the Year in 1983 and was the second most accurate NFL kicker in 1984.

Nielsen is a member of the NFIC Sports Council; Benirschke is its chairman.

Pearl Lewis, an NFIC employee and volunteer founder of the Maryland chapter, was diagnosed as having Crohn's when she was 21. The disease has cost Lewis 12 operations, including removal of her colon and rectum. She still has her disease, but treatment keeps her symptoms in check so that she can get on with her active, productive life—not the least part of which has been raising six children. Spurred on by success, Lewis—like Nielsen, Benirschke and other winners—is an advocate for people with IBD. She lobbies regularly on their behalf and offers empathy, advice on organizing self-help groups, and educational support.

From FIC, here are hints for dealing with IBD.

- *Find a physician who is an expert in the disease, one you believe in and feel comfortable with.*

- *Take time to understand your medicines.* It's important to take them only as directed and to tell the doctor about any physical changes, which could signal an adverse effect or the need for a dosage adjustment.

- *Become an expert on your nutrition.* A nourishing diet is important, but there is no perfect IBD diet. Pinpoint troublesome foods and be aware that the list may change with different stages of disease. Frequent offenders are insoluble fiber foods (like seeds, nuts and corn), fried or greasy foods, and caffeine. Switching to five or six smaller meals a day may produce few symptoms. A number of people find that lactose, found in milk and milk products, is a problem. When that is the case, there are milk substitutes, predigested milk, or commercially available lactase that can be added to milk to predigest the lactose.

- *Get enough rest and proper exercise.*

- *Reduce stress.* It's generally accepted that stress does not cause IBD. Anyone can get IBD, regardless of whether they're young, old, calm, tense, relaxed, compulsive, angry, or happy. Still, upsets can aggravate any illness. Some people give their emotional health a boost with physical activities, chats with a good listener, and simply putting things in proper perspective.

For more information about IBD, including such topics as complications, pregnancy, diet, special problems in childhood and adolescence, sex and IBD, ostomies, and emotional factors, write to:

American Digestive Disease Society, Inc.
7720 Wisconsin Ave.
Bethesda, MD 20814

National Digestive Diseases Information Clearinghouse
Box NDDIC
Bethesda, MD 20892

National Foundation for Ileitis and Colitis, Inc.
444 Park Avenue South
11th floor
New York, NY 10016

United Ostomy Association, Inc.
36 Executive Park
Suite 120
Irvine, CA 97214

*—by Dixie Farley, a member of FDA's public affairs staff.*

Chapter 27

# *Irritable Bowel Syndrome*

Irritable bowel syndrome (IBS) is a common disorder of the intestines that leads to crampy pain, gassiness, bloating, and changes in bowel habits. Some people with IBS have constipation (difficult or infrequent bowel movements); others have diarrhea (frequent loose stools, often with an urgent need to move the bowels); and some people experience both. Sometimes the person with IBS has a crampy urge to move the bowels but cannot do so.

Through the years, IBS has been called by many names: colitis, mucous colitis, spastic colon, spastic bowel, and functional bowel disease. Most of these terms are inaccurate. Colitis, for instance, means inflammation of the large intestine (colon). IBS, however, does not cause inflammation and should not be confused with ulcerative colitis, which is a more serious disorder.

The cause of IBS is not known, and as yet there is no cure. Doctors call it a functional disorder because there is no sign of disease when the colon is examined. IBS causes a great deal of discomfort and distress, but it does not cause permanent harm to the intestines and does not lead to intestinal bleeding of the bowel or to a serious disease such as cancer. Often IBS is just a mild annoyance, but for some people it can be disabling. They may be afraid to go to social events, to go out to a job, or to travel even short distances. Most people with IBS, however, are able to control their symptoms through diet, stress management, and sometimes with medications prescribed by their physicians.

---

NIH Pub. 92-693.

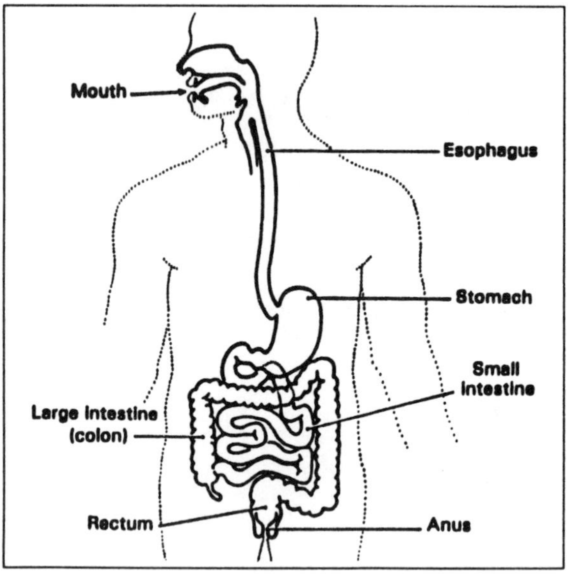


*Figure 27.1.*

## What Causes IBS?

The colon, which is about 6 feet long, connects the small intestine with the rectum and anus. The major function of the colon is to absorb water and salts from digestive products that enter from the small intestine. Two quarts of liquid matter enter the colon from the small intestine each day. This material may remain there for several days until most of the fluid and salts are absorbed into the body. The stool then passes through the colon by a pattern of movements to the left side of the colon, where it is stored until a bowel movement occurs.

Colon motility (contraction of intestinal muscles and movement of its contents) is controlled by nerves and hormones and by electrical activity in the colon muscle. The electrical activity serves as a "pacemaker" similar to the mechanism that controls heart function.

Movements of the colon propel the contents slowly back and forth but mainly toward the rectum. A few times each day strong muscle contractions move down the colon pushing fecal material ahead of them. Some of these strong contractions result in a bowel movement.

Because doctors have been unable to find an organic cause, IBS often has been thought to be caused by emotional conflict or stress.

While stress may worsen IBS symptoms, research suggests that other factors also are important. Researchers have found that the colon muscle of a person with IBS begins to spasm after only mild stimulation. The person with IBS seems to have a colon that is more sensitive and reactive than usual, so it responds strongly to stimuli that would not bother most people.

Ordinary events such as eating and distention from gas or other material in the colon can cause an overreaction in the person with IBS. Certain medicines and foods may trigger spasms in some people. Sometimes the spasm delays the passage of stool, leading to constipation. Chocolate, milk products, or large amounts of alcohol are frequent offenders. Caffeine causes loose stools in many people, but it is more likely to affect those with IBS. Researchers also have found that women with IBS may have more symptoms during their menstrual periods, suggesting that reproductive hormones can increase IBS symptoms.

## What Are the Symptoms of IBS?

If you are concerned about IBS, it is important to realize that normal bowel function varies from person to person. Normal bowel movements range from as many as three stools a day to as few as three a week. A normal movement is one that is formed but not hard, contains no blood, and is passed without cramps or pain.

People with IBS, on the other hand, usually have crampy abdominal pain with painful constipation or diarrhea. In some people, constipation and diarrhea alternate. Sometimes people with IBS pass mucus with their bowel movements. Bleeding, fever, weight loss, and persistent severe pain are not symptoms of IBS but may indicate other problems.

## How Is IBS Diagnosed?

IBS usually is diagnosed after doctors exclude more serious organic diseases. The doctor will take a complete medical history that includes a careful description of symptoms. A physical examination and laboratory tests will be done. A stool sample will be tested for evidence of bleeding. The doctor also may do diagnostic procedures such as x-rays or endoscopy (viewing the colon through a flexible tube inserted through the anus) to find out if there is organic disease.

## How Do Diet and Stress Affect IBS?

The potential for abnormal function of the colon is always present in people with IBS, but a trigger also must be present to cause symptoms. The most likely culprits seem to be diet and emotional stress. Many people report that their symptoms occur following a meal or when they are under stress. No one is sure why this happens, but scientists have some clues.

Eating causes contractions of the colon. Normally, this response may cause an urge to have a bowel movement within 30 to 60 minutes after a meal. In people with IBS, the urge may come sooner with cramps and diarrhea.

The strength of the response is often related to the number of calories in a meal, and especially the amount of fat in a meal. Fat in any form (animal or vegetable) is a strong stimulus of colonic contractions after a meal. Many foods contain fat, especially meats of all kinds, poultry skin, whole milk, cream, cheese, butter, vegetable oil, margarine, shortening, avocados, and whipped toppings.

Stress also stimulates colonic spasm in people with IBS. This process is not completely understood, but scientists point out that the colon is controlled partly by the nervous system. Mental health counseling and stress reduction (relaxation training) can help relieve the symptoms of IBS. However, doctors are quick to note that this does not mean IBS is the result of a personality disorder. IBS is at least partly a disorder of colon motility.

## How Does a Good Diet Help IBS?

For many people, eating a proper diet lessens IBS symptoms. Before changing your diet, it is a good idea to keep a journal noting which foods seem to cause distress. Discuss your findings with your doctor. You also may want to consult a registered dietitian, who can help you make changes in your diet. For instance, if dairy products cause your symptoms to flare up, you can try eating less of those foods. Yogurt might be tolerated better because it contains organisms that supply lactase, the enzyme needed to digest lactose, the sugar found in milk products. Because dairy products are an important source of calcium and other nutrients that your body needs, be sure to get adequate nutrients in the foods that you substitute.

Dietary fiber may lessen IBS symptoms in many cases. Whole grain breads and cereals, beans, fruits, and vegetables are good sources of fiber. Consult your doctor before using an over-the-counter fiber supplement. High-fiber diets keep the colon mildly distended, which may help to prevent spasms from developing. Some forms of fiber also keep water in the stools, thereby preventing hard stools that are difficult to pass. Doctors usually recommend that you eat just enough fiber so that you have soft, easily passed, painless bowel movements. High-fiber diets may cause gas and bloating, but within a few weeks, these symptoms often go away as your body adjusts to the diet.

Large meals can cause cramping and diarrhea in people with IBS. Symptoms may be eased if you eat smaller meals more often or just eat smaller portions. This should help, especially if your meals are low in fat and high in carbohydrates such as pasta, rice, whole-grain breads and cereals, fruits, and vegetables.

## Can Medicines Relieve IBS Symptoms?

There is no standard way of treating IBS. Your doctor may prescribe fiber supplements or occasional laxatives if you are constipated. Some doctors prescribe antispasmodic drugs or tranquilizers, which may relieve symptoms. Antidepressant drugs also are used sometimes in patients who are depressed.

The major concerns with drug therapy of IBS are the potential for drug dependency and the effects the disorder can have on lifestyle. In an effort to control their bowels or reduce stress, some people become dependent on laxatives or tranquilizers. If this happens, doctors try to withdraw the drugs slowly.

## How Is IBS Linked to More Serious Problems?

IBS has not been shown to lead to any serious, organic diseases. No link has been established between IBS and inflammatory bowel diseases such as Crohn's disease or ulcerative colitis. IBS does not lead to cancer. Some patients have a more severe form of IBS, and the fear of pain and diarrhea may cause them to withdraw from normal activities. In such cases, doctors may recommend mental health counseling.

## Additional Readings

Scanlon, D, Becnel, B. *Wellness Book of IBS*. New York: St. Martin's Press, 1989. "Practical Patient's Guide to Coping with IBS Written by a Registered Dietitian." Available in libraries and bookstores.

Shimberg, E. *Relief From IBS*. New York: M. Evans and Company, 1988. Practical book for patients offers information about IBS symptoms, diet, treatment, and self-care. Available in libraries and bookstores.

Steinhart, MJ. "Irritable Bowel Syndrome: How to Relieve Symptoms Enough to Improve Daily Function." *Postgraduate Medicine* 1992; 91(6): 315–321. Article for primary care physicians includes information about relief of IBS symptoms. Available in medical and university libraries.

Thompson, WG. *Gut Reactions: Understanding Symptoms of the Digestive Track*. New York: Plenum Publishing Corp., 1989. Clear, concise book by a digestive diseases specialist gives advice about diagnosis, diet, and treatment of IBS. Available in libraries and bookstores.

## National Digestive Diseases Information Clearinghouse

Box NDDIC
9000 Rockville Pike
Bethesda, MD 20892
(301) 468-6344

The National Digestive Diseases Information Clearinghouse is a service of the National Institute of Diabetes and Digestive and Kidney Diseases, part of the National Institutes of Health, under the U.S. Public Health Service. The clearinghouse was authorized by Congress to focus a national effort on providing information to the public, patients and their families, and doctors and other health care professionals. The clearinghouse works with organizations to educate people about digestive health and disease. The clearinghouse answers inquiries; develops, reviews, and distributes publications; and coordinates informational resources about digestive diseases.

Publications produced by the clearinghouse are reviewed carefully for scientific accuracy, appropriateness of content, and readability. Publications produced by sources other than the clearinghouse also are reviewed for scientific accuracy and are used, along with clearinghouse publications, to answer requests.

Chapter 28

# *Diarrhea: Diet Do's and Don'ts*

It's usually not life threatening, but two or three days of diarrhea sure can put a crimp in your lifestyle.

Adults average four bouts of diarrhea a year. Fortunately, most cases clear up on their own.

## *Is It a "Bug"?*

After you eat, most foods are digested in your small intestine. Then your colon absorbs the remaining liquid from digested food particles that pass through it, forming semi-solid stools.

But your system can become imbalanced in two ways:

1. Bacteria, commonly found in food or water that's contaminated, can make a toxin that triggers intestinal cells to secrete salt and water.

   This overwhelms the capacity of your lower small bowel and your colon to absorb fluid. The result: diarrhea.

2. More commonly, an invading virus, such as rotavirus or Norwalk, can damage the mucous membrane that lines your intestine. As a result, fluid absorption is disrupted.

---

This chapter originally appeared in the October 1993 *Mayo Clinic Health Letter*, published monthly by the Mayo Foundation for Medical Education and Research. Reprinted with permission.

Rotavirus frequently causes diarrhea in children less than 2 years old. Norwalk virus is more common in adults and is usually traced to drinking water or food, such as shellfish, that's contaminated.

## Home Remedy

For a mild case of diarrhea, here's how to manage your discomfort best at home:

- *Drink clear liquids*—The main liquid you need is water. Other options: broth, caffeine-free soft drinks, gelatin, popsicles, and fruit drinks or juices (except prune juice).
- *Drink lots of liquids*—Drink at least eight to 10 glasses of water and other liquids daily. This should prevent most complications that stem from substantial loss of fluids (dehydration) and electrolytes, such as sodium and potassium.
- *Eat low-fiber foods*—As your symptoms improve or your stools become formed, start to eat low-fiber foods, such as soda crackers, toast, eggs, rice, or chicken and other tender cuts of meat. Don't eat greasy or fatty foods, milk or highly seasoned foods for a few days.

Short-term diarrhea doesn't require antibiotics. And for most cases, you don't need an over-the-counter anti-diarrhea product. These may slow the elimination of the infectious agent and so actually prolong your diarrhea. Because situations vary, though, ask your doctor about your specific case.

## When Should You See Your Doctor?

Sometimes diarrhea is a sign of a more serious illness or can lead to complications.

See your doctor, if you have any of these conditions:

- Diarrhea lasting longer than three days.
- Severe abdominal or rectal pain.
- Fever of at least 102 degrees Fahrenheit.

- Blood in your stool.
- Signs of dehydration, such as dry mouth, anxiety or restlessness, excessive thirst, little or no urination, severe weakness, dizziness or lightheadedness.

# Chapter 29

# Constipation Fact Sheet

Constipation is the infrequent and difficult passage of stool. The frequency of bowel movements among healthy people varies greatly, ranging from three movements a day to three a week. As a rule, if more than 3 days pass without a bowel movement, the intestinal contents may harden, and a person may have difficulty or even pain during elimination. Stool may harden and be painful to pass, however, even after shorter intervals between bowel movements.

## What Are Some Common Misconceptions About Constipation?

Many false beliefs exist concerning proper bowel habits. One of these is that a bowel movement every day is necessary. Another common fallacy is that wastes stored in the body are absorbed and are dangerous to health or shorten the life span. These misconceptions have led to a marked overuse and abuse of laxatives. Every year, Americans spend $725 million on laxatives. Many are not needed and some are harmful.

## What Are Some of the Causes of Constipation?

Constipation is a symptom, not a disease. Like a fever, constipation can be caused by many different conditions. Most people have

NIH Pub. 92–2754.

experienced an occasional brief bout of constipation that has corrected itself with diet and time. The following is a list of some of the most common causes of constipation:

- *Poor Diet.* A main cause of constipation may be a diet high in animal fats (meats, dairy products, eggs) and refined sugar (rich desserts and other sweets), but low in fiber (vegetables, fruits, whole grains). Some studies have suggested that high-fiber diets result in larger stools, more frequent bowel movements, and therefore less constipation.

- *Imaginary Constipation.* This is very common and results from misconceptions about what is normal and what is not. If recognized early enough, this type of constipation can be cured by informing the sufferer that the frequency of his or her bowel movements is normal.

- *Irritable Bowel Syndrome (IBS).* Also known as spastic colon, IBS is one of the most common causes of constipation in the United States. Some people develop spasms of the colon that delay the speed with which the contents of the intestine move through the digestive tract, leading to constipation.

- *Poor Bowel Habits.* A person can initiate a cycle of constipation by ignoring the urge to have a bowel movement. Some people do this to avoid using public toilets, others because they are too busy. After a period of time a person may stop feeling the urge. This leads to progressive constipation.

- *Laxative Abuse.* People who habitually take laxatives become dependent upon them and may require increasing dosages until, finally, the intestine becomes insensitive and fails to work properly.

- *Travel.* People often experience constipation when traveling long distances, which may relate to changes in lifestyle, schedule, diet, and drinking water.

- *Hormonal Disturbances.* Certain hormonal disturbances, such as an underactive thyroid gland, can produce constipation.

- *Pregnancy*. Pregnancy is another common cause of constipation. The reason may be partly mechanical, in that the pressure of the heavy womb compresses the intestine, and may be partly due to hormonal changes during pregnancy.

- *Fissures and Hemorrhoids*. Painful conditions of the anus can produce a spasm of the anal sphincter muscle, which can delay a bowel movement.

- *Specific Diseases*. Many diseases that affect the body tissues, such as scleroderma or lupus, and certain neurological or muscular diseases, such as multiple sclerosis, Parkinson's disease, and stroke, can be responsible for constipation.

- *Loss of Body Salts*. The loss of body salts through the kidneys or through vomiting or diarrhea is another cause of constipation.

- *Mechanical Compression*. Scarring, inflammation around diverticula, tumors, and cancer can produce mechanical compression of the intestine and result in constipation.

- *Nerve Damage*. Injuries to the spinal cord and tumors pressing on the spinal cord can produce constipation by affecting the nerves that lead to the intestine.

- *Medications*. Many medications can cause constipation. These include pain medications (especially narcotics), antacids that contain aluminum, antispasmodic drugs, antidepressant drugs, tranquilizers, iron supplements, and anticonvulsants for epilepsy.

## What Causes Constipation in Children?

Constipation is common in children and may be related to any of the causes noted in the previous section. In a small number of children, constipation may be the result of physical problems. Children with such defects as the absence of normal nerve endings in portions of the bowel, abnormalities of the spinal cord, thyroid deficiency, mental retardation, and certain other inherited metabolic disorders often suffer symptoms of constipation. Constipation in children, however, usually is due to poor bowel habits.

Studies show that many children who suffer from constipation when they are older have a history of passing stools that are firmer than average in their early weeks of life. Because this occurs before there are significant variations in diet, habits, or attitudes, it suggests that many children who develop constipation have a normal tendency to have firmer stools. Such children suffer little from the tendency unless it is aggravated by poor bowel habits or poor diet.

Constipation may result in pain when the child has bowel movements. Cracks in the skin, called fissures, may develop in the anus. These fissures can bleed or increase pain, causing a child to withhold his or her stool.

Children may withhold their stools for other reasons as well. Some find it inconvenient to use toilets outside the home. Also, severe emotional stress caused by family crises or difficulties at school may cause children to withhold their stools. In these instances, the periods between bowel movements may become quite long, in some cases lasting longer than 1 or 2 weeks. These children may develop fecal impactions, a situation where the stool is packed so tightly in the bowel that the normal pushing action of the bowel is not enough to expel the stool spontaneously.

## What Causes Constipation in Older Adults?

Older adults are five times more likely than younger adults to report problems with constipation. Poor diet, insufficient intake of fluids, lack of exercise, the use of certain drugs to treat other conditions, and poor bowel habits can result in constipation. Experts agree, however, that too often older people become overly concerned with having a bowel movement and that constipation is frequently an imaginary ailment.

Diet and dietary habits can play a role in developing constipation. Lack of interest in eating—a problem common to many single or widowed older people—may lead to heavy use of convenience foods, which tend to be low in fiber. In addition, loss of teeth may force older people to choose soft, processed foods, which also tend to be low in fiber.

Older people sometimes cut back on fluids, especially if they are not eating regular or balanced meals. Water and other fluids add bulk to stools, making bowel movements softer and easier to pass.

Prolonged bedrest, for example, after an accident or during an illness, and lack of exercise may contribute to constipation. Also, drugs may contribute to constipation. Also, drugs prescribed for other conditions, such as antidepressants, antacids containing aluminum or calcium, antihistamines, diuretics, and antiparkinsonism drugs, can produce constipation in some people.

The preoccupation with bowel movements sometimes leads older people to depend heavily on laxatives, which can be habit-forming. The bowel begins to rely on laxatives to bring on bowel movements, and over time, the natural mechanisms fail to work without the help of drugs. Habitual use of enemas also can lead to a loss of normal function.

## What Diagnostic Tests Can Help Determine the Causes of Constipation?

Constipation may be caused by abnormalities or obstructions of the digestive system in some people. A doctor can perform tests to determine if constipation is the symptom of an underlying disorder.

In addition to routine blood, urine, and stool tests, a sigmoidoscopy may help detect problems in the rectum and lower colon. In this procedure, which can be done in the doctor's office, the doctor inserts a flexible, lighted instrument through the anus to examine the rectum and lower intestine. The doctor may perform a colonoscopy to inspect the entire colon. In colonoscopy, an instrument similar to the sigmoidoscope, but longer and able to follow the twists and turns of the entire large intestine, is used. A barium enema x-ray will provide similar information. If bleeding is present, a double-contrast barium enema is preferred. Other highly specialized techniques are available for measuring pressures and movements within the colon and its sphincter muscles, but these are used only in unusual cases.

## Is Constipation Serious?

Although it may be extremely bothersome, constipation itself usually is not serious. However, it may signal and be the only noticeable symptom of a serious underlying disorder such as cancer. Constipation can lead to complications, such as hemorrhoids caused by extreme straining or fissures caused by the hard stool stretching the sphincters. Bleeding can occur for either of these reasons and appears as bright red streaks on the surface of the stool. Fissures may be quite painful and can aggravate the constipation that originally caused them. Fecal impactions tend to occur in very young children and in older adults and may be accompanied by a loss of control of stool, with liquid stool flowing around the hard impaction.

Occasionally, straining causes a small amount of intestinal lining to push out from the rectal opening. This condition is known as rectal prolapse and may lead to secretion of mucus that may stain underpants. In children, mucus may be a feature of cystic fibrosis.

## When Is Medical Attention Needed?

The doctor should be notified when symptoms are severe, last longer than 3 weeks, or are disabling; or when any of the complications listed above occur. The doctor should be informed whenever a significant and prolonged change of usual bowel habits occurs.

## What Is the Treatment for Constipation?

The first step in treating constipation is to understand that normal frequency varies widely, from three bowel movements a day to three a week. Each person must determine what is normal to avoid becoming dependent on laxatives.

For most people, dietary and lifestyle improvements can lessen the chances of constipation. A well-balanced diet that includes fiber-rich foods, such as unprocessed bran, whole-grain breads, and fresh fruits and vegetables, is recommended. Drinking plenty of fluids and exercising regularly will help to stimulate intestinal activity. Special exercises may be necessary to tone up abdominal muscles after pregnancy or whenever abdominal muscles are lax.

Bowel habits also are important. Sufficient time should be set aside to allow for undisturbed visits to the bathroom. In addition, the urge to have a bowel movement should not be ignored.

If an underlying disorder is causing constipation, treatment will be directed toward the specific cause. For example, if an underactive thyroid is causing constipation, the doctor may prescribe thyroid hormone replacement therapy.

In most cases, laxatives should be the last resort and taken only under a doctor's supervision. A doctor is best qualified to determine when a laxative is needed and which type is best. There are various types of oral laxatives, and they work in different ways (see sidebar below). Above all, it is necessary to recognize that a successful treatment program requires persistent effort and time. Constipation does not occur overnight, and it is not reasonable to expect that constipation can be relieved overnight.

## Summary

The frequency of bowel movements among healthy people varies from three movements a day to three a week. Individuals must determine what is normal. As a rule, constipation should be suspected if more than 3 days pass between bowel movements or if there is difficulty or pain when passing a hardened stool. Most people experience occasional short bouts of constipation, but if a laxative is necessary for longer than 3 weeks, check with a doctor.

Doctors agree that prevention is the best approach to constipation. While there is no way to ensure never experiencing constipation, the following guidelines should help:

- Know what is normal and do not rely unnecessarily on laxatives.
- Eat a well-balanced diet that includes unprocessed bran, whole wheat grains, fresh fruits and vegetables.
- Drink plenty of fluids.
- Exercise regularly.
- Set aside time after breakfast or dinner for undisturbed visits to the toilet.
- Don't ignore the urge to defecate.
- Whenever there is a significant or prolonged change in bowel habits, check with a doctor.

## Additional Readings

Cummings M. "Overuse Hazardous: Laxatives Rarely Needed." *FDA Consumer* 1991; 25(3): 33–35. Article reprint available from the Food and Drug Administration, 5600 Fishers Lane, Rockville, MD 20857, or in libraries. This article discusses the dangers of the overuse of laxatives and suggests alternative methods for treating constipation.

*Diet, Nutrition, & Cancer Prevention: The Good News* (NIH Publication No. 87–2878). Pamphlet available from the Cancer Information Service, Office of Cancer Communications, National Cancer Institute, 9000 Rockville Pike, Bethesda, MD 20892. 1 (800) 4-CANCER. Discusses high-fiber diet and fiber-rich foods.

Larson DE, Editor-in-chief. *Mayo Clinic Family Health Book*. New York: William Morrow and Company, Inc., 1990. General medical guide that includes a section on constipation. Available in libraries and bookstores.

Marshall JB. "Chronic Constipation in Adults: How Far Should Evaluation and Treatment Go?" *Postgraduate Medicine*, 1990; 88(3): 49–51, 54–59, 63. This article for primary care physicians offers advice on diagnosis and treatment of constipation.

Murray FE, Bliss CM. "Geriatric Constipation: Brief Update on a Common Problem." *Geriatrics*, 1991; 46(3): 64–68. This article for health professionals discusses the causes and management of constipation in older adults.

## Oral Laxatives

- Bulk-forming laxatives are generally considered the safest laxative form but can interfere with the absorption of some drugs. These laxatives, which should be taken with 8 ounces of water, absorb water in the intestine and make the stool softer. Bulk laxatives include psyllium (Metamucil), methylcellulose (Citrucel), calcium polycarbophil (FiberCon), and bran (in food and supplements).

- Stimulants cause rhythmic muscular contractions in the small or large intestine. These agents can lead to dependency and can damage the bowel with prolonged daily use. These products include phenolphthalein (Correctol, Ex-Lax), bisacodyl (Dulcolax), castor oil (Purge, Neoloid), and senna (Senokot, Fletcher's Castoria).

- Stool softeners, or wetting agents, provide moisture to the stool and prevent excessive dehydration. These laxatives often are recommended after childbirth or surgery. Products include those with docusate (Colace, Dialose, and Surfak).

- Lubricants grease the stool and make it slip through the intestine more easily. Mineral oil is the most commonly used lubricant.

- Osmotics are salts or carbohydrates that cause water to remain in the intestine for easier movement of stool. Laxatives in this group include milk of magnesia, citrate of magnesia, lactulose, and Epsom salts.

## Chapter 30

# Age Page: Constipation

Constipation is a symptom, not a disease. It is defined as a decrease in the frequency of bowel movements, accompanied by prolonged or difficult passage of stools. There is no accepted rule for the correct number of daily or weekly bowel movements. "Regularity" may be a twice-daily bowel movement for some or two bowel movements a week for others.

Older people are five times as likely as younger people to report problems with constipation. But experts agree that too often older people become overly concerned with having a daily bowel movement and that constipation is frequently an overemphasized ailment.

## Who Has Constipation?

Some doctors suggest asking yourself these questions to decide if you are really constipated:

- Do you often have fewer than two bowel movements each week?
- Do you have difficulty passing stools?
- Is there pain?
- Are there other problems such as bleeding?

---

This chapter was originally published in September 1992 as *Age Page: Constipation* for the National Institute on Aging, National Digestive Diseases Education and Information Clearinghouse, National Institutes of Health.

Unless these are regular symptoms for you, then you are probably not constipated. And if you are constipated, there are steps you can take to improve your condition without resorting to harsh drug treatments.

## What Causes Constipation?

Doctors do not always know what causes constipation. But an older person who eats a poor diet, drinks too few fluids, or misuses laxatives can easily become constipated.

Drugs given for other conditions (for example, certain antidepressants, antacids containing aluminum or calcium, antihistamines, diuretics, and antiparkinsonism drugs) can produce constipation in some people, as can lack of exercise.

**The Role of Diet**—A shift in dietary habits away from high-fiber* foods (vegetables, fruits, and whole grains) to foods that are high in animal fats (meats, dairy products, and eggs) and refined sugars (rich desserts and other sweets) and low in fiber can contribute to constipation. Some studies have suggested that high-fiber diets result in larger stools, more frequent bowel movements, and therefore less constipation.

Lack of interest in eating—a common problem for many people who live alone—may lead to heavy use of convenience foods, which tend to be low in fiber. In addition, loss of teeth may force older people to choose soft, processed foods that also contain little, if any, fiber.

Older people sometimes cut back on liquids in their diet, especially if they are not eating regular or balanced meals. Water and other fluids add bulk to stools, making bowel movements easier.

**Misuse of Laxatives and Enemas**—It is estimated that Americans spend $250 million on over-the-counter (nonprescription) laxatives each year. Many people view them as the cure for constipation. But heavy use of laxatives is usually not necessary and often can be habit forming. The body begins to rely on the laxatives to bring on bowel movements and, over time, the natural "emptying" mechanisms fail to work without the help of these drugs. For the same reason, habitual use of enemas can also lead to a loss of normal bowel function. Another side effect of heavy laxative use is diarrhea.

Overuse of mineral oil—a popular laxative—may reduce the absorption of certain vitamins (A,D,E, and K). Mineral oil may also interact with drugs such as anticoagulants (given to prevent blood clots) and other laxatives, causing undesired side effects.

**Other Causes of Constipation**—Lengthy bedrest, for example after an accident or illness, and lack of exercise may contribute to constipation. For patients who stay in bed and who suffer from chronic constipation, drug therapy may be the best solution. But simply being more active is a better idea for individuals who are not bedfast.

Ignoring the natural urge to defecate (have a bowel movement) can result in constipation. Some people prefer to have their bowel movements only at home, but holding a bowel movement can cause ill effects if the delay is too long.

In some people, constipation may be caused by abnormalities or blockage of the digestive system. These disorders may affect either the muscles or nerves responsible for normal defecation. A doctor can perform a series of tests to determine if constipation is the symptom of an underlying (and often treatable) disorder.

## *Treatment*

If you become constipated, you should first see your doctor to rule out a more serious problem. If the results show that no intestinal disease or abnormality exists and your doctor approves, try these remedies:

- Eat more fresh fruits and vegetables, either cooked or raw, and more whole-grain cereals and breads. Dried fruits such as apricots, prunes, and figs are especially high in fiber. Try to cut back on highly processed foods (such as sweets) and foods high in fat.

- Drink plenty of liquids (1 to 2 quarts daily) unless you have heart, circulatory, or kidney problems. But be aware that some people become constipated from drinking large quantities of milk.

- Some doctors recommend adding small amounts of unprocessed bran** ("miller's bran") to baked goods, cereals, and fruits as a way of increasing the fiber content of the diet. If your diet is well-balanced and contains a variety of foods high in natural fiber, it is usually not necessary to add bran to other foods. But if you do use unprocessed bran, remember that some people suffer from bloating and gas for several weeks after adding bran to their diet. All changes in the diet should be made slowly, to allow the digestive system to adapt.

- Stay active. Even taking a brisk walk after dinner can help tone your muscles.
- Try to develop a regular bowel habit. If you have had problems with constipation, attempt to have a bowel movement shortly after breakfast or dinner.
- Avoid taking laxatives if at all possible. Although they will usually relieve the constipation, you can quickly come to depend on them and the natural muscle actions required for defecation will be impaired.
- Limit your intake of antacids, as some can cause constipation as well as other health problems.
- Above all, do not expect to have a bowel movement every day or even every other day. "Regularity" differs from person to person. If your bowel movements are usually painless and occur regularly (whether the pattern is three times a day or two times each week), then you are probably not constipated.

*Fiber is the nondigestible portion of plant foods. It retains water as it passes through the system, adding bulk to stools.

**Unprocessed bran is usually sold in health food stores or in the health foods section of supermarkets. It should not be confused with the packaged cereals that contain large amounts of bran or bran flakes.

# Chapter 31

# *Iron Metabolism and Hemochromatosis*

[Editor's Note: The information in this chapter is highly technical but may help those suffering from hemochromatosis understand their condition. We recommend discussing this material with your physician.]

*The complications of hemochromatosis can be prevented if the condition is recognized and treated early. Often, however, the diagnosis is missed. Treatment involves removal of excessive iron by phlebotomy or chelation.*

Hemochromatosis (HC) is a complex group of disorders in which progressively increasing total body iron stores result in iron deposition in the parenchymal cells of the liver, pancreas, and other organs. This excess iron deposition eventually causes tissue damage and insufficiency of the organs that are involved.

Although the gene frequency is high, and hereditary HC is one of the most commonly seen genetic disorders, the diagnosis is often missed. All physicians should be familiar with this common disease since the complications of iron overload can be prevented if HC is diagnosed and treated before clinical signs and symptoms start to develop.

---

This copyrighted document originally appeared in *Contemporary Gastroenterology* June/July 1992. Reprinted by permission.

## Iron Metabolism

Iron metabolism is crucial to the pathophysiology of HC.[1] Iron exists as two common oxidation states, $Fe^{2+}$ (ferrous) and $Fe^{3+}$ (ferric). In biological systems, the highly toxic free cation [positively charged ion] exists only transiently. Various proteins, such as hemoglobin, myoglobin, the cytochromes, ferritin, and transferrin (TF), bind or incorporate the iron cation into their structure, maintaining it in a soluble, nontoxic form.

The body can excrete only limited amounts of iron; absorption plays the key role in maintaining normal body iron content. The normal Western diet contains 10 to 20 mg of iron a day, 10% to 20% of this is heme iron. Only 1 to 2 mg of iron a day is absorbed to balance daily obligatory losses, primarily as exfoliated gastrointestinal mucosal cells. The total body iron content in a normal man is 4 gm; 60% is in hemoglobin, 10% in myoglobin, and 5% in enzyme systems, such as cytochromes. Twenty percent to 30% is stored in the liver, spleen, and bone marrow as ferritin and hemosiderin. About 7 mg is in transit, bound to TF in the extracellular fluid.

Although the stomach, ileum, and colon can absorb small amounts of iron salts, the proximal duodenum most actively absorbs both heme and nonheme iron. Normally, many factors govern the rate of iron absorption; two of the most important are total body iron stores and rate of erythropoiesis. Anemia, faster erythropoiesis, and rapid iron turnover all increase iron absorption. Bioavailability also influences iron absorption; heme iron is much more bioavailable (25% absorbed) than nonheme iron (3% absorbed). Gastric acid is important in absorbing ferric but not ferrous or heme iron. Pancreatic and biliary secretions play no significant role in iron absorption.

Small intestinal epithelial cells form a selective barrier between the lumen and serosal surfaces, which is fundamental to iron homeostasis. To enter the body, iron passes through the enterocyte and into the submucosal capillary network in three phases uptake, intracellular, and transfer (Figure 31.1).

## Iron Binding and Storage Proteins

Almost all serum iron is bound to TF, a glycoprotein.[2] One TF molecule can bind two ferric ions. Normally, TF is present in such excess that only 30% is saturated with iron. For most cells, serum TF is the most readily available source of iron. Cells requiring iron express cell

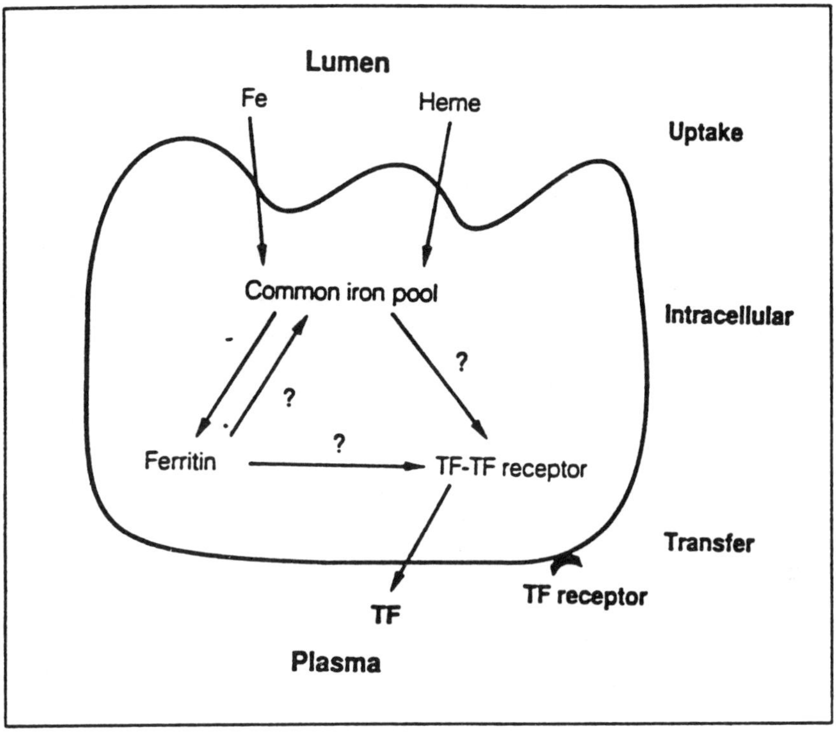


***Figure 31.1.*** *Enterocyte Iron Absorption. To enter the body, iron passes through the enterocyte and into the submucosal capillary network in three basic phases: (1) The uptake phase is iron entry into the enterocyte through its apical (lumenal) surface. (2) The intracellular phase is intracellular iron storage or transport to the basolateral surface. Heme oxygenase degrades intracellular heme to biliverdin and inorganic iron, which then enter a common iron pool. This phase is complex, but appears to involve at least ferritin and transferrin (TF). (3) The last phase of iron absorption, the transfer phase, is transfer of iron from the basolateral surface of the mucosal cell into the circulation. TF- receptor is expressed on the basolateral surface and is involved in receptor-mediated endocytosis of TF.*

surface receptors for TF. Transferrin receptor is a disulfide-linked dimeric glycoprotein whose expression depends on iron level and the degree of cellular proliferation and differentiation. TF transports ferric iron into cells by receptor-mediated endocytosis, a unique process by which TF and its receptor are reutilized repeatedly in iron delivery.

Although the TF gene is expressed in many organs, including the liver, brain, placenta, stomach, and spleen, the main source of TF synthesis is the liver. TF synthesis is increased by iron deficiency and estrogen and dexamethasone administration, and decreased by iron overload, fasting, and from protein malnutrition.[3]

Ferritin consists of a roughly spherical hollow protein shell, within which a substantial amount of ferric iron can be stored.[4] Iron represents 26% of the dry molecular mass of a fully loaded ferritin molecule. In the liver, the rate of ferritin synthesis is increased by increased iron levels and during inflammation. Partial degradation of ferritin protein may lead to the production of intralysosomal hemosiderin, an ill-defined entity consisting of clumps of partially degraded ferritin with varying amounts of protein, lipids, and sugars. Ferritin and hemosiderin are the major storage forms of iron.

## Role of the Liver

Normally, TF transports 80% to 85% of absorbed iron to the bone marrow; the remainder goes to liver or muscle.[5] The liver as a major storage organ and the principal site of TF synthesis serves an important function in maintaining whole body iron homeostasis. Hepatocytes store much of the excess body iron. Although TF is probably the major source of hepatic iron, it is also derived from heme-hemopexin, hemoglobin-haptoglobin, methemalbumin, ferritin, lactoferrin, and low-molecular-weight iron uptake. Ninety-eight percent of liver iron is stored primarily as ferritin within the hepatocyte. Hemosiderin exists predominantly in the lysosomes of the reticuloendothelial (RE) cells and gives the Prussian blue reaction. As hepatic iron content increases so does the amount of iron in RE cells. In pathologic iron overload, hemosiderin progressively becomes the predominant storage form of iron.

## Causes of HC

HC may be produced by inappropriately increased mucosal iron absorption, parental administration of iron, or grossly excessive dietary intake over a prolonged period. In iron storage disease, more than one mechanism may be relevant. The only well-documented cases of excessive oral intake occurred in a group of South African blacks (Bantus) who ingested large amounts of iron from beer fermented in iron pots. Some of them developed iron overload with features similar to those of hereditary HC except that their heavy deposition of hemosiderin began in the RE system. Alcoholic liver disease is not a cause of HC.[6,7] Hereditary HC and secondary HC, resulting from various anemias and ineffective erythropoiesis, are the most common causes of iron overload.

## Causes of Hemochromatosis.

*Hereditary (primary, idiopathic) Hemochromatosis*

*Secondary Hemochromatosis*

- Anemia and ineffective erythropoesis
  —Sideroblastic anemia
  —Thalassemia major
  —Pyruvate kinase deficiency

- Liver diseases
  —After portacaval anastomosis

- Excessive high oral intake
  —Intake of iron in brewed beverages as in the South African Bantus

## Hereditary HC

Hereditary HC is an autosomal recessive genetic disorder.[8] In 1975, Simon and coworkers first reported an association of HC with certain HLA antigens—A3, B7, and B14. Subsequently, the HC gene has been localized to the short arm of chromosome 6, close to the A locus. Frequency of HLA-A3 is 71% among patients with hereditary HC (versus 28% in normals). A3 is the only independent marker of the HC allele; the HLA-B7 and B14 associations are due to their linkage to A3.

Studies from Western countries have revealed that whites have a gene frequency of 5% to 7%, implying 10% of the general population are heterozygotes and 0.2% to 0.5% of the population are homozygotes.[8,9] Only homozygotes develop clinical manifestations of HC.[10] Expression depends on such factors as age, chronic blood loss, iron intake, and gender. Clinical and biochemical expression occurs in almost all men with HC, but in women, phenotypic expression is often mild, incomplete, or occasionally absent because of physiologic blood loss.

Heterozygotes develop no significant iron excess or toxicity without a secondary cause of iron overload, such as ineffective erythropoiesis. They have partial biochemical expression; 20% to 30% have abnormal iron and TF saturation. One third have increased hepatic iron content, but iron stores plateau at age 45 and seldom exceed 5 gm total. The increased heptic iron produces no histologically detectable alteration in hepatic architecture. Prospective studies of heterozygotes over two decades showed no evidence of progressively increased iron stores, even in subjects with excessive alcohol intakes.

## Pathophysiology

The basic metabolic defect in hereditary HC is unknown but probably involves regulation of iron absorption by the enterocytes.[11,12] Hepatic TF receptors,[13] uptake of TF, and ferritin expression function normally in hereditary HC. Serum TF is highly saturated in hereditary HC, and up to 30% of serum iron may be present in non-TF-bound (NTFB) low-molecular-weight iron. Hepatocytes take up NTFB iron more rapidly than TF-bound iron, and abnormal lysosomal iron accumulation occurs, which may increase lysosomal fragility.[14]

Excessive body iron clearly correlates with cellular injury after the cells' capacity for safe iron storage has been exceeded.[15] Irons damage living systems by forming toxic $O_2$ free radicals, such as the highly reactive hydroxyl radical. Iron and these free radicals stimulate lipid peroxidation, leading to organelle dysfunction, cell injury, and death. Iron salts, especially ferrous ion, are the toxic forms of iron. Bound iron ineffectively mediates lipid peroxidation.

The main hepatic pathologic findings in hereditary HC are fibrosis and cirrhosis, and the most feared complication is development of hepatocellular carcinoma. Bassett and colleagues reported that the development of hepatic fibrosis and cirrhosis depends on the hepatic iron concentration.[16] Without coexistent liver diseases, fibrosis and cirrhosis usually do not occur until the hepatic iron concentration reaches >22,000 μg/gm dry weight or 12-fold the normal level. Recently, Chojkier and associates showed that aldehydic byproducts of iron-induced lipid peroxidation increased collagen gene expression in cultured human fibroblasts, directly linking lipid peroxidation to fibrogenesis.[17] Hepatocellular carcinoma is seen much more commonly in cirrhosis induced by iron overload than in cirrhosis of other causes. The mechanisms are unclear.

## Clinical Manifestations

Increased iron absorption is a life-long event. When symptoms develop, total body iron stores are usually 20 to 40 gm. Patients usually present in the fifth to sixth decades with nonspecific symptoms like weakness and lassitude. Signs of organ failure, arthritis, and hyperpigmentation develop later. When severe overload develops in the second to fourth decades, cardiac arrhythmias, heart failure, and hypogonadism are the predominant manifestations.

Figure 31.2 illustrates the frequency of symptoms and signs in endstage HC. Major manifestations involve the hepatic, endocrine, skin, joint, and cardiac systems. Hepatomegaly is the most common sign. Liver tests become abnormal only in end-stage disease, with transaminases two to four times the normal level and mild increases in bilirubin levels. Cirrhosis is present in 40% to 80% of symptomatic patients undergoing liver biopsy. In most studies, hepatoma is seen in one third of patients with established cirrhosis secondary to HC.

Endocrinopathies occur in 80% of patients with end-stage disease, diabetes mellitus being the most common. The next most common is hypogonadism, primarily as a result of gonadotrophin insufficiency. Panhypopituitarism is seen in 6% of end-stage patients and does not improve with phlebotomy.

Hyperpigmentation occurs over the entire body but is most prominent over sun-exposed surfaces and in the axilla, groin, and scars. The bronze color is secondary to increased melanin in the basal layer of the epidermis. The gray hue represents hemosiderin deposits in fibroblasts of the corium near dermal gland appendages.

Arthropathy is seen in 50% of patients and is most commonly polyarticular and progressive. The second and third metacarpal phalangeal joints are most often involved. Radiographic studies sometimes show sclerosis in the subchondral bone, loss of articular cartilage, subchondral cyst formation, and chondrocalcinosis of the articular cartilage.

Heart disease, including arrhythmias and congestive heart failure, is reported in up to one third of patients with end-stage disease. Autopsy studies show that myocardial iron loads correlate with the severity of cardiac dysfunction. The cardiomyopathy seen in these patients is usually dilated congestive but may rarely be restrictive. Some studies suggest atrioventricular node but not sinoatrial node iron deposition.

**Figure 31.2** Signs and Symptoms in Patients with End-Stage Renal Failure.*

| Symptoms | Frequency (%) |
|---|---|
| Weakness | 50-70 |
| Weight loss | 50 |
| Arthralgias | 40-50 |
| Abdominal pain | 25-50 |
| Loss of libido and/or impotence | 25 |
| Cardiac complaints | 33 |
| Asymptomatic | 15-30 |
| **Physical and laboratory findings** | |
| Hepatomegaly | 50-90 |
| Cirrhosis | 40-90 |
| Hepatoma | 5-18 |
| Splenomegaly | 35-50 |
| Hyperpigmentation | 50-85 |
| Diabetes | 50-80 |
| Hypogonadism | 20-50 |
| Arthropathy | 50 |
| Cardiac arrhythmia | 25-30 |
| Congestive heart failure | 33 |
| Abnormal liver tests | 50-60 |

*Source: Edwards et al.[8] Based on four studies and a total of 1,173 patients.

## Diagnosis of HC

Because of relative preservation of hepatocyte integrity, routine liver tests are frequently normal despite cirrhosis. No single serologic test accurately diagnoses iron overload.

*Serum iron.* This is a poor screening test; 24% of patients with iron overload have normal levels where 10% of normal controls have increased levels. Diurnal variation is 25%, peaking in the morning. Levels can fall as a result of systemic stresses such as infection or inflammation.

*TF and % saturation.* Serum TF levels are slightly decreased as a result of down regulation by excess iron; iron saturation is high. These values must be obtained after an overnight fast. Nonfasting % saturation values may be falsely increased. Almost all HC patients older than 20 years of age have >50% saturation.

*Ferritin.* Ferritin correlates with total body as well as hepatic iron stores, but has a short half life and is an acute phase reactant. Patients with HC usually have levels >1,000 ng/mL. Levels may be normal in latent or precirrhotic HC, however, and very high in other liver diseases, including alcoholic hepatitis. Therefore, ferritin levels are not useful in differentiating HC from other liver diseases.

Increased % saturation (>50%) with increased serum ferritin more accurately diagnoses HC than either test alone. Older assays of total body iron stores, such as quantitative phlebotomy and chelation tests, are seldom done now.

*Liver biopsy.* Liver biopsy is the definitive test. It can quantitate hepatic iron and evaluate histology. Iron quantitation requires a 0.5- to 1.0-cm needle-biopsy specimen. This most objectively evaluates iron stores. The normal hepatic iron content is 400 mg or <1,500 μg/gm dry weight (<250 μg/gm wet weight). Patients with HC usually have >10,000 μg/gm dry weight (or >179 μmoles/gm dry weight because the molecular weight of iron is 55.8 gm). Recently, Summers and colleagues introduced the hepatic iron index (HII). which is the amount of liver iron in μmoles/gm dry weight/age.[18] Hepatic iron increases with age. Thus, a young homozygote may have a low hepatic iron level and an older heterozygote may have a higher level. The HII corrects for age. In the study by Summers and coworkers, all homozygotes had a HII >1.9 whereas all heterozygotes had a HII <1.5. Alcoholics with siderosis also had a HII <2.0. A cutoff of 2 is the best index to differentiate patients with HC from heterozygotes and patients with alcoholic siderosis.

Liver biopsy allows evaluation of hepatic architecture, presence of fibrosis and cirrhosis, and degree and location of iron staining. Degree of iron staining, or degree of siderosis, is graded on a scale of 0 to 4: 0 = no stainable iron; 1 = stainable iron in <25% of cells; 2 = stainable iron in 25% to 50% of cells; 3 = stainable iron in 50% to 75%; 4 = >75% of cells. Patients with HC all have 3 to 4 + iron staining, but degree of iron staining and hepatic iron concentration correlate crudely at high ranges (3 + can be 5,000 to 30,000 μg/gm dry weight). Early in HC, stainable iron is almost exclusively in the hepatic parenchyma, particularly in the periportal zones within the lobules, with relative sparing of the RE cells. This contrasts with secondary iron overload and alcoholic siderosis, in which iron deposits predominate in the Kupffer cells early on. As iron accumulates, the histology and stainable iron pattern in the various types of iron overload become indistinguishable.

Noninvasive imaging techniques like computed tomography and magnetic resonance imaging provide no information on histology and are not sensitive enough to screen or follow patients. These imaging studies are useful only in patients unwilling or unable to undergo liver biopsy.[19,20]

## Complications and Causes of Death

A retrospective analysis of 163 patients with HC followed for 1 to 24 years (mean, 10 years) elucidated complications and causes of death in HC [21] All patients underwent phlebotomy until liver biopsy documented iron depletion. Life expectancy fell in patients with cirrhosis compared with those without cirrhosis (20-year survival of 45% vs. 75%) and in diabetics compared with nondiabetics. Patients without cirrhosis had normal life expectancy. Those with major complications of liver cirrhosis had the worse prognosis. Seven percent died before iron depletion could be achieved.

Plasma iron levels, TF saturation, ferritin, and grade of liver iron staining were higher in patients with cirrhosis, but significant overlap precluded their usefulness as predictors. Fifty three patients died. Four causes of death were significantly higher in patients with HC: Hepatobiliary carcinoma occurred 219 times more frequently, cardiomyopathy 306 times more frequently, cirrhosis 13 times more frequently, and diabetic complications 7 times more frequently in these patients than in normal controls.

Iron overload also predisposes to infection by facilitating bacterial growth and virulence.[22,23] Also, patients with iron overload may have liver disease and diabetes, which may impair leukocyte chemotaxis. *Vibrio vulnificus* and *Yersinia enterocolitica*, which usually cause benign gastroenteritis in normal individuals, may cause highly fatal sepsis in patients with HC.

## Treatment

Treatment of HC involves removing excessive iron by phlebotomy (in hereditary HC) or chelation (in secondary HC).[8,24] Although no controlled studies have demonstrated benefits from phlebotomy, removing excessive iron probably improves prognosis in patients with and without cirrhosis.

*Treatment of hereditary HC*. The treatment protocol for hereditary HC is outlined in [the sidebar below]. Weekly or semiweekly phlebotomy, removing 250 mg of iron each time, removes the 20 gm of excessive iron found in the average newly diagnosed patient in 1 to 2 years. In patients with liver failure, diabetes, or heart failure, phlebotomy should be more frequent. The goal should be to normalize iron stores as quickly as possible.

During therapy, residual iron stores should be assessed by following ferritin levels, which may fluctuate during initial treatment. Later, the decrease should be steady and sustained. Serum iron lags behind ferritin and is not useful in evaluating progress.

Liver iron stores may remain high despite anemia and absent bone marrow iron. This residual iron probably is a storage form unavailable for erythropoiesis. Hepatic iron concentration should be measured soon after intensive therapy. If the concentration remains high, the frequency of phlebotomy should not be reduced unless worsening anemia or clinical symptoms of iron deficiency occur.

Maintenance therapy should remove one unit every 3 to 4 months to keep ferritin levels <200 ng/mL in women and <350 ng/mL in men. Most manifestations of HC improve dramatically with phlebotomy, except for hypogonadism, arthropathy, and hepatocellular carcinoma.

*Treatment of secondary HC*. Chelation therapy with deferoxamine is the preferred treatment for secondary HC. One molecule of deferoxamine chelates a single ferric iron. It does not chelate heme iron. Deferoxamine is contraindicated in pregnant patients or those with renal insufficiency. Simultaneous administration of ascorbate increases the potency of deferoxamine, but it can also exacerbate iron-induced toxicities, and, for this reason, many do not advocate routine use of ascorbate.

## Screening

TF saturation and ferritin should be measured in first-degree relatives of patients with hereditary HC.[25] HLA typing should also be done in siblings since sibs have a one fourth chance of being HLA identical. Screening should also include the spouse because high heterozygous frequency (10%) may necessitate genetic counseling. If saturation is >75% and serum ferritin is high, the family member being screened is probably a homozygote. Those identified by the initial screening to have increased iron stores should undergo liver biopsy. Those not iron overloaded should undergo repeat studies every 2 years. Measurement of TF saturation and ferritin is the most cost-effective way to screen.

## Summary

We have learned much about the pathophysiology of these disorders in the past few years. The gene frequency is relatively high, and HC has been underdiagnosed. Prompt recognition before development of irreversible damage is critical since removal of excess iron will prevent it. Increased awareness and screening should improve survival.

## Administration of Deferoxamine

Deferoxamine can be delivered by:

- IM or SQ injection. 0.5–1.0 gm/day removes approximately 20 mg of iron per day. Cost is $1,200 per patient per year.
- SQ pump. 1.5 gm delivered over 12 hours removes approximately 15–55 mg of iron per day. Cost is $4,800 per patient per year.
- Continuous IV infusion. Up to 4–6 gm delivered over 24 hours will remove up to 80 mg of iron per day.

Side effects of deferoxamine include systemic hypotension (during IV delivery), mild skin hypersensitivity, cataracts, and visual and auditory neurotoxicity in young patients. Deferoxamine is contraindicated in pregnancy and in renal insufficiency.

The potency of deferoxamine can be increased by simultaneously giving ascorbate. Patients with iron overload may be ascorbate deficient, probably as a result of accelerated oxidative catabolism of ascorbate to oxalate in the presence of large iron deposits. During deferoxamine treatment, repletion of tissue ascorbate stores increases iron excretion by 20% to 80% by mobilizing RE iron and causing internal redistribution. Ascorbate may, however, exacerbate iron-induced toxicities, like heart failure, because it promotes iron absorption by converting ferric to ferrous iron, which is more readily absorbed and more effective in creating free radical formation and lipid peroxidation. For these reasons, many do not advocate routine use of ascorbate.

## References


1. Powell LW, Halliday JW: Iron absorption and iron overload. *Clin Gastroenterol*, 1981;10:707.

2. Aisen P: Transferrin metabolism and the liver *Sem Liv Dis*, 1984;4:193.

3. Adrian GS, Bowman BH, Herbert DC, et al: Human transferrin. Expression and iron modulation of chimeric genes in transgenic mice. *J Biol Chem*, 1990; 265:13344.

4. Worwood M: Ferritin. *Blood Rev*, 1990; 4:259.

5. Bacon BR, Tavill AS: Role of the liver in normal iron metabolism. *Sem Liv Dis*, 1984;4:181.

6. Chapman RW, Morgan MY, Laulicht M, et al: Hepatic iron stores and markers of iron overload in alcoholics and patients with idiopathic hemochromatosis. *Dig Dis Sci*, 1982;27:909.

7. LeSage GD, Baldus WP, FairDanks VF, et al: Hemochromatosis: genetic or alcohol-induced? *Gastroenterology*, 1983;84:1471.

8. Edwards CQ, Dadone MM, Skolnick MH, et al: Hereditary hemochromatosis. *Clin Haematol*, 1982;11:411.

9. Edwards CQ. Griffin LM, Goldgar D, et al: Prevalence of hemachromatosis among 11,065 presumably healthy blood donors. *N Engl J Med*, 1988;318:1355.

10. Powell LW, Summers KM, Board PG, et al: Expression of hemochromatosis in homozygous subjects. Implications for early diagnosis and prevention. *Gastroenterology*, 1990;98:1625.

11. Fracanzani AL, Fargion S, Romano R, et al: Immunohistochemical evidence for a lack of ferritin in duodenal absorptive epithelial cells in idiopathic hemochromatosis. *Gastroenterology*, 1989;96:1071.

12. Lombard M, Bomford A, Poison RJ, et al: Differential expression of transferrin receptor in duodenal mucosa in iron overload. Evidence for a site-specific defect in genetic hemochromatosis. *Gastroenterology*, 1990;98:976.

13. Lombard M, Bomford A, Hynes M, et al: Regulation of the hepatic transferrin receptor in hereditary hemochromatosis. *Hepatology*, 1989;9:1.

14. Batey RG, Shamir S, Wilms J: Properties and hepatic metabolism of nontransferrin-bound iron. *Dig Dis Sci*, 1981;26:1084.

15. Bacon BR, Britton RS: The pathology of hepatic iron overload: a free radical-mediated process? *Hepatology*, 1990;11:127.

16. Basset ML, Halliday JW, Powell LW: Value of hepatic iron measurements in early hemochromatosis and determination of the critical iron level associated with fibrosis. *Hepatology*, 1986;6:24.

17. Chojkier M, Hougium K, Solis-Herruzo J. et al: Stimulation of collagen gene expression by ascorbic acid in cultured human fibroblasts. A role for lipid peroxidation? *J Biol Chem*, 1989;264:16957.

18. Summers KM, Halliday JW, Powell LW Identification of homozygous hemochromatosis subjects by measurement of hepatic iron index. *Hepatology*, 1990;12:20.

19. Guyader D, Gandon Y, Deugnier Y, et al: Evaluation of computed tomography in the assessment of liver iron overload. *Gastroenterology*, 1989;97:737.

20. Stark DD, Moseley ME, Bacon BR, et al: Magnetic resonance imaging and spectroscopy of hepatic iron overload. *Radiology*, 1985;154:137.

21. Niederau C, Fischer R, Sonnenberg A, et al: Survival and causes of death in cirrhotic and in noncirrhotic patients with primary hemochromatosis. *N EngL J Med*, 1985;313:1256.

22. Muench KH: Hemochromatosis and infection: alcohol and iron, oysters and sepsis. *Am J Med*, 1989;87:3.

23. Morris JG Jr, Black RE: Cholera and other vibrioses in the United States. *N Engl J Med*, 1985;312:343.

24. Cohen A, Witzleben C, Schwvartz E: Treatment of iron overload. *Sem Liv Dis*, 1984;4:228.

25. Basset ML, Halliday JW, Feris RA, et al: Diagnosis of hemochromatosis in young subjects: predictive accuracy of biochemical screening tests. *Gastroenterology*, 1984;87:628.

*—by Shelly C. Lu, MD, and Lawrence S. Maldonado, MD.*

Dr. Lu is assistant professor of medicine, University of Southern California School of Medicine, Los Angeles, California.

Dr. Maldonado is clinical assistant professor of medicine, UCLA School of Medicine and director, Medical Intensive Care Unit, Cedars-Sinai Medical Center, Los Angeles, Calif.

Chapter 32

# Lactose Intolerance

## What Is Lactose Intolerance?

Lactose intolerance is the inability to digest significant amounts of lactose, the predominant sugar of milk. This inability results from a shortage of the enzyme lactase, which is normally produced by the cells that line the small intestine (see figure 32.1). Lactase breaks down milk sugar into simpler forms that can then be absorbed into the bloodstream. When there is not enough lactase to digest the amount of lactose consumed, the results, although not usually dangerous, may be very distressing. While not all persons deficient in lactase have symptoms, those who do are considered to be lactose intolerant.

Common symptoms include nausea, cramps, bloating, gas, and diarrhea, which begin about 30 minutes to 2 hours after eating or drinking foods containing lactose. The severity of symptoms varies depending on the amount of lactose each individual can tolerate.

Some causes of lactose intolerance are well known. For instance, certain digestive diseases and injuries to the small intestine can reduce the amount of enzymes produced. In rare cases, children are born without the ability to produce lactase. For most people, though, lactase deficiency is a condition that develops naturally over time. After about the age of 2 years, the body begins to produce less lactase. However, many people may not experience symptoms until they are much older.

---

NIH 94-2751.

Between 30 and 50 million Americans are lactose intolerant. Certain ethnic and racial populations are more widely affected than others. As many as 75 percent of all African-Americans and Native Americans and 90 percent of Asian-Americans are lactose intolerant. The condition is least common among persons of northern European descent.

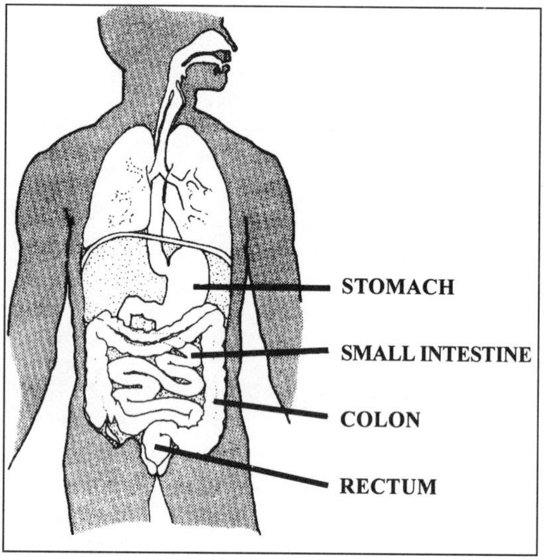


***Figure 32.1.*** *The Digestive Tract.*

## How Is Lactose Intolerance Diagnosed?

The most common tests used to measure the absorption of lactose in the digestive system are the lactose tolerance test, the hydrogen breath test, and the stool acidity test. These tests are performed on an outpatient basis at a hospital's clinic or doctor's office.

The lactose tolerance test begins with the individual fasting (not eating) before the test and then drinking a liquid that contains lactose. Several blood samples are taken over a 2-hour period to measure the person's blood glucose (blood sugar) level, which indicates how well the body is able to digest lactose.

Normally, when lactose reaches the digestive system, the lactase enzyme breaks down lactase into glucose and galactose. The liver then changes the galactose into glucose, which enters the bloodstream and raises the person's blood glucose level. If lactose is incompletely broken down the blood glucose level does not rise, and a diagnosis of lactose intolerance is confirmed.

The hydrogen breath test measures the amount of hydrogen in the breath. Normally, very little hydrogen is detectable in the breath. However, undigested lactose in the colon is fermented by bacteria, and various gases, including hydrogen, are produced. The hydrogen is absorbed from the intestines, carried through the bloodstream to the lungs, and exhaled. In the test, the patient drinks a lactose-loaded beverage, and the breath is analyzed at regular intervals. Raised levels of hydrogen in the breath indicate improper digestion of lactose. Certain foods, medications, and cigarettes can affect the test's accuracy and should be avoided before taking the test. This test is available for children and adults.

The lactose tolerance and hydrogen breath tests are not given to infants and very young children who are suspected of having lactose intolerance. A large lactose load may be dangerous for very young individuals because they are more prone to dehydration that can result from diarrhea caused by the lactose. If a baby or young child is experiencing symptoms of lactose intolerance, many pediatricians simply recommend changing from cow's milk to soy formula and waiting for symptoms to abate.

If necessary, a stool acidity test, which measures the amount of acid in the stool, may be given to infants and young children. Undigested lactose fermented by bacteria in the colon creates lactic acid and other short-chain fatty acids that can be detected in a stool sample. In addition, glucose may be present in the sample as a result of unabsorbed lactose in the colon.

## How Is Lactose Intolerance Treated?

Fortunately, lactose intolerance is relatively easy to treat. No treatment exists to improve the body's ability to produce lactase, but symptoms can be controlled through diet.

Young children with lactase deficiency should not eat any foods containing lactose. Most older children and adults need not avoid lactose completely, but individuals differ in the amounts of lactose they can handle. For example, one person may suffer symptoms after drinking a small glass of milk, while another can drink one glass but not two. Others may be able to manage ice cream and aged cheeses, such as cheddar and Swiss but not other dairy products. Dietary control of lactose intolerance depends on each person's learning through trial and error how much lactose he or she can handle.

For those who react to very small amounts of lactose or have trouble limiting their intake of foods that contain lactose, lactase enzymes are available without a prescription. One form is a liquid for use with milk. A few drops are added to a quart of milk, and after 24 hours in the refrigerator, the lactose content is reduced by 70 percent. The process works faster if the milk is heated first, and adding a double amount of lactase liquid produces milk that is 90 percent lactose free. A more recent development is a chewable lactase enzyme tablet that helps people digest solid foods that contain lactose. Three to six tablets are taken just before a meal or snack.

Lactose-reduced milk and other products are available at many supermarkets. The milk contains all of the nutrients found in regular milk and remains fresh for about the same length of time or longer if it is super-pasteurized.

## How Is Nutrition Balanced?

Milk and other dairy products are a major source of nutrients in the American diet. The most important of these nutrients is calcium. Calcium is essential for the growth and repair of bones throughout life. In the middle and later years, a shortage of calcium may lead to thin, fragile bones that break easily (a condition called osteoporosis). A concern, then, for both children and adults with lactose intolerance, is getting enough calcium in a diet that includes little or no milk.

The recommended dietary allowance (RDA) for calcium, revised in 1989 by the Food and Nutrition Board of the National Academy of Sciences, varies by age group. Infants up to 5 months need 400 mg per day, and from 5 months to 1 year, 600 mg. Children 1 to 10 years need 800 mg and 11- to 24-year-olds need 1,200 mg. Pregnant and nursing women also need 1,200 mg per day, and people age 25 and older need 800 mg per day. However, the results of a 1984 conference at the National Institutes of Health (NIH) suggest that women who have not yet reached menopause and older women who are taking the hormone estrogen after menopause should consume about 1,000 mg of calcium daily (roughly the amount in a quart of milk).

In planning meals, making sure that each day's diet includes enough calcium is important, even if the diet does not contain dairy products. Many nondairy foods are high in calcium. Green vegetables, such as broccoli and kale, and fish with soft, edible bones, such as salmon and sardines, are excellent sources of calcium. To help in planning a high-calcium and low-lactose diet, [the chart below] lists some common foods that are good sources of dietary calcium and shows about how much lactose the foods contain.

Recent research shows that yogurt with active cultures may be a good source of calcium for many people with lactose intolerance, even though it is fairly high in lactose. Evidence shows that the bacterial cultures used in making yogurt produce some of the lactase enzyme required for proper digestion.

Clearly, many foods can provide the calcium and other nutrients the body needs, even when intake of milk and dairy products is limited. However, factors other than calcium and lactose content should be kept in mind when planning a diet. Some vegetables that are high in calcium (Swiss chard, spinach, and rhubarb, for instance) are not listed in [the chart below] because the body cannot use their calcium content. They contain substances called oxalates, which stop calcium absorption. Calcium is absorbed and used only when there is enough vitamin D in the body. A balanced diet should provide an adequate supply of vitamin D. Sources of vitamin D include eggs and liver. However, sunlight helps the body naturally absorb or synthesize vitamin D, and with enough exposure to the sun, food sources may not be necessary.

Some people with lactose intolerance may think they are not getting enough calcium and vitamin D in their diet. Consultation with a doctor or dietitian may be helpful in deciding whether any dietary supplements are needed. Taking vitamins or minerals of the wrong kind or in the wrong amounts can be harmful. A dietitian can help in planning meals that will provide the most nutrients with the least chance of causing discomfort.

## *What Is Hidden Lactose?*

Although milk and foods made from milk are the only natural sources, lactose is often added to prepared foods. People with very low tolerance for lactose should know about the many food products that may contain lactose, even in small amounts. Food products that may contain lactose include:

- Bread and other baked goods.
- Processed breakfast cereals.
- Instant potatoes, soups, and breakfast drinks.
- Margarine.
- Lunch meats (other than kosher).
- Salad dressings.
- Candies and other snacks.
- Mixes for pancakes, biscuits, and cookies.

Some products labeled nondairy, such as powdered coffee creamer and whipped toppings, may also include ingredients that are derived from milk and therefore contain lactose.

Smart shoppers learn to read food labels with care, looking not only for milk and lactose among the contents but also for such words as whey, curds, milk by-products, dry milk solids, and nonfat dry milk powder. If any of these are listed on a label, the item contains lactose.

In addition, lactose is used as the base for more than 20 percent of prescription drugs and about 6 percent of over-the-counter medicines. Many types of birth control pills, for example, contain lactose, as do some tablets for stomach acid and gas. However, these products typically affect only people with severe lactose intolerance.

### *Calcium and Lactose in Common Foods*

#### Vegetables

- Broccoli (cooked), 1 cup
  - 94-177 mg calcium
  - 0 g lactose
- Chinese cabbage (bok choy, cooked), 1 cup
  - 158 mg calcium
  - 0 g lactose
- Collard greens (cooked), 1 cup
  - 148-357 mg calcium
  - 0 g lactose
- Kale (cooked), 1 cup
  - 94-179 mg calcium
  - 0 g lactose
- Turnip greens (cooked), 1 cup
  - 194-279 mg calcium
  - 0 g lactose

#### Dairy Products

- Ice cream/ice milk, 8 oz.
  - 176 mg calcium
  - 6-7 g lactose
- Milk (whole, low-fat, skim, buttermilk), 8 oz.
  - 291-316 mg calcium
  - 12-13 g lactose

Processed cheese, 1 oz.
159-219 mg calcium
2-3 g lactose
Sour cream, 4 oz.
134 mg calcium
4-5 g lactose
Yogurt (plain), 8 oz.
274-415 mg calcium
12-13 g lactose

**Fish/Seafood**

Oysters (raw), 1 cup
226 mg calcium
0 g lactose
Salmon with bones (canned), 3 oz.
167 mg calcium
0 g lactose
Sardines, 3 oz.
371 mg calcium
0 g lactose
Shrimp (canned), 3 oz.
98 mg calcium
0 g lactose

**Other**

Molasses, 2 tbs.
274 mg calcium
0 g lactose
Tofu (processed with calcium salts), 3 oz.
225 mg calcium
0 g lactose

(Calcium content represents the nutritive value of the food cited. Actual value varies according to the method of food preparation. Lactose contents are derived from *Lactose Intolerance: A Resource Including Recipes,* Food Sensitivity Series, American Dietetic Association, 1991.)

## Summary

Even though lactose intolerance is widespread, it need not pose a serious threat to good health. People who have trouble digesting lactose can learn which dairy products and other foods they can eat without discomfort and which ones they should avoid. Many will be able to enjoy milk, ice cream, and other such products if they take them in small amounts or eat other food at the same time. Others can use lactase liquid or tablets to help digest the lactose. Even older women at risk for osteoporosis and growing children who must avoid milk and foods made with milk can meet most of their special dietary needs by eating greens, fish, and other calcium-rich foods that are free of lactose. A carefully chosen diet (with calcium supplements if the doctor or dietitian recommends them) is the key to reducing symptoms and protecting future health.

## Additional Readings

*American Dietetic Association. Lactose Intolerance: A Resource Including Recipes, Food Sensitivity Series* (1991). American Dietetic Association, 216 West Jackson Blvd. Chicago, IL 60606. (312) 899-0040. Resource book provides recipes and information about food products.

Kidder B. *The Milk-Free Kitchen: Living Well Without Dairy Products. 450 Family-Style Recipes*. New York: Henry Holt and Company, 1991. Cookbook with 450 lactose-free recipes.

Montes RG, Perman JA. Lactose intolerance: pinpointing the source of nonspecific gastrointestinal symptoms. *Postgraduate Medicine* 1991;89 (8): 175–184. Article for health care professionals explains diagnosis and treatment of lactose intolerance.

Zukin J. *Dairy-Free Cookbook*. New York: St. Martin's Press, 1989. Commercial Writing Service, P.O. Box 3074, Iowa City, IA 52244. Book contains more than 150 recipes and practical information for living with lactose intolerance.

Zukin J. *The Newsletter For People With Lactose Intolerance and Milk Allergy*. Commercial Writing Service, P.O. Box 3074, Iowa City, IA 52244. Newsletter provides practical information, resources, and recipes.

**National Digestive Diseases Information Clearinghouse**
Box NDDIC
9000 Rockville Pike
Bethesda, MD 20892
(301) 654-3810

The National Digestive Diseases Information Clearinghouse is a service of the National Institute of Diabetes and Digestive and Kidney Diseases, part of the National Institutes of Health, under the U.S. Public Health Service. The clearinghouse, authorized by Congress in 1980, is designed to increase knowledge and understanding about digestive diseases and health among people with digestive diseases and their families, health care professionals, and the public. The clearinghouse answers inquiries; develops, reviews, and distributes publications; and works closely with professional and patient organizations and government agencies to coordinate informational resources about digestive diseases.

Publications produced by the clearinghouse are reviewed carefully for scientific accuracy, content, and readability. Publications produced by sources other than the clearinghouse are also reviewed for scientific accuracy and are used, along with clearinghouse publications, to answer requests.

# Chapter 33

# Hemorrhoids

## What Are Hemorrhoids?

Hemorrhoids are swollen but normally present blood vessels in and around the anus and lower rectum that stretch under pressure, similar to varicose veins in the legs.

The increased pressure and swelling may result from straining to move the bowel. Other contributing factors include pregnancy, heredity, aging, and chronic constipation or diarrhea.

Hemorrhoids are either inside the anus (internal) or under the skin around the anus (external).

## What Are the Symptoms of Hemorrhoids?

Many anorectal problems, including fissures, fistulae, abscesses, or irritation and itching (pruritus ani), have similar symptoms and are incorrectly referred to as hemorrhoids.

Hemorrhoids usually are not dangerous or life threatening. In most cases, hemorrhoidal symptoms will go away within a few days.

Although many people have hemorrhoids, not all experience symptoms. The most common symptom of internal hemorrhoids is bright red blood covering the stool, on toilet paper, or in the toilet bowl. However, an internal hemorrhoid may protrude through the anus outside the body, becoming irritated and painful. This is known as a protruding hemorrhoid.

---

NIH Pub. 94–3021.

Symptoms of external hemorrhoids may include painful swelling or a hard lump around the anus that results when a blood clot forms. This condition is known as a thrombosed external hemorrhoid.

In addition, excessive straining, rubbing, or cleaning around the anus may cause irritation with bleeding and/or itching, which may produce a vicious cycle of symptoms. Draining mucus may also cause itching.

## How Common Are Hemorrhoids?

Hemorrhoids are very common in men and women. About half of the population have hemorrhoids by age 50. Hemorrhoids are also common among pregnant women. The pressure of the fetus in the abdomen, as well as hormonal changes, cause the hemorrhoidal vessels to enlarge. These vessels are also placed under severe pressure during childbirth. For most women, however, hemorrhoids caused by pregnancy are a temporary problem.

## How Are Hemorrhoids Diagnosed?

A thorough evaluation and proper diagnosis by the doctor is important any time bleeding from the rectum or blood in the stool lasts more than a couple of days. Bleeding may also be a symptom of other digestive diseases, including colorectal cancer.

The doctor will examine the anus and rectum to look for swollen blood vessels that indicate hemorrhoids and will also perform a digital rectal exam with a gloved, lubricated finger to feel for abnormalities.

Closer evaluation of the rectum for hemorrhoids requires an exam with an anoscope, a hollow, lighted tube useful for viewing internal hemorrhoids, or a proctoscope, useful for more completely examining the entire rectum.

To rule out other causes of gastrointestinal bleeding, the doctor may examine the rectum and lower colon (sigmoid) with sigmoidoscopy or the entire colon with colonoscopy. Sigmoidoscopy and colonoscopy are diagnostic procedures that also involve the use of lighted, flexible tubes inserted through the rectum.

## What Is the Treatment?

Medical treatment of hemorrhoids initially is aimed at relieving symptoms. Measures to reduce symptoms include:

- Warm tub or sitz baths several times a day in plain, warm water for about 10 minutes.
- Ice packs to help reduce swelling.
- Application of a hemorrhoidal cream or suppository to the affected area for a limited time.

Prevention of the recurrence of hemorrhoids is aimed at changing conditions associated with the pressure and straining of constipation. Doctors will often recommend increasing fiber and fluids in the diet. Eating the right amount of fiber and drinking six to eight glasses of fluid (not alcohol) result in softer, bulkier stools. A softer stool makes emptying the bowels easier and lessens the pressure on hemorrhoids caused by straining. Eliminating straining also helps prevent the hemorrhoids from protruding.

Good sources of fiber are fruits, vegetables, and whole grains. In addition, doctors may suggest a bulk stool softener or a fiber supplement such as psyllium (Metamucil) or methylcellulose (Citrucel).

In some cases, hemorrhoids must be treated surgically. These methods are used to shrink and destroy the hemorrhoidal tissue and are performed under anesthesia. The doctor will perform the surgery during an office or hospital visit.

A number of surgical methods may be used to remove or reduce the size of internal hemorrhoids. These techniques include:

- Rubber band ligation—A rubber band is placed around the base of the hemorrhoid inside the rectum. The band cuts off circulation, and the hemorrhoid withers away within a few days.

- Sclerotherapy—A chemical solution is injected around the blood vessel to shrink the hemorrhoid.

Techniques used to treat both internal and external hemorrhoids include:

- Electrical or laser heat (laser coagulation) or infrared light (infrared photo coagulation)—Both techniques use special devices to burn hemorrhoidal tissue.

- Hemorrhoidectomy—Occasionally, extensive or severe internal or external hemorrhoids may require removal by surgery known as hemorrhoidectomy. This is the best method for permanent removal of hemorrhoids.

## How Are Hemorrhoids Prevented?

The best way to prevent hemorrhoids is to keep stools soft so they pass easily, thus decreasing pressure and straining, and to empty bowels as soon as possible after the urge occurs. Exercise, including walking, and increased fiber in the diet help reduce constipation and straining by producing stools that are softer and easier to pass. In addition, a person should not sit on the toilet for a long period of time.

## Additional Readings

*Bleeding in the Digestive Tract*. 1992. Fact sheet discusses many common causes of bleeding in the digestive tract and related diagnostic procedures and treatment. Available from the National Digestive Diseases Information Clearinghouse, Box NDDIC, 9000 Rockville Pike, Bethesda, Maryland 20892.

Cocchiara, J.L. Hemorrhoids: A practical approach to an aggravating problem. *Postgraduate Medicine* 1991; 89(1): 149–152. Article for health care professionals discusses causes, symptoms, and treatments.

Sohn, N. Hemorrhoids: Etiology, pathogenesis, classification, and medical therapy. *Practical Gastroenterology* 1991; XV(9): 21–24. General article for physicians.

Stehlin, D. No strain no pain: The bottom line in treating hemorrhoids. *FDA Consumer* 1992; 26(2): 31–33. General information article for patients and the public.

# Chapter 34

# *Small Intestine and Combined Liver–Small Intestine Transplantation*

Health Technology Reviews *are brief evaluations of health technologies prepared by the Office of Health Technology Assessment, Agency for Health Care Policy and Research (OHTA/AHCPR) of the Public Health Service. Reviews may be composed in lieu of a technology assessment because: the medical or scientific questions are limited and do not warrant the resources required for a full assessment; the available evidence is lirnited and the published medical or scientific literature is insufficient in quality or quantity for an assessment; or the time frame available precludes utilization of the full, formal assessment process. This review has been prepared in response to a request from the Civilian Health and Medical Program of the Uniformed Services (CHAMPUS).*

The reacquisition of bowel functions by transplantation of the small intestines was demonstrated to be technically feasible in dogs in 1966.[1] However, unlike the successful transplantation of the heart, lung, liver, and kidney, transplantation of the small bowel in humans was unsuccessful through the 1980s, mainly because of the failure of immunosuppressive therapy to prevent graft rejections and graft versus host disease.[2-5] Typically, reports described stormy postoperative courses for small intestine graft recipients, with lengthy periods of intensive care before rejection of the grafts. The substantial lymphoid

---

AHCPR Pub. 93-0067. Individual copies of this document are available from the AHCPR Clearinghouse, P.O. Box 8547, Silver Spring, MD 20907. (800) 358-9295.

components in the small intestines are thought to contribute to making the control of immunological reactions that generally occur between graft and host more difficult in small bowel transplant than in other organ transplants. With the use of newer immunosuppressive agents, such as FK 506, transplantation of the small intestine may show improved outcomes as is currently being reported by investigators in Pittsburgh, Pennsylvania.[6]

## Background

The first successful small intestine transplantation was performed by Goulet et al[7] in 1989; the recipient was a 5-month-old infant. After being successfully treated for episodes of rejection, the infant was released from the hospital 10 months after surgery and was reported to be on an enteral diet and growing normally 30 months after transplantation. The only other report of successful small intestine transplantations was that by Todo et al.[6] Of the eight small intestines transplanted, one failed at 22 months and the others were reported to be surviving at 3 weeks to 5 months posttransplant. Four of the surviving recipients did not require parenteral nutrition at 2 to 5 months posttransplant, while the other three, at 1 month or less posttransplant, continued to be partially supported by parenteral nutrition.

All recipients of small intestine transplants have had short-bowel syndromes as the result of massive small bowel resections for conditions such as volvulus, enterocolitis, Crohn's disease, mesenteric vascular disease, or trauma. These patients had received total parenteral nutrition (TPN) for varying lengths of time.

Many patients receiving TPN develop complications such as severe infections caused by permanent intravenous catheters or metabolic disturbances of the liver caused by parenterally administered nutrition. Some TPN recipients with signs of liver dysfunction have received combined liver-small intestine grafts. Except for the recent success reported for small intestine transplants, recipients of these combined grafts appeared to have had better graft survival outcomes than those who received only the small intestine grafts.[8,9] The possible protective effect of the liver[10] was reminiscent of findings in animal studies showing that a simultaneous liver graft seemed to exert a protective effect that appeared to enhance the survival of other organ grafts.[11-13]

## Discussion

The first successful combined liver-small intestine transplantation in a patient was reported in 1990 by Grant et al,[8] who transplanted a combined graft into a 41 year-old woman who had a short-bowel syndrome secondary to mesenteric thrombosis and had signs of liver failure as manifested by an antithrombin III deficiency. Episodes of graft rejection and transient acute graft versus host disease in the first few months posttransplant were overcome by administration of immunosuppressant agents including cyclosporine A, OKT3, steroid, and azathioprine. Two months after transplantation, the liver showed no clinical or biochemical evidence of liver rejection and was functioning to maintain liver enzyme values, bilirubin concentrations, and prothrombin times within the normal range. Since the eighth week posttransplant, the patient's entire nutrient, fluid, and electrolyte requirements were satisfied by an enteral diet. The patient was discharged from the hospital 8 months after surgery, after recovering from complications that resulted from a Hickman catheter infection, and was leading a normal lifestyle that included an unrestricted oral diet a year after grafting. In a subsequent report,[14] this patient was again noted to be in good health and on a normal diet 23 months posttransplant. This later report also described two additional liver-small intestine transplant recipients, one of whom died 9 weeks posttransplant with biopsy-proved cytomegalovirus enteritis. The other recipient was reported to be surviving and on a normal diet 11 months posttransplant.

In Pittsburgh, eight patients underwent combined liver-small intestine transplantation in 1990–1991.[6] All recipients (two adults and six children) had advanced hepatic disease with elevated serum total bilirubin concentrations and had been receiving TPN because of shortgut syndrome. An infant recipient died 23 days posttransplant of sepsis and graft versus host disease. The remaining seven recipients were reported to be well, at home, and consuming normal oral diets 7–20 months posttransplant. Except for very brief notations that liver-rejection episodes occurring in some of the patients were treated successfully and that the livers resumed normal function before the grafted intestine,[15] none of the reports presented any data to evaluate functional status of the transplanted livers in these patients. Recently a report from Wisconsin[16] described a 14 month-old child with short-gut syndrome, cirrhosis, and variceal bleeding, who received a combined liver-small intestine transplant. The child's postoperative course was apparently satisfactory, and biopsy showed that the intestines were histologically normal and viable. However, severe coagulopathy and renal failure developed, and the patient died on the 52nd postoperative day.

## Summary

Recent published accounts of experiences with either small intestine or combined liver-small intestine transplants indicate that both types of transplantations may be feasible, with some expectation of successful outcome in terms of graft survival and benefit to the patient. Clinical and outcome data for recipients of small intestine transplants are presented in Table 34.1, and data for recipients of combined liver-small intestine grafts are presented in Table 34.2. Only the Pittsburgh group has reported successful transplantations and survival of recipients of small intestine (eight patients, one graft failure) and combined liver-small intestine transplants (eight patients, one death).[6] Aside from these patients, there have been reports of a few other recipients with generally poorer outcomes at other transplant centers. In Ontario, Canada, two of three patients who received combined liver-small intestine grafts were reported to be surviving, and the only recipient of a small intestine transplant died 10 weeks after surgery.[14] In Paris, France, of five patients who received small intestine grafts, only one child is surviving with a functioning graft.[17] An unsuccessful combined liver-small intestine transplantation was done at one other center,[16] and unsuccessful small intestine transplantations were attempted at three other centers.[18–21] The total experience reported in the literature numbers 18 small intestine transplantations with eight surviving, functioning grafts. Twelve combined liver-small intestine transplantations have been done, with nine recipients surviving with functional grafts. Perhaps with improvements in immunosuppressive therapy, satisfactory long-term outcomes might be expected. Although the results with the use of FK 506 reported from Pittsburgh are encouraging, the small number of cases so far, the short period of follow-up, and the lack of similar successful transplantation experiences at other transplant centers preclude the ascertainment of whether transplantation of the small intestine or the combined liver-small intestine is a generally beneficial treatment procedure at this time. The short period of follow-up is of concern in view of the reported failure of one of the grafts after 17 months and another after 22 months.

**Table 34.1.** *Small intestine transplantation.*

| Patient age, y | Short-bowel syndrome etiology | Reported results | References |
|---|---|---|---|
| 8 | Congenital neuromyopathy | Graft fail, 2 wk | 14,32,34 |
| 26 | Gardner's syndrome | Graft fail, died day 11 | 18,19 |
| 5 | Volvulus | Graft fail, day 12 | 20-23* |
| 34 | Aortic embolism | Died, day 12 | 24 |
| 12 | Volvulus | Died, day 5 | 24 |
| 3 | Total bowel resection | Graft fail, 2 mo | 17,25 |
| 6 | Total bowel resection | Graft fail, 17 mo | 17,25 |
| 0.8 | Total bowel resection | Graft fail, 3 wk | 17,25 |
| 9 | Total bowel resection | Graft fail, 6 mo | 17,26 |
| 0.5 | Total bowel resection | Surviving at 30 mo | 7,17,27 |
| 2.5 | Microvillus including disease | Graft functional, 5 mo | 6 |
| 1.3 | Intestinal atresia | Graft functional, 3.2 mo | 6 |
| 50 | Crohn's disease | Graft functional, 3.1 mo | 6 |
| 34 | Gardner's syndrome | Graft functional, 2.0 mo | 6 |
| 38 | Crohn's disease | Parenteral support, 0.9 mo | 6 |
| 10.2 | Chronic intestinal obstruction | Parenteral support, 0.8 mo | 6 |
| 23 | Crohn's disease | Parenteral support, 0.7 mo | 6 |
| 31 | Gunshot wound | Graft fail, 22 mo | 6,9,15,28-31 |

Total No. of patients = 18
Number of grafts surviving = 8
Follow-up for surviving grafts: median = 3 months
mean = 5 months
range = 0.7-30 months

* Data not available for a 43-year-old small intestine recipient mentioned in References 22 and 23.

***Table 34.2.*** *Combined liver-small intestine transplantation.*

| Patient age, y | Short-bowel syndrome etiology | Reported results | References |
|---|---|---|---|
| 3.2 | Necrotizing enterocolitis | Home, normal diet, 20.2 mo | 6,9,15,28-31 |
| 26.7 | SMA thrombosis | Home, normal diet, 19.9 mo | 6,9,15,28-31 |
| 4.3 | Gastroschisis | Home, normal diet, 16.2 mo | 6,9,15,28-31 |
| 2.8 | Intestinal atresia | Home, normal diet, 12.3 mo | 6,9,15,28-31 |
| 1.1 | Volvulus | Home, normal diet, 7.7 mo | 6,9,15,28-31 |
| 1.7 | Volvulus | Home, normal diet, 7.6 mo | 6,9,15,28-31 |
| 21 | Traffic accident | Home, normal diet, 7.3 mo | 6,9,15,28-31 |
| 0.6 | Intestinal atresia | Died day 23 (sepsis and GVHD) | 6,9,15,28-31 |
| 41 | SMA thrombosis | Home, normal diet, 23 mo | 8,14,32-34 |
| 36 | Recurrent ulcer/stenosis | Home, normal diet, 11 mo | 14,34 |
| 46 | Not specified | Died at 9 wk (stroke, renal failure) | 14,34 |
| 1.2 | Volvulus | Died day 52 (coagulopathy, renal failure) | 16 |

Total No. of patients = 12
Number of recipients surviving = 9
Follow-up for surviving grafts: median = 11 months
mean = 11.5 months
range = 7 - 23 months

Abbreviations: SMA, superior mesenteric artery; GVHD, graft versus host disease.

## References


1. Lillehei RC, Manax WG, Lyons GW, et al. Transplantation of gastrointestinal organs, including small intestine and stomach. *Gastroenterology* 1966;51:936–948.

2. Watson AJM, Lear PA. Current status of intestinal transplantation. *Gut* 1989;30:1771–1782.

3. Martinelli GP, Knight RK, Schanzer H. Smallbowel transplantation: An overview. *Mt Sinai J Med* 1987;54:475–480.

4. First MR. Annual review of transplantation. *Clin Transpl* 1990:357–373.

5. Wood RFM. Small bowel transplantation. *Br J Surg* 1992;79:193–194.

6. Todo S, Tzakis AG, Abu-Elmagd K, et al. Intestinal transplantation in composite visceral grafts or alone. *Ann Surg* 1992;216:223–234.

7. Goulet O, Revillon Y, Canioni D, et al. Two and one-half-year follow-up after isolated cadaveric small bowel transplantation in an infant. *Transplant Proc* 1992;24: 1224–1225.

8. Grant D, Wall W, Mimeault R, et al. Successful small-bowel/liver transplantation. *Lancet* 1990;335: 181–184.

9. Todo S, Tzakis A, Reyes J, et al. Clinical small bowel or small bowel plus liver transplantation under FK 506. *Transplant Proc* 1991;23:3093–3095.

10. Johnston C. Protective benefits of liver key to successful bowel transplants, surgeon says. *Can Med Assoc J* 1992;146:1441–1444.

11. Zhong R, He G, Sakai Y, et al. Combined small bowel and liver transplantation in the rat: Possible role of the liver in preventing intestinal allograft rejection. *Transplantation* 1991;52:550–552.

12. Murase N, Demetris AJ, Kim DG, et al. Rejection of multivisceral allografts in rats: A sequential analysis with comparison to isolated orthotopic small-bowel and liver grafts. *Surgery* 1990;108:880–889.

13. Murase N, Demetris AJ, Matsuzaki T, et al. Long survival in rats after multivisceral versus isolated small-bowel allotransplantation under FK 506. *Surgery* 1991 ;110(1):87–98.

14. Bach DB, Hurlbut DJ, Romano WM, et al. Human orthotopic small intestine transplantation: Radiologic assessment. *Radiology* 1991;180(1):3741.

15. Tzakis AG, Todo S, Reyes J, et al. Clinical intestinal transplantation: Focus on complications. *Transplant Proc* 1992;24: 1238–1240.

16. D'Alessandro AM, Kalayoglu M, Sollinger HW, et al. Liver-intestinal transplantation: Report of a case. *Transplant Proc* 1992;24: 1228–1229.

17. Goulet O, Revillon Y, Jan D, et al. Small-bowel transplantation in children. *Transplant Proc* 1990;22:2499–2500.

18. Cohen Z, Silverman RE, Wassef R, et al. Small intestinal transplantation using cyclosporine: Report of a case. *Transplantation* 1986;42:613–621.

19. Cohen Z, Silverman R, Levy G, et al. Clinical small intestinal transplantation using cyclosporine A and methylprednisolone. *Transplant Proc* 1987;19:2588–2590.

20. Deltz E, Mengel W, Hamelmann H. Small bowel transplantation: Report of a clinical case. *Prog Pediatr Surg* 1990;25:90–96.

21. Hansmann ML, Deltz E, Gundlach M, et al. Small bowel transplantation in a child: Morphologic, immunohistochemical, and clinical results. *Am J Clin Pathol* 1989;92:686–692.

22. Deltz E, Schroeder P, Gundlach M, et al. Successful clinical small-bowel transplantation. *Transplant Proc* 1990;22:2501.

23. Schroeder P, Gebhardt H, Gundlach M, et al. Diagnosis and treatment of graft rejection in experimental and clinical small bowel transplantation. *Transplant Proc* 1990;22:2326.

24. Okumura M, Mester M. The coming of age of small bowel transplantation: A historical perspective. *Transplant Proc* 1992;24: 1241–1242.

25. Brousse N, Canioni D, Rambaud C, et al. Intestinal transplantation in children: Contribution of immunohistochemistry. *Transplant Proc* 1990;22:2495–2496.

26. Goulet OJ, Revillon Y, Cerf-Bensussan N, et al. Small intestinal transplantation in a child using cyclosporine. *Transplant Proc* 1988;20:288–296.

27. Goulet O, Revillon Y, Brousse N, et al Successful small bowel transplantation in an infant. *Transplantation* 1992;53:940-943.

28. Casavilla A, Selby R, Abu-Elmagd K, et al Logistics and technique for combined hepaticintestinal retrieval. *Ann Surg* 1992;216(5): 605–609.

29. Abu-Elmagd K, Fung JJ, Reyes J, et al. Management of intestinal transplantation in humans. *Transplant Proc* 1992;24: 1243–1244.

30. Todo S, Tzakis AG, Abu-Elmagd K, et al. Cadaveric small bowel and small bowel-liver transplantation in humans. *Transplantation* 1992;53:369–376.

31. Reyes J, Abu-Elmagd K, Tzakis A, et al. Infectious complications after human small bowel transplantation. *Transplant Proc* 1992;24:1249-1250.

32. Grant D, Garcia B, Wall W, et al. Graft-versushost disease after clinical small bowel/liver transplantation. *Transplant Proc* 1990;22:2464.

33. Grant D, Wall W, Zhong R, et al. Experimental clinical intestinal transplantation: Initial experience of a Canadian center. *Transplant Proc* 1990;22:2497–2498.

34. McAlister V, Wall W, Ghent C, et al. Successful small intestine transplantation. *Transplant Proc* 1992;24:1236-1237.

*—by S. Steven Hotta, M.D., Ph.D.*

# *Part Five*

# *Liver, Pancreatic, and Gallbladder Diseases and Disorders*

# Chapter 35

# *Autoimmune Hepatitis Fact Sheet*

## *What Is Autoimmune Hepatitis?*

Autoimmune hepatitis or autoimmune chronic hepatitis is a progressive inflammation of tho liver that has been identified by a number of different names, including autoimmune chronic active hepatitis (CAH), idiopathic chronic active hepatitis, and lupoid hepatitis. The reason for this inflammation is not certain, but it is associated with an abnormality of the body's immune system and is often related to the production of antibodies that can be detected by blood tests.

Autoimmune hepatitis was first described in 1950 as a disease of young women, associated with increased gamma globulin in the blood and chronic hepatitis on liver biopsy. The presence of antinuclear antibodies (ANA) and the resemblance of some symptoms to "systemic lupus erythematosus" (SLE) led to the label "lupoid hepatitis." It later became evident that this disease was not related to SLE. The disease is now called autoimmune hepatitis.

## *What Are the Symptoms?*

The typical patient with autoimmune hepatitis is female (70%). The disease may start at any age, but is most common in adolescence or early adulthood. Blood tests identify ANA or smooth muscle antibodies

---

This chapter originally appeared as *Autoimmune Hepatitis* in the American Liver Foundation Fact Sheet, July 1993. Reprinted with permission.

(SMA) in the majority of patients (60%). More than 80% of affected individuals have increased gamma globulin in the blood. Some patients have other autoimmune disorders such as thyroiditis, ulcerative colitis, diabetes mellitus, vitiligo (patchy loss of skin pigmentation), or Sjogren's syndrome (a syndrome that causes dry eyes and dry mouth). Other liver diseases such as viral hepatitis, Wilson's disease, hemochromatosis, and alpha-1-antitrypsin deficiency should be excluded by appropriate blood tests, and the possibility of drug-induced hepatitis is ruled out by careful questioning.

The most common symptoms of autoimmune hepatitis are fatigue, abdominal discomfort, aching joints, itching, jaundice, enlarged liver, and spider angiomas (tumors) on the skin. Patients may also have complications of more advanced chronic hepatitis with cirrhosis, such as ascites (abdominal fluid) or mental confusion called encephalopathy. A liver biopsy is important to confirm the diagnosis and provide a prognosis. Liver biopsy may show mild chronic active hepatitis, more advanced chronic active hepatitis with scarring (fibrosis), or a fully developed cirrhosis.

## How Is Autoimmune Hepatitis Treated?

The 10-year survival rate in untreated patients is approximately 10%. The treatment of autoimmune hepatitis is immunosuppression with prednisone alone or prednisone and azathioprine (Imuran). This medical therapy has been shown to decrease symptoms, improve liver tests, and prolong survival in the majority of patients. Therapy is usually begun with prednisone 30 to 40 mg per day and then this dosage is reduced after a response is achieved.

The standard dosage used in the majority of patients is prednisone 10-15 mg per day, either alone or with azathioprine 50 mg per day. Higher doses of prednisone given long-term are associated with an increase in serious side effects, including: hypertension, diabetes, peptic ulcer, bone thinning, and cataracts. Lower doses of prednisone may be used when combined with azathioprine.

The goal of treatment of autoimmune hepatitis is to cure or control the disease. In two-thirds to three-quarters of the patients, liver tests fall to within the normal range. Long-term follow-up studies show that autoimmune hepatitis appears more often to be a controllable rather than a curable disease, because the majority of patients relapse within six months after therapy is ended. Therefore, most patients need long-term maintenance therapy.

Not all patients with autoimmune hepatitis respond to prednisone treatment. Approximately 15-20% of patients with severe disease continue to deteriorate despite initiation of appropriate therapy. This is most common in patients with advanced cirrhosis on initial liver biopsy. Such patients are unlikely to respond to further medical therapy, and liver transplantation should be considered.

American Liver Foundation
1425 Pompton Avenue
Cedar Grove, New Jersey 07009
1-800-223-0179

## Chapter 36

# *Autoimmune Hepatitis: Current Approaches*

*Successful management [of autoimmune hepatitis] depends on an accurate estimate of the immediate prognosis, a full understanding of the early and late consequences of treatment, and an appreciation of alternative measure to handle unsatisfactory results.*

The unresolving inflammation of the liver of at least 6 months' duration known as autoimmune hepatitis is characterized by periportal hepatitis (piecemeal necrosis) and the presence of organ- or nonorgan-specific autoantibodies in serum. Unfortunately, no immunoserologic marker is pathognomonic of the disease. Its clinical and histologic features at presentation may resemble those of other chronic hepatocellular diseases.[1] Indeed, the various immunoserologic markers required for diagnosis may occur in acute and chronic liver diseases of a viral, drug, toxic (alcohol), or immunologic (primary biliary cirrhosis) nature. The histologic features of periportal hepatitis also lack disease specificity.[2] Consequently, the diagnosis is one of exclusion, implying the absence of epidemiologic and serologic evidence of viral infection, lack of exposure to hepatotoxic drugs, and exclusion of hereditary disorders such as Wilson's disease, hemochromatosis, and $\alpha_1$-antitrypsin deficiency.[3,4] Table 1 lists the minimum requirements for diagnosis; Table 2 summarizes the differential diagnosis.

---

This article originally appeared in *Contemporary Gastroenterology*, February/March 1992. Reprinted with permission.

Multiple controlled clinical trials have demonstrated that prednisone (Deltasone, Meticorten, Orasone) alone or in combination with azathioprine (Imuran) ameliorates symptoms, improves biochemical and histologic features, and enhances survival in patients with severe disease. [1,4] Not all patients respond to therapy, however, and not all of those with the correct diagnosis have a benefit-risk ratio that favors treatment.[1,4]

## Subclassifications

Only now are efforts being made to subgroup patients with autoimmune hepatitis into homogeneous subpopulations with distinctive clinical, immunoserologic, and prognostic features.[5] Three subclassifications have been proposed (Table 3). Their validity as distinct clinical entities has not been proved, however.

In the United States, at least 80% of cases in adults can be classified as type 1 autoimmune hepatitis (classical or lupoid variety). This type is characterized by the presence of smooth-muscle or antinuclear antibodies, hypergammaglobulinemia, concurrent immunologic disorders, HLA positivity for A1, B8, and DR3, and responsiveness to corticosteroid therapy.[2,4,6] Antiactin antibodies should be sought, because they enhance the specificity of smooth-muscle antibodies. In fact, type 1 disease has been referred to as "antiactin hepatitis."[7,8] Typically, 71% of patients in this category are women, and 48% of them are younger than 40 years.[6] Onset of illness is acute in 40%; patients may be misdiagnosed as having acute viral hepatitis.[1,9,10] The presence of hypoalbuminemia, hypergammaglobulinemia, or features of portal hypertension, such as thrombocytopenia, ascites, or esophageal varices, however, should raise the suspicion of autoimmune hepatitis.[10]

Concomitant immunologic diseases are seen in 17% of patients in this category. These include thyroiditis or Graves' disease (41%), ulcerative colitis (24%), and rheumatoid arthritis (12%).[6] In patients with chronic ulcerative colitis, cholangiography is mandatory, since primary sclerosing cholangitis may resemble autoimmune hepatitis or coexist with it. HLA-B8 positivity can be demonstrated in 58% of patients, a group who are younger (an average of 38 years compared with 48 years) and have more inflammatory activity at presentation than their HLA-B8 negative counterparts.[11]

Type 2 (anti-LKM1) autoimmune hepatitis is characterized by the presence of antibodies to liver/kidney microsome type 1.[8] This antibody reacts strongly by immunofluorescence with murine kidney proximal tubules and not with distal tubules, a response that distinguishes it from antimitochondrial antibodies (AMA). Additionally, anti-LKM1 positivity requires uniform staining of the cytoplasm of murine hepatocytes. Antibodies in sera react on Western blot with a 50-kD hepatic microsomal protein; this major antigen of anti-LKM1 is cytochrome P450db1, a drug metabolizing system.[12,13] Clear understanding of the different patterns of immunofluorescence of antiLKM1 and AMA is essential, since recent studies have indicated that 27% of patients with autoimmune hepatitis and seropositivity for AMA (overlap or hybrid syndromes) actually are anti-LKM1 rather than AMA positive.[14] Such patients can respond fully to corticosteroid therapy with loss of their immunoserologic markers.[14,15]

Most patients with type 2 autoimmune hepatitis are children between the ages of 2 and 14 years, but adults can also be afflicted.[8] Associated immunologic disorders, seen in 40% of cases, include vitiligo, thyroiditis, insulin-dependent diabetes, autoimmune hemolytic anemia, idiopathic thrombocytopenic purpura, pernicious anemia, rheumatoid arthritis, and ulcerative colitis.[8] Hypergammaglobulinemia is less pronounced than in type 1 disease, and serum immunoglobulin A levels may be low. Nonorgan-specific autoantibodies are rare, while organ-specific antibodies are common (30%), including antithyroid microsome, antithyroglobulin, anti-islets of Langerhans, and antiparietal cell antibodies.[8] Preliminary experience suggests that type 2 autoimmune hepatitis progresses more rapidly to cirrhosis than does type 1 disease (82% vs. 43% within 3 years).

Type 3 autoimmune hepatitis is the most recent, least well-established of the subclassifications.[17] It is characterized by the presence of antibodies to soluble liver antigen (anti-SLA), which probably are directed against cytokeratin.[12,16] Of these patients, 91% are women with a mean age of 37 years (range, 17 to 67 years). They lack antibodies to nuclear antigens (ANA), LKM1, thyroglobulin, and thyroid microsome, but only 26% are seronegative for all markers except anti-SLA.[17] Indeed, smooth-muscle antibodies (35%), antibodies to liver membrane antigen (26%), and AMA (22%) may be present in these patients, who may have serologic similarities to type 1 disease. Consequently, it is still uncertain whether anti-SLA is the hallmark of a disease with a variety of nonspecific immunoserologic manifestations or an unusual but nonspecific marker of type 1 disease.

***Table 36.1. Diagnostic Features of Autoimmune Hepatitis***

≥6 months' duration
Multisystemic expression
- Synovitis
- Thyroiditis/Graves' disease

Nonorgan-specific antibodies*
- Anti-actin (smooth muscle)
- Anti-DNA
- Anti-LKM1
- Antinuclear
- Anti-SLA

Organ-specific antibodies
- Acetylcholine receptor
- Asialoglycoprotein receptor
- Liver-membrane antigen
- Liver-specific antigen
- Thyroid (microsome, thyroglobulin)

HLA-A1, B8, DR3 positive
- Periportal hepatitis (piecemeal necrosis)*
- Exclusion of drug and viral causes and hereditary diseases*

*Minimal requirements for diagnosis

***Table 36.2. Differential Diagnosis***

Alcoholic liver disease
$a_1$-antitrypsin deficiency
Drug-induced (resembles type 1 hepatitis)
- α-methyldopa
- Nitrofurantoin
- Oxyphenisatin
- Propylthiouracil

Hemochromatosis
Hereditary diseases
Nonalcoholic steatohepatitis
Primary biliary cirrhosis
Primary sclerosing cholangitis
Viral diseases
Wilson's disease

**Table 36.3.** *Subclassifications of autoimmune hepatitis.*

| Features | Type 1 (Classical) | Type 2 (Anti-LKM1) | Type 3 (Anti-SLA) |
|---|---|---|---|
| Age (years): Mean | 39 | 25 | 37 |
| Age (years): Range | 1–81 | 0.5–77 | 17–67 |
| Age (years): Predominant | 30–45 | 2–14 | Uncertain |
| Sex (% female) | 71 | 89 | 91 |
| Immunologic disorders (%) | 17 | 40 | Uncertain |
| Autoantibodies (%) | | | |
| AMA | 20 | 0 | 22 |
| ANA | 60 | 2 | 0 |
| Anti-LKM1 | 5 | 100 | 0 |
| Organ-specific | 4 | 30 | 26 |
| SMA | 70 | 0 | 35 |
| γ-globulin (mean, g/L) | 3.7 | 2.3 | 3.2 |
| Steroid-responsive (%) | 70 | Uncertain | 100 |

LKM1: Liver/kidney/microsome type 1
SLA: Soluble liver antigen

Since type 3 autoimmune hepatitis afflicts mainly adults who may lack the conventional immunoserologic markers of type 1 autoimmune hepatitis, it is a diagnostic consideration in those patients now classified by conventional screening methods as having idiopathic or cryptogenic chronic active hepatitis.[17] Type 3 autoimmune hepatitis is associated with hypergammaglobulinemia and corticosteroid responsiveness. The presence of anti-SLA in patients with severe cryptogenic chronic active hepatitis justifies corticosteroid therapy.[16,17]

None of the antibodies that characterize the various subgroups of autoimmune hepatitis have been shown to be liver-specific or pathogenic.[2] Theoretically, liver-specific antibodies should be of greater diagnostic value and pathogenic significance than nonorgan-specific varieties. Unfortunately, however, liver-specific antibodies have not enhanced diagnostic specificity or been established as primary target antigens.[2,18] Other organ-specific antibodies, including microsomal thyroid, thyroglobulin, parietal cell, and acetylcholine receptor antibodies, facilitate differentiation from viral hepatitis, but they are insensitive markers of autoimmune hepatitis.[2]

To establish the autoimmune nature of autoimmune hepatitis, a target antigen that is associated with a disease-specific antibody must be identified. This target antigen must consistently produce the antibody and the disease in immunized animals, and the disease must be transferable to nonimmunized animals by antibodies or lymphoid cells.[19] Until these requirements are met, the autoimmune basis of autoimmune hepatitis is presumptive, and the various immunoserologic markers of the disease must be regarded as epiphenomena of diagnostic value but of no pathogenic significance.[2]

## Prognostic Factors

The prognosis depends on the severity of the inflammatory activity at the time of presentation and the presence or absence of cirrhosis (Table 4). Anticipate a 3-year mortality of 50% and a 10-year mortality of 90% when the serum aspartate aminotransferase (AST) level remains elevated to at least ten times normal or five times normal in conjunction with at least a two-fold elevation of the gamma globulin level.[1] In patients with histologic features of bridging or multilobular necrosis, expect an 82% frequency of cirrhosis within 5 years and a mortality of 45%.[20] Patients with bridging necrosis between portal tract and central vein are more likely to develop cirrhosis than are those with bridging necrosis between portal tract and portal tract (29% vs. 10%), but these distinctions are often difficult to make with certainty. A 5-year mortality of 58% has been reported when a patient has cirrhosis at presentation.[20] Esophageal varices develop in 54% of these patients within 2 years, and death from hemorrhage occurs in 20% of those with varices.[1]

In contrast, patients with less severe biochemical and histologic findings have better prognoses. Their 15-year survival exceeds 80%, and the probability of progression to cirrhosis is 49%.[22] Patients with periportal hepatitis have a normal 5-year life-expectancy and a 17% frequency of cirrhosis.[21] Spontaneous resolution or improvement may occur in 13% to 20%, regardless of disease severity.[22]

Other features that augur a poor prognosis include abrupt onset of disease, encephalopathy, ascites, and ulcerative colitis.[1] Cholangiography is warranted in all patients with sustained cholestasis, pruritus, and ulcerative colitis.

| **Features** | **Consequences** |
|---|---|
| Biochemical features | |
| AST ≥ 10 × normal | 50% 3-year mortality |
| AST ≥ 5 × normal and GG ≥ 2 × normal | 90% 10-year mortality |
| Histologic findings | |
| Bridging necrosis | 82% cirrhosis |
| Cirrhosis | 58% 5-year mortality |
| Multilobular necrosis | 45% 5-year mortality |
| Clinical findings | |
| Abrupt onset | |
| Development of varices | 20% 2-year mortality |
| Ascites, Cholestasis, Encephalopathy, Ulcerative colitis | Poor prognosis |

***Table 36.4.*** *Prognosis in untreated autoimmune hepatitis.*

## Treatment Regimens

Indications for corticosteroid therapy are severe sustained aminotransferase (AST) and gamma globulin (GG) elevations (AST level of at least ten times normal or at least five times normal in conjunction with a GG level of at least twice normal) or the presence of bridging or confluent necrosis.[24] Relative indications for treatment are incapacitating symptoms attributable to inflammatory activity or relentless progression of the liver disease. All other patients are best managed expectantly or enrolled in a prospective treatment trial evaluating the benefit-risk ratio of corticosteroid therapy.[22]

A combination of prednisone and azathioprine is the preferred treatment schedule unless the latter is contraindicated by cytopenia, pregnancy, or malignant disease (Table 5).[23] A higher dose of prednisone alone is equally effective, but drug-related side effects occur more frequently. It is useful in patients in whom only a short trial of treatment (3 to 6 months) is proposed and in young, fertile women who are contemplating pregnancy.[23]

Treatment is continued until remission is achieved, until the patient's condition deteriorates despite compliance with the treatment regimen, until drug toxicity develops, or until protracted therapy has failed to induce remission.[1] After 3 years of continuous therapy has failed to induce remission, the benefit-risk ratio diminishes. Consider empiric therapy with low-dose or alternate-day prednisone.[22,23] Conventional therapy continued beyond 3 years has a probability of only 7% a year of inducing remission, and the likelihood of drug-related complications increases.[22,23]

Cosmetic changes (obesity, facial puffiness, acne, or hirsutism) develop in 80% of patients after 2 years of therapy, regardless of the regimen.[25] Severe, potentially debilitating complications (osteoporosis with vertebral compression, diabetes, cataracts, hypertension, and psychosis) usually develop only after 18 months of continuous therapy and at doses that exceed 10 mg daily.[24] Severe side effects occur less often with prednisone in combination with azathioprine (10%) than with a higher dose of prednisone alone (44%).[24] During therapy, only 13% of treated patients develop complications that necessitate dose reduction or premature drug withdrawal.[25] Patients with cirrhosis at presentation are most often afflicted (25% vs. 08%), presumably because of increased serum levels of unbound prednisolone resulting from prolonged hypoalbuminemia or hyperbilirubinemia.[25] Surprisingly, postmenopausal women tolerate initial therapy as well as their premenopausal counterparts, and their outcomes after initial therapy are also similar.[26] Consequently, these patients can be treated as vigorously as others at the time of presentation.

| Prednisone and azathioprine* | Prednisone alone |
|---|---|
| **Dosage** | |
| Prednisone: | |
| 30 mg/day for 1 week | 60 mg/day for 1 week |
| 20 mg/day for 1 week | 40 mg/day for 1 week |
| 15 mg/day for 2 weeks | 30 mg/day for 2 weeks |
| 10 mg/day thereafter | 20 mg/day thereafter |
| Azathioprine: 50 mg/day | |
| **Contraindications (relative)** | |
| Cytopenia | Brittle diabetes |
| Malignant disease | Cushingoid features |
| Pregnancy | Labile hypertension |
| Short-term trial | Osteoporosis |
| | Also postmenopausal patients |
| **Ideal candidates** | |
| Obese patients | Patients with cytopenia |
| Patients with acne | Patients with malignant disease |
| Patients with diabetes | Pregnant patients |
| | Patients who need a short-term trial |
| Patients with osteoporosis | |
| Postmenopausal patients | |

*Preferred regimen

***Table 36.5.*** *Treatment regimens for severe autoimmune hepatitis.*

## Treatment Outcome

Prednisone alone or in combination with azathioprine induces clinical, biochemical, and histologic remission in 70% of patients within 2 years.[1] The 5- and 10-year life expectancies of patients without cirrhosis at presentation exceed 90%, while those with cirrhosis at presentation have a 5-year life expectancy of 80% and a 10-year life expectancy of 65%.[4] Only those with severe, rapidly progressive disease have been studied in a controlled fashion. Thus, they are the only ones for whom there are firmly set treatment guidelines.

The major problem is relapse after drug withdrawal. Inflammatory activity returns in 50% of patients within 6 months and in 70% within 3 years.[27] Reinstituting treatment reliably induces remission, but drug withdrawal usually is followed by another relapse. Although the causes of relapse are unknown, premature discontinuation of medication may be a factor. When treatment is continued until the hepatic architecture has reverted to normal, relapse occurs in only 20% of cases. It occurs in 50% of cases when inflammatory activity is nonspecific or does not disrupt the limiting plate of the portal tract.[28] Frequency of relapse in patients with cirrhosis at entry or who develop it during treatment is 87% to 100% despite treatment to inactive cirrhosis.[25,29] Because the histologic end point may not be reflected by the biochemical changes, an examination of liver biopsy tissue is desirable before the medication is withdrawn.[30]

The HLA status also influences the likelihood of relapse. Patients who are HLA-B8 negative or HLA-A1 positive, relapse less frequently than their counters who are HLA-B8 positive.[11] Recent studies also have indicated that patients with autoimmune hepatitis who undergo liver transplantation are younger and have a higher frequency of HLA-A1, B8, and DR3 than their counterparts who do not require transplantation. This finding suggests the presence of more aggressive or corticosteroid-resistant disease in these patients.[31]

The major consequences of relapse and retreatment are drug-related side effects. The frequency of side effects after initial therapy is 29%; after the first relapse and retreatment it is 33%. With subsequent relapses and retreatments, however, the complication frequency is 70%.[32] Patients who have relapsed many times are best managed by long-term, low-dose prednisone.[33] The dose should be reduced to the lowest level that will control symptoms and maintain the serum AST level below five times normal. All such patients can be managed in this fashion on less-than-conventional doses (median dose of prednisone, 7.5 mg daily), and 87% can be treated with 10 mg daily or less. Side effects that had accrued during conventional treatment improve in 85%, new side effects do not develop, and mortality is unaffected (9% vs. 10%).[33] Similar results may be obtainable using indefinite low-dose azathioprine therapy (2 mg/kg/day), but the uncertain long-term oncogenic and teratogenic effects of such treatment dampen enthusiasm for this regimen.[34]

Unfortunately, corticosteroids do not prevent cirrhosis from developing eventually in some patients. In the Mayo experience, 40% of patients developed cirrhosis within 10 years.[29] Patients who developed cirrhosis during or after treatment, however, had 5- and 10-year survivals of 90%, suggesting that the prognosis of cirrhosis is related to the stage of the disease at presentation and the degree of inflammatory activity that accompanies the process.[29]

Deterioration despite therapy (treatment failure) occurs in 9% of patients.[3] High-dose prednisone (60 mg/day) alone or a lower dose (30 mg/day) in conjunction with azathioprine (150 mg/day) induces biochemical remission in more than 60% of these patients within 2 years, but histologic remission is achieved in only 20%.[4] Patients who fail to respond to conventional therapy may eventually become candidates for liver transplantation. At Mayo, the 5-year survival after liver transplantation of patients with autoimmune hepatitis is 96%, and serial liver biopsy evaluations have not disclosed evidence of recurrent disease as yet.[35]

The optimal timing for liver transplantation remains uncertain, since there are no findings at presentation that reliably predict response to corticosteroid therapy and survival. Consequently, the decision for transplantation must be based on an assessment of the response to conventional treatment. In patients with multilobular necrosis at presentation, the transplant decision need only be deferred for 2 weeks, as failure to document biochemical improvement (especially a reduction in the hyperbilirubinemia) identifies patients with a dismal immediate prognosis.[36] It is highly likely that patients who are unable to achieve remission after 4 years of therapy will need liver transplantation, especially if they are young, HLA-B8 positive, and develop ascites late in their disease.[35]

Hepatocellular cancer occurs in 7% of patients with cirrhosis of at least 5 years' duration; the probability rises to 30% after 13 years.[37] A cancer surveillance program that includes regular determination of the serum α-fetoprotein level and hepatic ultrasonography can be justified in such patients.

Unfortunately, the risk of extrahepatic malignant disease increases slightly in patients with autoimmune hepatitis on long-term immunosuppressive therapy.[38] The frequency of extrahepatic malignant disease is 5% in patients with a cumulative duration of treatment of 42 months. The average duration to malignancy has been 116 months: the risk is 1.4 (range, 0.6 to 2.9) times that of an age- and sex-matched normal population. and no specific cell type has been noted.[39] The risk of neoplasm does not contraindicate the use of immunosuppressive therapy, but it does underscore the importance of carefully selecting patients for such treatment.

## Other Considerations

A viral etiology for autoimmune hepatitis cannot be excluded, but recent studies have suggested that the hepatitis C virus (HCV) is either an infrequent cause or a coincidental finding in patients with type 1 autoimmune hepatitis.[39] The enzyme immunoassay for antibodies to HCV (anti-HCV) may be positive in autoimmune hepatitis (44% to 84%), especially in patients with anti-LKM1.[40-42] Hypergammaglobulinemia, cross-reacting polyclonal antibodies, or other serum factors, however, may confound the enzyme immunoassay and produce false-positive results.[43]

At Mayo, only 6% of patients with severe autoimmune hepatitis are seropositive for anti-HCV, and only 40% of these have specific antibodies against HCV-encoded antigens by recombinant immunoblot assay (RIBA).[39] In patients who are seropositive for anti-HCV by enzyme immunoassay but nonreactive by RIBA, corticosteroid therapy may actually suppress expression of anti-HCV and reduce seronegativity.[44] In contrast, RIBA-reactive seropositive patients retain their seropositivity during corticosteroid therapy, and the strength of the reactivity may actually increase with treatment.[44] Preliminary studies suggest that patients with nonspecific seropositivity for anti-HCV may respond fully to corticosteroid therapy, while the administration of recombinant interferon to patients with autoimmune hepatitis and false seropositivity may be detrimental.[45] Consequently, it is essential to document RIBA-reactivity in patients with anti-HCV and immunoserologic markers before instituting interferon therapy.

The relationship between chronic HCV infection and anti-LKM production has not been fully defined. The assessment of patients with chronic active hepatitis type C for anti-LKM1 seropositivity is typically negative, and yet the assessment of anti-LKM1 patients for HCV infection is commonly positive. not just for anti-HCV but also for HCV RNA in serum by polymerase chain reaction. These findings suggest that HCV infection in some patients may be immunogenic and thereby stimulate anti-LKM1 production.

Use of cyclosporine (Sandimmune), 3 to 6 mg/kg/day, has been reported anecdotally in patients with corticosteroid resistance or drug-related complications.[46,47] Favorable results have been reported in these isolated cases, but the drug is not established as a treatment for this condition. FK-506 is a new immunosuppressive agent that may be more potent and safer than cyclosporine. Its efficacy and safety in liver transplantation must be demonstrated, however, before it can be considered in any immunologically mediated chronic liver disease such as autoimmune hepatitis.[48]

Ursodeoxycholic acid (Actigall), administered daily for 2 months in doses of 250 mg, 500 mg, and 750 mg, has been able to reduce serum aminotransferase levels in patients with chronic active hepatitis.[49] Most of the patients treated in this fashion have had viral disease, however, and these preliminary experiences may not apply to patients with autoimmune hepatitis. Nevertheless, the drug may have promise in the treatment of hepatocellular diseases, and this application deserves additional investigation.

## *In Summary*

Autoimmune hepatitis is a chronic inflammatory disorder of the liver whose cause is unknown. It has an aggressive potential that can result in cirrhosis and premature death from the complications of portal hypertension or liver failure. Satisfactory treatment regimens are available, however, for patients with severe disease.

Prednisone alone or in combination with azathioprine induces remission and enhances life expectancy in the majority of patients, although cirrhosis may still develop, and relapse after drug withdrawal remains a common problem. Long-term low-dose corticosteroid therapy may be necessary in patients who relapse frequently. New therapies are being evaluated for those who deteriorate during treatment, have an incomplete response, or develop drug toxicities. Liver transplantation is an option for patients with advanced or decompensated disease. The 5-year survival is excellent, with no evidence of recurrent disease. Subclassifications of autoimmune hepatitis by specific immunoserologic markers promise to improve the understanding of pathogenic mechanisms and refine treatment strategies.

*—by Albert J. Czaja, MD*

Dr. Czaja is a professor of medicine, Mayo Medical School, and consultant in Gastroenterology, Mayo Clinic, Rochester, Minn.

## *References*

1. Czaja AJ: Current problems in the diagnosis and management of chronic active hepatitis. *Mayo Clin Proc* 1981;56:311.

2. Czaja AJ: Autoimmune chronic active hepatitis—a specific entity? The negative argument. *J Gastro Hepatology* 1990;5:343.

3. Czaja AJ: Diagnosis and treatment of chronic hepatitis. *Compr Ther* 1984;10:58.

4. Czaja AJ: Natural history, clinical features and treatment of autoimmune hepatitis. *Semin Liv Dis* 1984;4:1.

5. Maddrey WC: Subdivisions of idiopathic autoimmune chronic active hepatitis. *Hepatology* 1987;7:1372.

6. Czaja AJ, Davis GL, Ludwig J, et al: Autoimmune features as determinants of prognosis in steroid-treated chronic active hepatitis of uncertain etiology. *Gastroenterology* 1983;85:713.

7. Lidman K, Biberfield G, Fagraeus A, et al: Anti-actin specificity of human smooth muscle antibodies in chronic active hepatitis. *Clin Exp Immunol* 1976;24:266.

8. Hombero J-C, Abuaf N, Bernard O, et al: Chronic active hepatitis associated with antiliver/ kidney microsome antibody type 1: a second type of "autoimmune" hepatitis. *Hepatology* 1987;7:1333.

9. Amontree JS, Stuart TD, Bredfeldt JE: Autoimmune chronic active hepatitis masquerading as acute hepatitis. *J Clin Gastroenterol* 1981;11:303.

10. Davis GL, Czaja AJ, Baggenstoss AH, et al: Prognostic and therapeutic implications of extreme serum aminotransferase elevation on chronic active hepatitis *Mayo Clin Proc* 1982;57:303.

11. Czaja AJ, Rakela J, Hay JE, et al: Clinical and prognostic implications of human leukocyte antigen B8 in corticosteroid-treated severe autoimmune chronic active hepatitis. *Gastroenterology* 1990;98:1587.

12. Meyer zum Buschenfelde K-H, Lohse AW, Manns M, et al: Autoimmunity and liver disease. *Hepatology* 1990;12:354.

13. Manns MP, Johnson EF, Griffin KJ, et al: Major antigen of liver kidney microsomal auto-antibodies in idiopathic autoimmune hepatitis is cytochrome P45Qdb1 *J Clin Invest* 1989;83:1066.

14. Czaja AJ, Manns M, Homburger HA: Specificity of antibodies to liver/kidney microsome type 1 for type 2 autoimmune chronic active hepatitis: evidence against overlapping syndromes and hepatitis B and C viruses as important immunogenic stimuli. *Hepatology* 1991;14:134A.

15. Kenny RP, Czaja AJ, Ludwig J, et al: Frequency and significance of antimitochondrial antibodies in severe chronic active hepatitis. *Dig Dis Sci* 1986;31:705.

16. Manns M, Gerken G, Kyriatsoulis A, et al: Characterization of a new subgroup of autoimmune chronic active hepatitis by antibodies against a soluble liver antigen. *Lancet* 1987;1:292.

17. Czaja AJ, Hay JE, Rakela J: Clinical features and prognostic implications of severe corticosteroid-treated cryptogenic chronic active hepatitis. *Mayo Clin Proc* 1990;65:23.

18. Mackay IR: Immunological aspects of chronic active hepatitis. *Hepatology* 1983;3:724.

19. Witebsky E, Rose NR, Terplan K, et al: Chronic thyroiditis and autoimmunization. *JAMA* 1957;164:1439.

20. Schaim Sw, Korman MG, Summerskill WHJ, et al: Severe chronic active liver disease: prognostic significance of initial morphologic patterns. *Am J Dig Dis* 1977;22:973.

21. Cooksley WGE, Bradbear RA, Robinson W, et al: The prognosis of chronic active hepatitis without cirrhosis in relation to bridging necrosis. *Hepatology* 1984;6:345.

22. Czaja AJ: Strategies in the management of chronic active hepatitis. *Surv Dig Dis* 1984;2:233.

23. Czaja AJ: Chronic active hepatitis, in Lichtenstein LM, Fauci AS (eds): *Current Therapy in Allergy and Immunology* 1983-1984. Burlington, Ont 1983 BC Decker Inc. pp. 239–244.

24. Summerskill WHJ, Korman MG, Ammon HV, et al: Prednisone for chronic active liver disease: dose titration, standard dose, and combination with azathioprine compared. *Gut* 1975;16:876.

25. Czaja AJ, Davis GL, Ludwig J, et al: Complete resolution of inflammatory activity following corticosteroid treatment of HBsAg-negative chronic active hepatitis. *Hepatology* 1984;4:622.

26. Wang KK, Czaja AJ: Prognosis of corticosteroid-treated hepatitis B surface antigen-negative chronic active hepatitis in postmenopausal women: a retrospective analysis. *Gastroenterology* 1989;97:1288.

27. Czaja AJ, Ammon HV, Summerskill WHJ: Clinical features and prognosis of sever chronic active liver disease (CALD) after corticosteroid-induced remission. *Gastroenterology* 1980;78:518.

28. Czaja AJ, Ludwig J, Baggenstoss AH, et al: Corticosteroid-treated chronic active hepatitis in remission: uncertain prognosis of chronic persistent hepatitis *N Engl J Med* 1981;304:5.

29. Davis GL, Czaja AJ, Ludwig J: The development and prognosis of histologic cirrhosis in corticosteroid-treated HBsAg-negative chronic hepatitis. *Gastroenterology* 1984;87:1222.

30. Czaja A, Wolf AM, Baggenstoss AH: Laboratory assessment of severe chronic active liver disease (CALD): correlation of serum transaminase and gamma globulin levels with histologic features. *Gastroenterology* 1981;80:687.

31. Donaldson PT, Doherty DG, Hayliar KM, et al: Susceptibility to autoimmune chronic active hepatitis: human leukocyte antigens DR4 and A1-B8-DR3 are independent risk factors. *Hepatology* 1991;13:701.

32. Czaja AJ, Beaver SJ, Shiels MT: Sustained remission following corticosteroid therapy of severe HBsAg-negative chronic active hepatitis. *Gastroenterology* 1987;92:215.

33. Czaja AJ: Low dose corticosteroid therapy after multiple relapses of sever HBsAg-negative chronic active hepatitis. *Hepatology* 1990;11:1044.

34. Stellon AJ, Keating JJ, Johnson PJ, et al: Maintenance of remission in autoimmune chronic active hepatitis with azathioprine after corticosteroid withdrawal. *Hepatology* 1990;12:970.

35. Sanchez-Urdazpal L, Czaja AJ, Van Hoek B, et al: Prognostic factors in severe autoimmune chronic active hepatitis: role of orthotopic liver transplantation. *Hepatology* 1990;12:970.

36. Czaja AJ, Rakela J, Ludwig J: Features reflective of early prognosis in corticosteroid-treated severe autoimmune chronic active hepatitis. *Gastroenterology* 1988;95:448.

37. Wang KK, Czaja AJ: Hepatocellular cancer in corticosteroid-treated severe autoimmune chronic active hepatitis. *Hepatology* 1988;8:1679.

38. Wang KK, Czaja AJ, Beaver SJ, et. al.: Extrahepatic malignancy following long-term immunosuppressive therapy of severe hepatitis B surface antigen-negative chronic active hepatitis. *Hepatology* 1989;10:39.

39. Czaja AJ, Taswell HF, Rakela J, et. al.: Frequency and significance of antibody to hepatitis C virus in severe corticosteroid-treated autoimmune chronic active hepatitis. *Mayo Clin Proc* 1991;66:572.

40. Esteban JI, Esteban R, Validomiu L, et. al.: Hepatitis C virus among risk groups in Spain. *Lancet* 1989;2:294.

41. Lenzi M, Vallardini G, Fusconi M, et. al.: Type 2 autoimmune hepatitis and hepatitis C virus infection. *Lancet* 1990;335:258.

42. Sanchez-Tapias JM, Barrera JM, Costa J, et. al.: Hepatitis C virus infection in patients with nonalcoholic chronic liver disease. *Ann Intern Med* 1990;112:921.

43. McFarlane IG, Smith HM, Johnson PJ, et. al.: Hepatitis C virus antibodies in chronic active hepatitis pathogenetic factor or false-positive result? *Lancet* 1990;335:754.

44. Czaja AJ, Taswell HF, Rakela J, et. al.: Duration and specificity of antibodies to hepatitis C virus in chronic active hepatitis effect of corticosteroid therapy. *Hepatology* 1990;2:877 Abstract.

45. Vento S, DiPerri G, Garofano T, et. al.: Hazards of interferon therapy for HBV-seronegative chronic hepatitis. *Lancet* 1989;2:926.

46. Mistilis SP, Vickers CR, Darroch MH, et. al.: Cyclosporin, a new treatment for autoimmune chronic active hepatitis. *Med J Aus* 1985;143:463.

47. Hyams JS, Ballow M, Leichtner AM, Cyclosporine treatment of autoimmune chronic active hepatitis. *Gastroenterology* 1987;93:890.

48. Thompson AW, FK-506: profile of an important new immunosuppressant. *Transplant Rev* 1990;4:1.

49. Crosignani A, Battezzati PM, Setcheil KDR, et. al.: Effects of ursodeoxycholic acid on serum liver enzymes and bile acid metabolism in chronic active hepatitis: a dose-response study. *Hepatology* 1991;13:339.

Chapter 37

# *Diagnosis and Management of Autoimmune Hepatitis*

*Abstract: Autoimmune hepatitis is a syndrome of idiopathic, chronic hepatitis of unknown etiology characterized by the presence of serum autoantibodies. The symptoms and clinical manifestations vary widely, and there are clinical subgroups based on the pattern of autoantibodies present. The disease may progress to cirrhosis and death in patients with significant liver injury. The prognosis is greatly improved for patients with severe disease who are recognized early in the course of their disease and who receive appropriate treatment with prednisone, immunosuppressive agents, or both.*

## *Introduction*

Autoimmune chronic active hepatitis (CAH) is an uncommon syndrome that includes several subcategories of patients having chronic hepatitis, evidence of autoimmunity, and absence of other definable causes of hepatitis. The first descriptions of the syndrome were of young women with severe, rapidly progressive hepatitis: however, it is now clear that the spectrum of disease is broad and includes patients with mild or even asymptomatic disease.

When confronted with a patient who may have autoimmune hepatitis, it is important to carry out a diagnostic plan that will quickly distinguish autoimmune hepatitis from the many other much more

This article originally appeared in *Practical Gastroenterology*, December 1993. Vol. 17, No. 12. Used by permission.

common causes of chronic hepatitis. Accurate diagnosis of the syndrome is important for several reasons: 1) treatment with corticosteroids, when indicated, leads to a very favorable outcome; 2) inappropriate treatment with certain drugs, such as alpha interferon for viral hepatitis, may be deleterious for patients with autoimmune hepatitis; 3) corticosteroid treatment of patients who have other chronic liver diseases may be ineffective or harmful; and 4) providing appropriate prognostic information for the patient requires accurate diagnosis.

## Background

The first detailed description of the syndrome is attributed to Waldenstrom and Kunkel[1], who identified young women with severe chronic hepatitis and hypergammaglobulinemia, with a progressive fatal course. Shortly thereafter, the system features of the disease were recognized[2] and the first direct evidence of autoimmunity was identified, the presence of the LE cell phenomenon. The presence of the LE phenomenon and antinuclear antibodies (ANA) in this disease of young women led Mackay et. al.[4] to suggest the term "lupoid hepatitis," which gained widespread use. Unfortunately, the term has led to considerable confusion, since this disease is not thought to have any relationship to systemic lupus erythematosus; it was soon recognized that the clinical features and the presence of other autoantibodies, such as smooth muscle antibody,[5] distinguish these diseases. The next crucial development was the demonstration in controlled trials that treatment with corticosteroids and immunosuppressive drugs could be life-saving for patients with severe autoimmune hepatitis.[6-8] Further advances include, first, the recognition that the syndrome may have a broad spectrum of activity and that subcategories exist.[9] Second, better methods to diagnose viral hepatitis and other causes of chronic hepatitis have left only a relatively small number of patients who clearly fit the syndrome of autoimmune hepatitis. Nonetheless, there is continuing interest in the role of hereditary factors and autoantigens in autoimmune hepatitis as a motel to understand pathogenetic mechanisms in chronic liver disease.[10]

**Table 37.1. Typical Clinical Features of Autoimmune Hepatitis.**

*Symptoms*
- May be asymptomatic
- Insidious onset
- Fatigue, malaise
- Anorexia
- Low-grade fever
- Jaundice
- Amenorrhea
- Symptoms of advanced liver disease: ascites, bleeding, hepatic encephalopathy
- Arthralgia

*Physical findings*
- Female sex predominates
- Mild disease: no physical abnormalities
- Moderate, severe disease: hepatomegaly; splenomegaly; jaundice; signs of cirrhosis, liver failure

*Laboratory*
- Frequently positive ANA, anti-SMA

*Liver biopsy*
- Wide spectrum of abnormalities: mild periportal chronic inflammation, piecemeal necrosis; bridging necrosis; fibrosis and cirrhosis

(ANA = antinuclear antibodies: anti SMA = anti smooth muscle) antibody.

## Clinical Features

### *Typical Autoimmune ("Lupoid") Hepatitis (Type 1)*

Autoimmune hepatitis predominantly affects women, with a female:male ratio of about 4:1. Although classically described as a disease of young women, with a peak age of onset between the ages of 15 and 25, the disease may have an onset at any age, and there is a second peak of incidence at about the age of 50. The typical symptoms (Table 37.1) are nonspecific, and include the insidious onset of fatigue, malaise, anorexia, and arthralgias. Initial presentation with symptoms of severe liver disease, such as nausea, vomiting, and jaundice, and complications of advanced liver disease such as ascites, encephalopathy, or bleeding is uncommon. Associated syndromes such as amenorrhea, cushingoid appearance, hyperthyroidism, and Coombs-positive hemolytic anemia may be found. The typical physical features range from no physical abnormalities in mild cases to hepatomegaly and other signs of active liver disease in moderately active disease to typical signs of cirrhosis in advanced cases.

Standard laboratory tests reveal an elevation of aspartate aminotransferase (AST) that may correlate well with the degree of ongoing liver injury. The level of aminotransferase elevation is often greater than 10 times normal. Other abnormalities may be found that are also features of chronic liver disease or cirrhosis of other etiologies, including elevations of gamma-glutamyltransferase (GGT) and bilirubin, hypoalbuminemia, and prolonged prothrombin time. Hypergammaglobulinemia, which may be quite marked, is often found in cases of active disease. The elevation is primarily due to an increase in immunoglobulin G levels, but this finding has no diagnostic specificity.

The frequency with which specific serologic abnormalities are found in typical autoimmune hepatitis varies and depends in part on arbitrary diagnostic criteria (Table 37.2). While the typical case of classical "lupoid" hepatitis is associated with high titers of ANA in serum, overall only from one-third to two-thirds of patients who have other typical features of CAH have this antibody. Chronic active hepatitis does not appear to be associated with any one specific pattern of nuclear reactivity, and the antigens recognized have not been defined.[11]

Typical or type I autoimmune hepatitis is by definition associated with the presence of another non-organ-specific autoantibody anti-smooth muscle antibody (anti-SMA). The major antigen recognized by anti-SMA is actin, a major cytoskeletal component of cells. In many cases, however, antigens other than actin are the target of the antibody, and these have yet to be identified. While the presence of this antibody is necessary for diagnosis, its presence has no diagnostic specificity, since anti-SMA is frequently found in many forms of chronic liver injury.

Antimitochondrial antibodies, which are typically found in high titer in patients with primary biliary cirrhosis (PBC), can also be found in a minority of patients with CAH. Sometimes, patients with this antibody may have an overlap syndrome of CAH and PBC.[12] One distinguishing feature of the overlap syndrome is that it behaves clinically like CAH in that the response to corticosteroids is good, whereas in PBC the response to corticosteroids is poor.

***Table 37.2.*** *Serologic Abnormalities in Autoimmune Hepatitis and Other Causes of Chronic Hepatitis and Hepatobiliary Inflammation.*

| Disease | Autoantibodies | | | | | Viral antibodies | |
|---|---|---|---|---|---|---|---|
| | ANA | anti-SMA | anti-LKM | SLA | AMA | anti-HB core | anti-HCV |
| Autoimmune hepatitis | | | | | | | |
| Classic | + | + | – | – | – | – | – |
| LKM antibody type | – | – | + | – | – | – | ± |
| Soluble liver antigen type | – | – | – | + | – | – | – |
| Viral hepatitis | | | | | | | |
| HBV | – | ± | – | – | – | + | – |
| HCV | – | ± | – | – | – | – | + |
| Primary biliary cirrhosis | ± | ± | – | – | + | – | – |
| Sclerosing cholangitis | – | ± | – | – | – | – | – |

ANA = antinuclear antibodies; anti-SMA = anti-smooth muscle antibody; anti-LKM = antibodies to liver-kidney microsomes; SLA = soluble liver antigens; AMA = antimitochondrial antibodies; HB = hepatitis B; HCV = hepatitis C virus.

Patients of European origin with autoimmune CAH have a greatly increased incidence of the HLA phenotype HLA B8-DR3. Recent work has shown that this association may be due to specific sequences in the HLA genes.[13] Patients who present later in life tend to have a different HLA phenotype, HLA-DR4. In other countries such as Japan where the genetic background is different, autoimmune CAH is associated with other HLA phenotypes.

### *Type 2 (Anti LKM) Autoimmune Hepatitis*

Type 2 autoimmune CAH is an infrequent syndrome that has distinctive clinical and laboratory features. The age of onset is typically less than 15 years, and it has been found primarily in European countries. The disease is more often associated with other autoimmune syndromes such as insulin-dependent diabetes, autoimmune thyroid disease, and vitiligo. The presentation may be acute and have a rapidly progressive course to cirrhosis. Usually, non organ-specific autoantibodies such as ANA and anti-SMA are absent, but patients characteristically have antibodies to liver-kidney microscomes (anti-LKM).[14] The target antigen has been identified by Manns et. al.[15] as cytochrome P450 db1 (now termed P-450 IID6).

The relationship of type 2 CAH to chronic hepatitis C is an interesting and as yet unresolved problem. About one-third of patients with type 2 CAH have anti-hepatitis C antibodies, usually in low titer, which initially raised the suspicion that these were false-positive reactions associated with autoimmunity. The fact that the majority of such patients respond to treatment with prednisone, and that some patients with the syndrome treated with alfa interferon deteriorate, has tended to support this argument. However, some patients have viral RNA in their circulation, indicating that they do not have hepatitis C virus infection. In such patients, whether the viral infection is the trigger of the apparent autoimmune disease or whether hepatitis C virus infection is the etiology of the syndrome is unclear. It has been suggested that type 2 CAH be divided into two subgroups, type 2a and type 2b, on the basis of the absence or presence respectively of hepatitis C virus markers, since it seems likely that at least in some patients hepatitis C virus infection is important in the pathogenesis of the syndrome.

### *SLA-Antibody-Positive Chronic Active Hepatitis*

Recently, a new subgroup of CAH that is characterized by the lack of ANA, anti-SMA, or anti-LKM and the presence of serum antibodies that react with cytosolic fractions of hepatocytes (soluble liver antigens [SLA]) has been identified.[16] Clinically, the small number of patients found to date with this syndrome are similar to patients with type 1 CAH in that they are predominantly female and respond well to immunosuppressive treatment.

### *Other Autoantibodies in Autoimmune Hepatitis*

Recently, antibody to hepatic asialoglycoprotein receptor (anti-ASGP-R) has been detected.[17] This antibody can be found in at least some patients with many acute and chronic liver diseases,[18] suggesting that the autoreactivity to this protein is a secondary consequence of liver injury. Titers of anti-ASGP-R are much higher in autoimmune CAH, consistent with other possibility of a primary pathogenetic role of a secondary epiphenomenon.

### *Cryptogenic Chronic Active Hepatitis and Cirrhosis*

New methods for diagnosis of viral hepatitis, including improved serological and polymerase chain reaction (PCR) methods, have shown that many patients previously classified as having "cryptogenic" cirrhosis have viral hepatitis. However, subgroups of patients remain in whom no etiology can be identified. Some of these patients, although lacking autoantibodies such as ANA, anti-SMA, anti-LKM, and SLA, have clinical features that otherwise resemble those of patients with classic autoimmune hepatitis, including hypergammaglobulinemia, typical liver biopsy features, and favorable responses to corticosteroids.[9,19] Although generally indistinguishable from patients with typical CAH, they tend to present at an older age and are more likely to have cirrhosis at the time of presentation. It has been suggested that these patients may have had autoantibodies early in the course of their disease that have been lost.

## *Liver Histologic Abnormalities*

Although serum biochemical and serological studies are helpful in making the diagnosis of autoimmune hepatitis. Liver biopsy remains an essential diagnostic procedure and guide for treatment. There are no histopathological features of CAH that are pathognomonic. The main feature is periportal lymphocytic infiltration with ballooning and lytic necrosis of hepatocytes, which results in an acinar arrangement of hepatocytes in periportal regions (piecemeal necrosis) and broad areas of collapse connecting portal triads (bridging necrosis). While these features are important criteria for the diagnosis of autoimmune CAH, they are not specific for this disease, being found in other forms of chronic liver disease, in particular chronic vital hepatitis. Piecemeal necrosis alone is not a good predictor of the likelihood of progression to cirrhosis. Patients who have only piecemeal necrosis seldom have progression to cirrhosis. On the other hand, bridging necrosis, in which bands of inflammation and necrosis connect portal triads, is thought to be the direct histologic predecessor of cirrhosis.[20] Liver biopsy is needed to exclude other important diseases that may mimic CAH. Autoimmune hepatitis is not characterized by the presence of granulomas, prominent plasma cell infiltrates or germinal centers, or prominent changes in bile ducts, fatty changes, or Mallory bodies; all of these features suggest other diagnostic possibilities. Special stains are not necessary to establish the diagnosis of autoimmune CAH, although they are useful in excluding other diagnostic possibilities (see below).

***Table 37.3. Differential Diagnosis of Autoimmune Chronic Hepatitis.***

*Causes of typical chronic hepatitis syndrome*

Common
- —Hepatitis B (with or without hepatitis D)
- —Hepatitis C

Uncommon
- —Autoimmune chronic hepatitis
- —Chronic drug reactions (alpha-methyldopa, oxyphenisatin, itrofurantoin, isoniazid, tienilic acid)

Rare
- —Wilson's disease

*Diseases that may have features of chronic hepatitis*

Metabolic
- —Diabetes
- —Hemochromatosis
- —Nonalcoholic steatonecrosis
- —Alpha-1 anetrypsin deficiency

Toxic
- —Alcoholic liver disease
- —Industrial exposure to toxins

Infectious
- —Liver disease associated with AIDS
- —Vira, bacterial, and fungal infections

Autoimmune
- —Primary biliary cirrhosis (especially with chronic active hepatitis overlap syndrome)
- —Sclerosing cholangitis

## Differential Diagnosis

Making an accurate diagnosis is essential for a number of reasons. First, other treatable causes of chronic hepatitis may mimic autoimmune hepatitis. Second, the diagnosis of autoimmune CAH involves commitment to lifelong observation and prolonged, possibly lifelong treatment. Finally, it is important to make the correct diagnosis of autoimmune CAH and initiate appropriate treatment, when necessary, to prevent progression to liver failure. Since there are no pathognomonic features of autoimmune hepatitis, the diagnosis depends on the presence of typical clinical, biochemical, serologic, and histologic abnormalities and the exclusion of other causes of chronic liver injury (Table 37.3).

The major cause of chronic hepatitis is infectious with hepatitis viruses (B, C, and D), which are much more common diseases than autoimmune hepatitis. The presence of typical viral serologic and histologic abnormalities usually assures the diagnosis of viral hepatitis, although, as mentioned above, the relationship of chronic hepatitis C virus infection to autoimmunity is uncertain. More problematic is the recent observation, using PCR technology, that occasional patients with chronic hepatitis B or C virus infection may lack all serologic markers of viral hepatitis. Occasional patients with hepatitis B virus infection may have only anti-hepatitis-B core antigen positivity, without circulating HBsAg. Clearly, such patients would previously have been diagnosed as having idiopathic CAH. A previous history of blood product transfusion, IV drug abuse, or sexual promiscuity should certainly raise the suspicion of chronic viral infection in a patient with abnormal liver function tests.

Other chronic systemic infections, such as Epstein-Barr virus infection, may rarely be causes of chronic abnormalities of liver function tests but do not ordinarily lead to significant liver injury. Patients with human immunodeficiency virus (HIV) infection very frequently have abnormalities of liver enzymes, which are typically due to any one of the numerous infectious or drug-induced complications of the disease. A careful history must be taken of both prescription and nonprescription drug use, as medications can occasionally lead to chronic hepatitis. Wilson's disease may present with chronic or fulminant hepatitis, and this diagnosis must not be missed, because of the potential for specific, life-saving therapy. The diagnosis of alcoholic liver disease is usually straightforward on the basis of careful history and, when indicated, liver biopsy. Toxic industrial exposures, which may cause chronic liver injury through a direct toxic effect or through hypersensitivity mechanisms, are probably uncommon but require careful history and removal of the exposure for diagnosis. The most common metabolic disease that involves the liver is diabetes. Diabetic steatonecrosis has features that most closely resemble alcoholic liver disease, but in the absence of alcohol use the disease may be confused with autoimmune liver disease if the diagnosis of diabetes is not recognized. Occasionally, obese patients without overt diabetes may have a similar syndrome. Other inherited metabolic liver diseases such as hemochromatosis and alpha 1-antitrypsin deficiency are usually easy to diagnose on the basis of serum biochemical changes (ferritin, alpha 1 antitrypsin levels) and liver histology.

Other autoimmune liver diseases, particularly PBC and sclerosing cholangitis, may initially present with features similar to autoimmune chronic hepatitis. Primary biliary cirrhosis typically presents with insidious symptoms in women, but the great majority of patients have antimitochondrial antibodies and hepatic histologic features that usually allow for the correct diagnosis. Sclerosing cholangitis can occasionally be confused with chronic hepatitis. The symptoms are nonspecific, but the biochemical picture is usually dominated by cholestatic changes and absence of autoantibodies. Although the liver biopsy classically shows relatively distinct features of biliary disease, sometimes in early disease the findings may resemble those of CAH. Sclerosing cholangitis is much more common in men, and the presence of associated inflammatory bowel disease should strongly suggest this diagnosis. Endoscopic retrograde cholangiopancreatography should be done if this diagnosis can not be excluded on the basis of serum biochemical, serologic, and histologic features.

## Treatment

The classic controlled trials of corticosteroid drugs for treatment of autoimmune CAH have unequivocally demonstrated that anti-inflammatory and immunosuppressive therapy is potentially life-saving. However, previous controlled studies primarily involved patients with severe illness who entered trials in referral centers. As indicated above, the absence of bridging necrosis carries a good prognosis, and there is still uncertainty as to whether patients in good prognostic groups benefit from treatment with corticosteoids.[9,20]

The usual starting dose is prednisone 20 To 40 mg/day. Most patients respond dramatically, with marked symptomatic improvement within several weeks. Aminotransferase levels also tend to decease rapidly and may return to normal within a few weeks of beginning therapy. Patients with more severe disease may have a delayed response. After the appropriate clinical and laboratory response is achieved, prednisone can usually be gradually tapered over 2 to 3 months to a maintenance dose of 10 to 20 mg/day, Aminotransferases should be followed with each dose reduction.

The combination of prednisone and azathioprine can be steroid-sparing, allowing the majority of patients to discontinue prednisone to avoid the potential long-term side effects of chronic steroid use. Azathioprine is started at a dose of 1.5 mg/kg/day and generally takes approximately 2 to 4 months to exert its therapeutic effects. Subsequently, prednisone can be further tapered and stopped. The majority of patients can be maintained on aziathioprine alone. Up to 75% of patients may require chronic therapy to prevent relapse but some patients may enter a prolonged remission without continued medical therapy.

A significant proportion of patients have cirrhosis at the time of diagnosis or may progress to cirrhosis before having adequate therapy. Such patients require conventional measures for management of cirrhosis, and may be candidates for liver transplantation for advanced liver failure. When patients die of this disease, it is invariably of the complications of cirrhosis. Interestingly, hepatocellular carcinoma appears to be a rare complication, possibly because of the autoimmune rather than viral etiology of cirrhosis.

## References


1. Kunkle HG, Ahrens EH Jr., Eisaunenger WJ, et. al.: Extreme hypergammagloubulinemia in young women with liver disease of unknown etiology (abstract). *J Clin Invest* 1951;30:654.

2. Bearn AG, Concede HG, Slater RG: The problem of chronic liver disease in young women. *Am J Med* 1956;21:3–15.

3. Joske RA, King WE: The L.E.-cell phenomenon in active chronic viral hepatitis. *Lancet* 1955;2:477–480.

4. Mackay IR, Taft U, Cowling DC: Lupoid hepatitis. *Lancet* 1956;2:1323–1326.

5. Whittingham SF, Irwin J, Mackay IR, Smalley M: Smooth muscle autoantibody in “auto immune” hepatitis. *Gastroenterology* 1966;51 :499-505.

6. Cook GC, Mulligan R, Sherlock S: Controlled prospective trial of corticosteroid therapy in active chronic hepatitis. *Q J Med* 1971;40:159–185.

7. Soloway RD, Summerskill WHJ, Baggenstoss A, et. al.: Clinical, biochemical and histological remission in severe chronic active liver disease: A controlled study of treatments and early prognosis. *Gastroenterology* 1972;63:820–833.

8. Murray-Lyon IM, Stern RB, Williams R: Controlled trial of prednisone and azathioprine in active chronic hepatitis. *Lancet* 1973;1:735–737.

9. Johnson PJ, McFarlane IG, Eddleston ALWF: The natural course and heterogeneity of autoimmune-type active hepatitis. *Semin Liver Dis* 1991;11:187–196.

10. Manns MP: Cytoplasmic autoantigens in autoimmune hepatitis: Molecular analysis and clinical relevance. *Semin Liver Dis* 1991;11:205–214.

11. Mackay IR: The hepatitis-lupus connection. *Semin Liver Dis* 1991;11:234–247.

12. Berg PA, Wiedmann KH, Sayers T, et. al.: Serologic classifications of chronic cholestatic liver disease by the use of two different types of antimitochondrial antibodies. *Lancet* 1980;1:1329–1332.

13. Doherty DG, Donaldson PT, Underhill JA, et. al.: Susceptibility to autoimmune hepatitis is associated with a specific amino acid substitution in the HLA-DR molecule (abstract) *Hepatology* 1992;16:63A.

14. Rizerto M, Swana G, Doniach D: Microsomal antibodies in active chronic hepatitis and other disorders. *Clin Exp Immunol* 1973;15:331–344.

15. Manns MP, Johnson EF, Griffen KJ, et. al.: Major antigen of liver kidney microsomal antibody in idiopathic autoimmune hepatitis is cytochrome P450dlb. *J Clin Invest* 1989;83:1066–1072.

16. Manns M, Gerken G, Kyriatsoulis A, et. al.: Characterization of a new subgroup of autoimmune chronic active hepatitis by autoantibodies against a soluble liver antigen. *Lancet* 1987;1:292–294.

17. McFarlane IG, McFarlane BM, Major GN, et. al.: Identification of the hepatic asialoglycoprotein receptor (hepatic lectin) as a component of liver specific membrane lipproein (LSP). *Clin Exp Immunol* 1984;55:347–354.

18. Poralla T, Treichel U, Lohr H, Fleischer B: The asialoglycoprotein receptor as target structure in autoimmune liver diseases. *Semin Liver Dis* 1991;11:215–222.

19. Czaja AJ, Hay JE, Rakeb J: Clinical features and prognostic implications of severe corticosteroid treated cryptogenic chronic active hepatitis. *Mayo Clin Prac* 1990;65:23–30.

20. Davies GL, Czaja AJ, Ludwig J: Development and prognosis of histologic cirrhosis in corticosteroid treated hepatitis B surface antigen negative chronic active hepatitis. *Gastroenterology* 1984–87;122–127.

21. Wright EC, Seeff LB, Berk PD, et. al.: Treatment of chronic active hepatitis. An analysis of three controlled trials. *Gastroenterology* 1977;73:1422–1430.

*—by George T. Fantry, M.D.*
*and Stephen P. James, M.D.:*
*Gastroenterology Division.*
*University of Maryland*
*at Baltimore.*
*Baltimore, Maryland.*

Chapter 38

# *Cirrhosis of the Liver*

The liver weighs about 3 pounds and is the largest organ in the body. It is located in the upper right side of the abdomen, below the ribs (see Figure 38.1). When chronic diseases cause the liver to become permanently injured and scarred, the condition is called cirrhosis.

The scar tissue that forms in cirrhosis harms the structure of the liver, blocking the flow of blood through the organ. The loss of normal liver tissue slows the processing of nutrients, hormones, drugs, and toxins by the liver. Also slowed is production of proteins and other substances made by the liver.

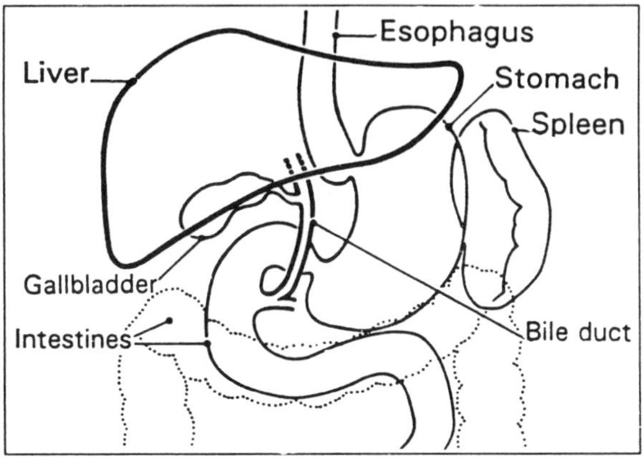


***Figure 38.1.***

NIH Pub. No. 9211–34.

## What Is the Impact of Cirrhosis?

Cirrhosis is the seventh leading cause of death by disease. About 25,000 people die from cirrhosis each year. There also is a great toll in terms of human suffering, hospital costs, and the loss of work by people with cirrhosis.

## What Are the Major Causes of Cirrhosis?

Cirrhosis has many causes. In the United States, chronic alcoholism is the most common cause. Cirrhosis also may result from chronic viral hepatitis (types B, C, and D). Liver injury that results in cirrhosis also may be caused by a number of inherited diseases such as cystic fibrosis, alpha-1 antitrypsin deficiency, hemochromatosis, Wilson's disease, galactosemia, and glycogen storage diseases.

Two inherited disorders result in the abnormal storage of metals in the liver leading to tissue damage and cirrhosis. People with Wilson's disease store too much copper in their livers, brains, kidneys, and in the corneas of their eyes.

In another disorder, known as hemochromatosis, too much iron is absorbed, and the excess iron is deposited in the liver and in other organs, such as the pancreas, skin, intestinal lining, heart, and endocrine glands.

If a person's bile duct becomes blocked, this also may cause cirrhosis. The bile ducts carry bile formed in the liver to the intestines, where the bile helps in the digestion of fat (see Figure 38.1). In babies, the most common cause of cirrhosis due to blocked bile ducts is a disease called biliary atresia. In this case, the bile ducts are absent or injured, causing the bile to back up in the liver. These babies are jaundiced (their skin is yellowed) after their first month in life. Sometimes they can be helped by surgery in which a new duct is formed to allow bile to drain again from the liver.

In adults, the bile ducts may become inflamed, blocked, and scarred due to another liver disease, primary biliary cirrhosis. Another type of biliary cirrhosis also may occur after a patient has gallbladder surgery in which the bile ducts are injured or tied off. Other, less common, causes of cirrhosis are severe reactions to prescribed drugs, prolonged exposure to environmental toxins, and repeated bouts of heart failure with liver congestion.

## What Are the Symptoms of Cirrhosis?

People with cirrhosis often have few symptoms at first. The two major problems that eventually cause symptoms are loss of functioning liver cells and distortion of the liver caused by scarring. The person may experience fatigue, weakness, and exhaustion. Loss of appetite is usual, often with nausea and weight loss.

As liver function declines, less protein is made by the organ. For example, less of the protein albumin is made, which results in water accumulating in the legs (edema) or abdomen (ascites). A decrease in proteins needed for blood clotting makes it easy for the person to bruise or to bleed.

In the later stages of cirrhosis, jaundice (yellow skin) may occur, caused by the buildup of bile pigment that is passed by the liver into the intestines. Some people with cirrhosis experience intense itching due to bile products that are deposited in the skin. Gallstones often form in persons with cirrhosis because not enough bile reaches the gallbladder.

The liver of a person with cirrhosis also has trouble removing toxins, which may build up in the blood. These toxins can dull mental function and lead to personality changes and even coma (encephalopathy). Early signs of toxin accumulation in the brain may include neglect of personal appearance, unresponsiveness, forgetfulness, trouble concentrating, or changes in sleeping habits.

Drugs taken usually are filtered out by the liver, and this cleansing process also is slowed down by cirrhosis. The liver does not remove the drugs from the blood at the usual rate, so the drugs act longer than expected, building up in the body. People with cirrhosis often are very sensitive to medications and their side effects.

A serious problem for people with cirrhosis is pressure on blood vessels that flow through the liver. Normally, blood from the intestines and spleen is pumped to the liver through the portal vein (see Figure 38.2). But in cirrhosis, this normal flow of blood is slowed, building pressure in the portal vein (portal hypertension). This blocks the normal flow of blood, causing the spleen to enlarge. So blood from the intestines tries to find a way around the liver through new vessels.

Some of these new blood vessels become quite large and are called "varices" (see Figure 38.3). These vessels may form in the stomach and esophagus (the tube that connects the mouth with the stomach). They have thin walls and carry high pressure. There is great danger

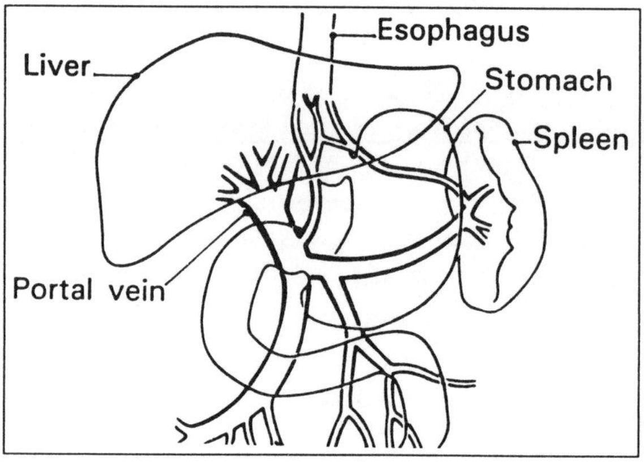


*Figure 38.2.*

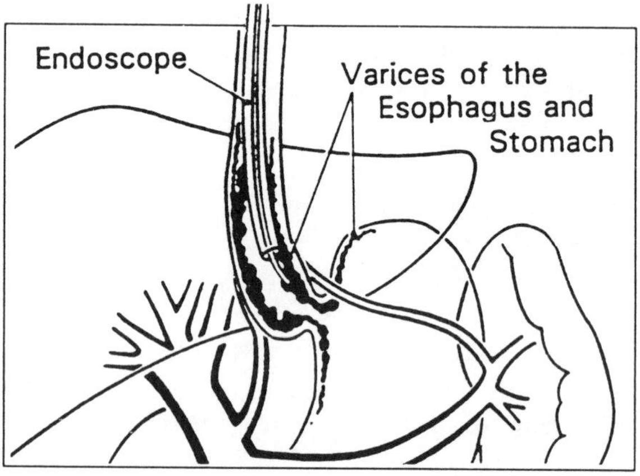


*Figure 38.3.*

that they may break, causing a serious bleeding problem in the upper stomach or esophagus. If this happens, the patient's life is in danger, and the doctor must act quickly to stop the bleeding.

## How Is Cirrhosis Diagnosed?

The doctor often can diagnosis cirrhosis from the patient's symptoms and from laboratory tests. During a physical exam, for instance, the doctor could notice a change in how your liver feels or how large it is. If the doctor suspects cirrhosis, you will be given blood tests. The purpose of these tests is to find out if liver disease is present. In some cases, other tests that take pictures of the liver are performed such as the computerized axial tomography (CAT) scan, ultrasound, and the radioisotope liver/spleen scan.

The doctor may decide to confirm the diagnosis by putting a needle through the skin to take a sample of tissue (a process called "biopsy") from the liver. In some cases, cirrhosis is diagnosed during surgery when the doctor is able to see the entire liver. The liver also can be inspected through a laparoscope, a viewing device that is inserted through a tiny incision in the abdomen.

## What Are the Treatments for Cirrhosis?

Treatment of cirrhosis is aimed at stopping or delaying its progress, minimizing the damage to liver cells, and reducing complications. In alcoholic cirrhosis, for instance, the person must stop drinking alcohol to halt progression of the disease. If a person has hepatitis, the doctor may administer steroids or antiviral drugs to reduce liver cell injury.

Medications may be given to control the symptoms of cirrhosis, such as itching. Edema and ascites (fluid retention) are treated by reducing salt in the diet. Drugs called "diuretics" are used to remove excess fluid and to prevent edema from recurring. Diet and drug therapies can help to improve the altered mental function that cirrhosis can cause. For instance, decreasing dietary protein results in less toxin formation in the digestive tract. Laxatives such as lactulose may be given to help absorb toxins and speed their removal from the intestines.

The two main problems in cirrhosis are liver failure, when liver cells just stop working, and the bleeding caused by portal hypertension. The doctor may prescribe blood pressure medication, such as a beta blocker, to treat the portal hypertension. If the patient bleeds from the varices of the stomach or esophagus, the doctor can inject these veins with a sclerosing agent administered through a flexible tube (endoscope) that is inserted through the mouth and esophagus (see Figure 38.3). In critical cases, the patient may be given a liver transplant or another surgery (such as a portacaval shunt) that is sometimes used to relieve the pressure in the portal vein and varices. Patients with cirrhosis often live healthy lives for many years. Even when complications develop, they usually can be treated. Many patients with cirrhosis have undergone successful liver transplantation.

## Additional Readings

*Biliary Atresia*. This fact sheet presents information on biliary atresia and cirrhosis, including discussions of diagnosis, treatment, and complications. Available from the American Liver Foundation. 1428 Pompton Avenue, Cedar Grove. NJ 07009. (201) 256-2550 or (800) 223-0179.

*Cirrhosis: Many Causes*. This fact sheet presents general information on cirrhosis of the liver, research, and the work of the American Liver Foundation. Available from the foundation.

Clayman CB, ed. *The American Medical Association Encyclopedia of Medicine*. New York: Random House. 1989. Authoritative reference guide for patients, with sections on cirrhosis, hepatitis, and other disorders affecting the liver. Widely available in libraries and bookstores.

*Primary Biliary Cirrhosis*. This fact sheet presents information on PBC and cirrhosis, including discussions of diagnosis, treatment, and liver transplantation. Available from the American Liver Foundation.

Rosenfeld I. *Second Opinion: Your Comprehensive Guide to Treatment*. New York: Bantam Books, 1988. General medical guide with sections on cirrhosis and other disorders affecting the liver. Widely available in libraries and bookstores.

## Resources

The Children's Liver Foundation, Inc. 14245 Ventura Boulevard, Suite 201, Sherman Oaks, CA 91423. (818) 906-3021 or (800) 526-1593.

United Network for Organ Sharing. 1100 Boulders Parkway, Suite 500, P.O. Box 13770, Richmond, VA 23225-8770. (804) 330-8500.

**National Digestive Diseases Information Clearinghouse**
Box NDDIC
9000 Rockville Pike
Bethesda, MD 20892
(301) 468-4344

The National Digestive Diseases Information Clearinghouse is a service of the National Institute of Diabetes and Digestive and Kidney Diseases, part of the National Institutes of Health, under the U.S. Public Health Service.

The clearinghouse was authorized by Congress to focus a national effort on providing information to the public, patients and their families, and doctors and other health care professionals. The clearinghouse works with organizations to educate people about digestive health and disease. The clearinghouse answers inquiries; develops, reviews, and distributes publications; and coordinates informational resources about digestive diseases.

Publications produced by the clearinghouse are reviewed carefully for scientific accuracy, appropriateness of content, and readability. Publications produced by sources other than the clearinghouse also are reviewed for scientific accuracy and are used, along with clearinghouse publications, to answer requests.

# Chapter 39

# *Primary Biliary Cirrhosis*

## *What Is Primary Biliary Cirrhosis?*

Primary biliary cirrhosis (PBC) is a chronic liver disease that causes slow, progressive destruction of bile ducts in the liver. This destruction interferes with the excretion of bile. Continued liver inflammation causes scarring and eventually leads to cirrhosis. Cirrhosis is present only in the later stage of the disease. In the early stages of the illness, the main problem is the build up of substances (like acids, cholesterol) in the blood, which are normally excreted into the bile.

## *Presentation*

Women are affected 10 times more frequently than men. The disease usually is first diagnosed in people 30 to 60 years old. Many patients have no symptoms of disease and are diagnosed by finding an abnormality on routine liver blood tests. Itching and fatigue are common symptoms. Other signs include jaundice, cholesterol deposits in the skin, fluid accumulation and darkening of the skin. Several other disorders are often associated with PBC. The most common are impaired functioning of the tear and salivary glands, causing dry eyes or mouth. Arthritis and thyroid problems may also be present. Bone

---

Originally published as *Primary Biliary Cirrhosis Fact Sheet* by the American Liver Foundation. Reprinted with permission.

softening and fragility leading to fractures can occur in late stages of the disease.

## Diagnosis

PBC diagnosis is based on several pieces of information. The patient may have symptoms (itching) suggesting bile duct damage. Laboratory tests, such as the alkaline phosphatase activity test, may confirm this. The test for mitochondrial antibodies is particularly useful as it is positive in nearly all patients. Often, the bile ducts are X-rayed to rule out possibilities of other causes of biliary tract disease, such as obstruction. A liver biopsy is useful in confirming the diagnosis and in giving information on the severity and extent of liver damage.

## Cause

Although the cause of the initial bile duct damage in PBC is unknown, there are certain clues that may be important. Strictly speaking, the disease is not inherited, but it is more common among siblings and in families where one member has previously been affected. Multiple disturbances of the immune system have been found in persons with PBC and may be an important factor. Hormones may also play a role given that this illness is so much more common in women.

## Prognosis

PBC advances slowly. Many patients lead active and productive lives for ten to fifteen years after diagnosis. Patients who show no symptoms at the time of diagnosis often remain symptom-free after ten years. Jaundice appears to be a sign of diminishing liver reserve and may be an important indication of the progress of the disease. The illness is chronic and may lead to life-threatening complications, especially after cirrhosis develops.

## Treatment

Treatment may be useful in several ways. Proper advice will ensure the elimination of potentially harmful drugs, foods or toxins. If the patient is deficient in vitamin D, then this should be corrected.

The thyroid function should be tested and if low, treated with a thyroid hormone. Symptoms may be successfully relieved. Itching is often reduced by using cholestyramine and rifampin. Salt restriction may be effective in reducing fluid accumulation. The diet should be well-balanced. Corticosteroids have been found ineffective in most patients. Few drugs such as Actigall and methotrexate have shown some promise in improving liver tests, but their impact on the survival rate remains unclear. Colchicine improves liver tests but does not slow the progression of the disease.

## Liver Transplantation

When medical treatment no longer controls the disease and the patient has severe liver failure, transplantation is indicated. Signs of liver failure include accumulation of fluid in the abdomen, malnutrition, gastrointestinal bleeding, intractable itching, jaundice, and bone fractures. Transplantation may be recommended before all these events occur. The outcome for patients with PBC who have undergone transplantation is excellent. The survival rate for two or more years is about 60–80 percent. The use of new drugs to suppress rejection has made transplantation even more successful. The disease's slow progress makes it possible to plan elective transplant surgery.

## The Future

PBC has been known for more than 100 years. This knowledge has led doctors to make earlier diagnoses. Many clues to the cause have been supplied by careful observation of patients over the last 25 years, but the basic cause is unknown. Research is following two paths:

- (1) Basic investigation of the causes and development of the disease.

- (2) Drug therapy trials, involving a large number of patients around the world, are exploring the potential use of several medications to lessen the symptoms and control liver damage.

American Liver Foundation
1425 Pompton Avenue
Cedar Grove, NJ 07009

## Chapter 40

# Liver Biopsy

### What Is a Liver Biopsy?

Liver biopsy is a diagnostic procedure used to obtain a small amount of liver tissue, which can be examined under a microscope to help identify the cause or stage of liver disease.

### What Are the Different Ways Liver Biopsy Can Be Performed?

The most common way this liver sample is obtained is by inserting a needle into the liver for a fraction of a second. This can be done in the hospital and the patient may be sent home within 3-6 hours if there are no complications. The physician determines the best site, depth, and angle of the needle puncture by physical examination or ultrasound. The skin and area under the skin is anesthetized, and a needle is passed quickly into and out of the liver. Approximately half of individuals have no pain afterwards, while another half will experience brief localized pain that may spread to the right shoulder.

Another technique used is guiding the needle to the liver through the abdomen or chest using images. This approach is used when there are localized tumors identified by images created by ultrasound or computed tomography (CT). Either ultrasound or CT scanning is used

---

Originally published as *Liver Biopsy Fact Sheet* by the American Liver Foundation. Reprinted with permission.

to pinpoint the site of the tumor and guide the needle to this specific area through the abdomen or chest. After this procedure, the patient is usually allowed to go home the same day.

Less commonly used are laparoscopy, transvenous or transjugular liver biopsy, and surgical liver biopsy. With laparoscopy, a lighted, narrow tubular instrument is inserted through a small incision in the abdominal wall. The internal organs are moved away from the abdominal wall by gas that is introduced into the abdomen. Instruments may be passed through this lighted instrument or through separate puncture sites to obtain tissue samples from several different areas of the liver. Patients who undergo this procedure may be discharged several hours later. Transvenous or transjugular liver biopsy may be performed by a radiologist in special circumstances, e.g. when the patient has a significant problem with blood clotting (coagulopathy) or a large amount of fluid within the abdomen (ascites). With this procedure, a small tube is inserted into the internal jugular vein in the neck and radiologically guided into the hepatic vein, which drains the liver. A small biopsy needle is then inserted through the tube and directly into the liver to obtain a sample of tissue. Finally, liver biopsy may be done at the time a patient undergoes an open abdominal operation, enabling the surgeon to inspect the liver and take one or more tissue samples as needed.

## When Is a Liver Biopsy Used?

Liver biopsy is often used to diagnose the cause of chronic liver disease that results in elevated liver tests or an enlarged liver. It is also used to diagnose liver tumors identified by imaging tests. In many cases the specific cause of the chronic liver disease is highly suspected on the basis of blood tests, but a liver biopsy is used to both confirm the diagnosis as well as the amount of damage to the liver. Liver biopsy is also used after liver transplantation to determine the cause of elevated liver tests and determine if rejection is present.

## What Are the Dangers of Liver Biopsy?

The primary risk of liver biopsy is bleeding from the site of needle entry into the liver, although this occurs in less than 1% of patients. Other possible complications include the puncture of other organs, such as the kidney, lung or colon. Biopsy, by mistake, of the gallbladder rather than the liver may be associated with leakage of bile into the abdominal cavity, causing peritonitis. Fortunately, the risk of death from liver biopsy is extremely low, ranging from 0.1% to 0.01%.

## *Are There Alternatives to Liver Biopsy?*

The primary alternative to a liver biopsy is to make the diagnosis of a liver disease based on the physical examination of the patient, medical history, and blood testing. In some cases, blood testing is quite accurate in giving the doctor the information to diagnose chronic liver disease, while in other circumstances a liver biopsy is needed to assure an accurate diagnosis.

## *Do Liver Biopsies Ever Need to Be Repeated?*

In most circumstances, a liver biopsy is only performed once to confirm a suspected diagnosis of chronic liver disease. Occasionally, liver biopsy is repeated if the clinical condition changes or to assess the results of medical therapy, such as interferon treatment of chronic viral hepatitis, or the use of the drug prednisone to treat autoimmune hepatitis. Patients who have undergone liver transplantation often require numerous liver biopsies in the early weeks to months following the surgery to allow accurate diagnoses of whether the new liver is being rejected or whether other problems have developed.

## Chapter 41

# *Primary Sclerosing Cholangitis*

Primary sclerosing cholangitis is a disease in which the bile ducts inside and outside the liver become narrowed due to inflammation and scarring. This causes bile to accumulate in the liver and can result in damage to liver cells. Although the exact cause of primary sclerosing cholangitis is unknown, genetic and immunologic factors appear to play a role. Primary sclerosing cholangitis has been considered a rare disease, but recent studies suggest that it is more common than previously thought. It may occur alone, but approximately 70% of patients have associated inflammatory bowel disease, particularly ulcerative colitis.

Primary sclerosing cholangitis is more common in men than women. Initially, many individuals have no symptoms and the disease is detected because of abnormal laboratory test results, particularly an enzyme test called alkaline phosphatase. It usually begins in the 30s, 40s, and 50s, and is commonly associated with fatigue, itching and jaundice. Episodes of fever and chills from superimposed infection in the bile ducts occasionally occur and can be distressing symptoms. The diagnosis of primary sclerosing cholangitis is made by cholangiography, an X-ray test involving injection of dye into the bile ducts. This is usually accomplished by an endoscopic procedure called ERCP (endoscopic retrograde cholangiopancreatography) but also may be done radiologically or surgically.

The course of the disease is unpredictable for the patient, but is generally slowly progressive. The patient may have the disease for

---

Reprinted with permission from the American Liver Foundation.

many years before symptoms develop. Symptoms may persist at a stable level, be intermittent, or progress gradually. Liver failure may occur after 7-15 years of disease or even longer. Approximately 10% of patients who have the disease on a longstanding basis may develop a superimposed tumor of the bile ducts called cholangiocarcinoma.

There is currently no specific treatment for primary sclerosing cholangitis. Research is under way to determine the effectiveness of a number of medications. The various symptoms of primary sclerosing cholangitis often respond effectively to medications that control itching, antibiotics when recurrent infections occur, and vitamins to replace those that are deficient. In some instances, endoscopic, radiologic, or surgical techniques may be employed to open major blockages in the common bile duct and improve bile flow. When progressive liver failure occurs in spite of these measures, liver transplantation may be indicated. It is associated with a survival rate of 75% or more and a good quality of life after recovery.

# Chapter 42

# *Tacrolimus and Liver Transplants*

The Food and Drug Administration said [on April 12, 1994] that it had approved the marketing of a new drug to help prevent rejection of transplanted livers. It became the third immunosuppressant drug licensed for organ transplant surgery in this country.

The new drug, called FK-506 during its investigational stages, is now known as tacrolimus. Its manufacturer, Fujisawa U.S.A., Inc. of Deerfield, Illinois, will sell it as Prograf.

Tacrolimus is derived from a fungus found in soil samples dug near the parent company's laboratory in Tsukuba, Japan, in 1984. The fungus was developed as a drug largely through the efforts of Dr. Thomas E. Starzl, the organ transplant pioneer, at the University of Pittsburgh in the late 1980s.

## *Studies Continued Despite Setbacks*

Dr. Starzl's team plunged into the research after scientists in England found tacrolimus too toxic for dogs and declared it too hazardous to test in humans. With additional research, Dr. Starzl's team found that the drug prolonged the survival of transplanted organs in other animals. He also saw hints that tacrolimus could rescue transplanted organs that were being rejected in humans despite the use

---

This chapter originally appeared as "Government Approves New Drug to Assist in Liver Transplants" in *The New York Times*, April 13, 1994. ©The New York Times. Used by permission.

of cyclosporine, the major antirejection drug now prescribed for organ transplants.

Cyclosporine is approved for heart, liver and kidney transplants and is sold as Sandimmune by Sandoz Pharmaceuticals of East Hanover, New Jersey. The other antirejection drug on the market, azathioprine, is approved for kidney transplants and is sold as Imuran by the Burroughs Wellcome Company of Research Triangle Park, North Carolina.

The package insert for tacrolimus says that "only physicians experienced in immunosuppressive therapy and management of organ transplants should prescribe Prograf."

## *Approval Comes Quickly*

Tacrolimus is administered initially by injection into a vein. It is taken as a pill as soon as the patient's condition permits, usually within two to three days after surgery.

The Government's approval of tacrolimus was relatively quick following a unanimous recommendation by an advisory committee to the FDA in November. The committee recommended approval because tacrolimus provides another alternative for preventing rejection of the 3,000 livers transplanted in the United States each year.

In approving the drug, the FDA relied on assessments of tacrolimus's efficacy and safety in two large clinical trials in Europe and the United States. Each study involved about 500 liver transplant patients.

Reports from early clinical trials suggested that tacrolimus might be safer and better tolerated than the other two anti-rejection drugs. In its recommendation last fall, though, the advisory committee agreed that the United States European studies showed tacrolimus to be equivalent to cyclosporine in safety and efficacy for liver transplants, but not safer and more effective.

The two trials examined survival of both the patients and the transplanted liver after one year. The combined, one-year patient-survival rate for tacrolimus and cyclosporine was 88 percent in the United States study and 78 percent in the European study. The overall one-year survival rate for the transplanted organs using the two drugs was 81 percent in the United States and 73 percent in the European study.

The adverse effects of both drugs were similar; the major risk was damage to the kidneys and nervous system. The principal adverse reactions of tacrolimus are tremors, headache, insomnia, diarrhea, high blood pressure, nausea and kidney impairment. The problems tend to occur early in treatment and tend to subside with time, the drug agency said.

The drug agency has asked Fujisawa to continue tracking the clinical and side effects of the drug after it is marketed, a customary step following approval of a new drug. Fujisawa, a subsidiary of Fujisawa Pharmaceutical Company Ltd., in Osaka, Japan, said it had not set a price for the drug and did not yet have enough of the drug available for commercial sale.

*—by Lawrence K. Altman*

# Chapter 43

# *Liver Function Tests*

The term "liver function tests" and its abbreviated form "LFTs" is a commonly used term that is applied to a variety of blood tests that assess the general state of the liver and biliary system. Routine blood tests can be divided into those tests that are true LFTs, such as serum albumin or prothrombin time, and those tests that are simply markers of liver or biliary tract disease, such as the various liver enzymes. In addition to the usual liver tests obtained on routine automated chemistry panels, physicians may order more specific liver tests such as viral serologic tests or autoimmune tests that, if positive, can determine the specific cause of a liver disease.

There are two general categories of "liver enzymes." The first group includes the alanine aminotransferase (ALT) and the aspartate aminotransferase (AST), formerly referred to as the SGPT and SGOT. These are enzymes that are indicators of liver cell damage. The other frequently used liver enzymes are the alkaline phosphatase and gammaglutamyltranspeptidase (GGT and GGTP) that indicate obstruction to the biliary system, either within the liver or in the larger bile channels outside the liver.

The ALT and AST are enzymes that are located in liver cells and leak out and make their way into the general circulation when liver cells are injured. The ALT is thought to be a more specific indicator of liver inflammation, since the AST may be elevated in diseases of other organs such as heart disease or muscle disease. In acute liver

---

This text originally appeared as a February 1993 publication by the American Liver Foundation. Reprinted with permission.

injury, such as acute viral hepatitis, the ALT and AST may be elevated to the high 100s or over 1,000 U/L. In chronic hepatitis or cirrhosis, the elevation of these enzymes may be minimal (less than 2-3 times normal) or moderate (100-300 U/L). Mild or moderate elevations of ALT or AST are nonspecific and may be caused by a wide range of liver diseases. ALT and AST are often used to monitor the course of chronic hepatitis and the response to treatments, such as prednisone and interferon.

The alkaline phosphatase and the GGT are elevated in a large number of disorders that affect the drainage of bile, such as a gallstone or tumor blocking the common bile duct, or alcoholic liver disease or drug-induced hepatitis, blocking the flow of bile in smaller bile channels within the liver. The alkaline phosphatase is also found in other organs, such as bone, placenta, and intestine. For this reason, the GGT is utilized as a supplementary test to be sure that the elevation of alkaline phosphatase is indeed coming from the liver or the biliary tract. In contrast to the alkaline phosphatase, the GGT tends not to be elevated in diseases of bone, placenta, or intestine. Mild or moderate elevation of GGT in the presence of a normal alkaline phosphatase is difficult to interpret and often caused by changes in the liver cell enzymes induced by alcohol or medications, but without causing injury to the liver.

Bilirubin is the main bile pigment in humans which, when elevated, causes the yellow discoloration of the skin and eyes called jaundice. Bilirubin is formed primarily from the breakdown of a substance in red blood cells called "heme." It is taken up from blood processed through the liver, and then secreted into the bile by the liver. Normal individuals have only a small amount of bilirubin circulating in blood (less than 1.2 mg/dL). Conditions which cause increased formation of bilirubin, such as destruction of red blood cells, or decrease its removal from the blood stream, such as liver disease may result in an increase in the level of serum bilirubin. Levels greater than 3 mg/dL are usually noticeable as jaundice. The bilirubin may be elevated in many forms of liver or biliary tract disease, and thus it is also relatively nonspecific. However, serum bilirubin is generally considered a true test of liver function (LFT), since it reflects the liver's ability to take up, process, and secrete bilirubin into the bile.

Two other commonly used indicators of liver function are the serum albumin and prothrombin time. Albumin is a major protein which is formed by the liver, and chronic liver disease causes a decrease in the amount of albumin produced. Therefore, in liver disease, particularly more advanced liver disease, the level of the serum albumin is reduced (less than 3.5 mg/dL). The prothrombin time, which is also called protime or PT, is a test that is used to assess blood clotting. Blood clotting factors are proteins made by the liver. When the liver is significantly injured, these proteins are not normally produced. The prothrombin time is also a useful LFT, since there is a good correlation between abnormalities in coagulation measured by the prothrombin time and the degree of liver dysfunction. Prothrombin time is usually expressed in seconds and compared to a normal control patient's blood.

Finally, specific and specialized tests may be used to make a precise diagnosis of the cause of liver disease. Elevations in serum iron, the percent of iron saturated in blood, or the storage protein ferritin may indicate the presence of hemochromatosis, a liver disease associated with excess iron storage. In another disease involving abnormal metabolism of metals, Wilson's disease, there is an accumulation of copper in the liver, a deficiency of serum ceruloplasmin and excessive excretion of copper into the urine. Low levels of serum $alpha_1$-antitrypsin may indicate the presence of lung and/or liver disease in children or adults with $alpha_1$-antitrypsin deficiency. A positive antemitochondrial antibody indicates the underlying condition of primary biliary cirrhosis. Striking elevations of serum globulin, another protein in blood, and the presence of antinuclear antibodies or antismooth muscle antibodies are clues to the diagnosis of autoimmune chronic hepatitis. Finally, there are specific blood tests that allow the precise diagnosis of hepatitis A, hepatitis B, hepatitis C, and hepatitis D.

In summary, blood tests are used to diagnose or monitor liver disease. They may be simply markers of disease (e.g., ALT, AST, alkaline phosphatase, and GGT), more true indicators of overall liver function (serum bilirubin, serum albumin, and prothrombin time) or specific tests that allow the diagnosis of an underlying cause of liver disease. Interpretation of these liver tests is a sophisticated process that your physician will utilize in the context of your medical history, physical examination, and other tests such as X-rays or imaging studies of the liver.

American Liver Foundation
1425 Pompton Avenue
Cedar Grove, NJ 07009
1-800-223-0179

# Chapter 44

# *Pancreatitis*

Your pancreas is a large gland behind your stomach and close to your duodenum. (See figure 44.1.) The pancreas secretes powerful digestive enzymes that enter the small intestine through a duct. These enzymes help you digest fats, proteins, and carbohydrates. The pancreas also releases the hormones insulin and glucagon into the bloodstream. These hormones play an important part in metabolizing sugar.

Pancreatitis is a rare disease in which the pancreas becomes inflamed. Damage to the gland occurs when digestive enzymes are activated and begin attacking the pancreas. In severe cases, there may be bleeding into the gland, serious tissue damage, infection, and cysts. Enzymes and toxins may enter the bloodstream and seriously injure organs, such as the heart, lungs, and kidney.

There are two forms of pancreatitis. The acute form occurs suddenly and may be a severe, life-threatening illness with many complications. Usually, the patient recovers completely. If injury to the pancreas continues, such as when a patient persists in drinking alcohol, a chronic form of the disease may develop, bringing severe pain and reduced functioning of the pancreas that affects digestion and causes weight loss.

## *What Is Acute Pancreatitis?*

An estimated 50,000 to 80,000 cases of acute pancreatitis occur in the United States each year. This disease occurs when the pancreas

---

NIH Pub. 92-1596.

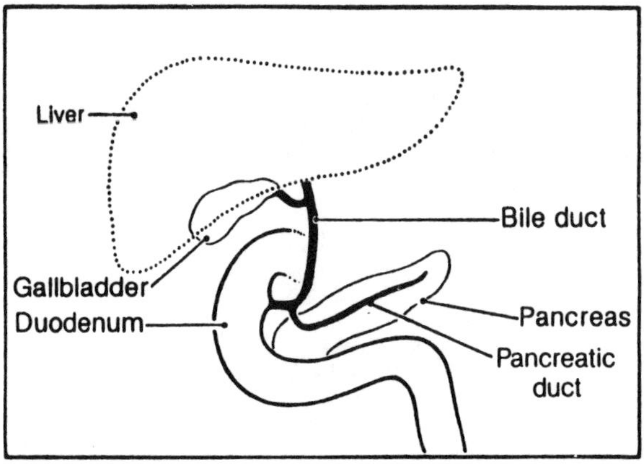


*Figure 44.1.*

suddenly becomes inflamed and then gets better. Some patients have more than one attack but recover fully after each one. Most cases of acute pancreatitis are caused either by alcohol abuse or by gallstones. Other causes may be use of prescribed drugs, trauma or surgery to the abdomen, or abnormalities of the pancreas or intestine. In rare cases, the disease may result from infections, such as mumps. In about 15 percent of cases, the cause is unknown.

## What Are the Symptoms of Acute Pancreatitis?

Acute pancreatitis usually begins with pain in the upper abdomen, that may last for a few days. The pain is often severe. It may be constant pain, just in the abdomen, or it may reach to the back and other areas. The pain may be sudden and intense, or it may begin as a mild pain that is aggravated by eating and slowly grows worse. The abdomen may be swollen and very tender. Other symptoms may include nausea, vomiting, fever, and an increased pulse rate. The person often feels and looks very sick.

About 20 percent of cases are severe. The patient may become dehydrated and have low blood pressure. Sometimes the patient's heart, lungs, or kidneys fail. In the most severe cases, bleeding can occur in the pancreas, leading to shock and sometimes death.

## How Is Acute Pancreatitis Diagnosed?

During acute attacks, high levels of amylase (a digestive enzyme formed in the pancreas) are found in the blood. Changes also may occur in blood levels of calcium, magnesium, sodium, potassium, and bicarbonate. Patients may have high amounts of sugar and lipids (fats) in their blood too. These changes help the doctor diagnose pancreatitis. After the pancreas recovers, blood levels of these substances usually return to normal.

## What Is the Treatment for Acute Pancreatitis?

The treatment a patient receives depends on how bad the attack is. Unless complications occur, acute pancreatitis usually gets better on its own, so treatment is supportive in most cases. Usually the patient goes into the hospital. The doctor prescribes fluids by vein to restore blood volume. The kidneys and lungs may be treated to prevent failure of those organs. Other problems, such as cysts in the pancreas, may need treatment too.

Sometimes a patient cannot control vomiting and needs to have a tube through the nose to the stomach to remove fluid and air. In mild cases, the patient may not have food for 3 or 4 days but is given fluids and pain relievers by vein. An acute attack usually lasts only a few days, unless the ducts are blocked by gallstones. In severe cases, the patient may be fed through the veins for 3 to 6 weeks while the pancreas slowly heals.

Antibiotics may be given if signs of infection arise. Surgery may be needed if complications such as infection, cysts, or bleeding occur. Attacks caused by gallstones may require removal of the gallbladder or surgery of the bile duct. (See figure 44.1.)

Surgery is sometimes needed for the doctor to be able to exclude other abdominal problems that can simulate pancreatitis or to treat acute pancreatitis. When there is severe injury with death of tissue, an operation may be done to remove the dead tissue.

After all signs of acute pancreatitis are gone, the doctor will determine the cause and try to prevent future attacks. In some patients the cause of the attack is clear, but in others further tests need to be done.

## What If the Patient Has Gallstones?

Ultrasound is used to detect gallstones and sometimes can provide the doctor with an idea of how severe the pancreatitis is. When gallstones are found, surgery is usually needed to remove them. When they are removed depends on how severe the pancreatitis is. If it is mild, the gallstones often can be removed within a week or so. In more severe cases, the patient may wait a month or more, until he improves, before the stones are removed. The CAT (computer axial tomography) scan also may be used to find out what is happening in and around the pancreas and how severe the problem is. This is important information that the doctor needs to determine when to remove the gallstones. After the gallstones are removed and inflammation subsides, the pancreas usually returns to normal. Before patients leave the hospital, they are advised not to drink alcohol and not to eat large meals.

## What Is Chronic Pancreatitis?

Chronic pancreatitis usually follows many years of alcohol abuse. It may develop after only one acute attack, especially if there is damage to the ducts of the pancreas. In the early stages, the doctor cannot always tell whether the patient has acute or chronic disease. The symptoms may be the same. Damage to the pancreas from drinking alcohol may cause no symptoms for many years, and then the patient suddenly has an attack of pancreatitis. In more than 90 percent of adult patients, chronic pancreatitis appears to be caused by alcoholism. This is more common in men than women and often develops between 30 and 40 years of age. In other cases, pancreatitis may be inherited. Scientists do not know why the inherited form occurs. Patients with chronic pancreatitis tend to have three kinds of problems: pain, malabsorption of food leading to weight loss, or diabetes.

Some patients do not have any pain, but most do. Pain may be constant in the back and abdomen, and for some patients, the pain attacks are disabling. In some cases, the abdominal pain goes away as the condition advances. Doctors think this happens because pancreatic enzymes are no longer being made by the pancreas.

Patients with this disease often lose weight, even when their appetite and eating habits are normal. This occurs because the body does not secrete enough pancreatic enzymes to break down food, so nutrients are not absorbed normally. Poor digestion leads to loss of fat, protein, and sugar into the stool. Diabetes may also develop at this stage if the insulin-producing cells of the pancreas (islet cells) have been damaged.

## How Is Chronic Pancreatitis Diagnosed?

Diagnosis may be difficult but is aided by a number of new techniques. Pancreatic function tests help the physician decide if the pancreas still can make enough digestive enzymes. The doctor can see abnormalities in the pancreas using several techniques (ultrasonic imaging, endoscopic retrograde cholangiopancreatography (ERCP), and the CAT scan). In more advanced stages of the disease, when diabetes and malabsorption (a problem due to lack of enzymes) occur, the doctor can use a number of blood, urine, and stool tests to help in the diagnosis of chronic pancreatitis and to monitor the progression of the disorder.

## How Is Chronic Pancreatitis Treated?

The doctor treats chronic pancreatitis by relieving pain and managing the nutritional and metabolic problems. The patient can reduce the amount of fat and protein lost in stools by cutting back on dietary fat and taking pills containing pancreatic enzymes. This will result in better nutrition and weight gain. Sometimes insulin or other drugs must be given to control the patient's blood sugar.

In some cases, surgery is needed to relieve pain by draining an enlarged pancreatic duct. Sometimes, part or most of the pancreas is removed in an attempt to relieve chronic pain.

Patients must stop drinking, adhere to their prescribed diets, and take the proper medications in order to have fewer and milder attacks.

## Additional Reading

Banks PA, Frey CF, Greenberger NJ. The spectrum of chronic pancreatitis. *Patient Care*, 1989; 23(9): 163–96. This review article for physicians is written in technical language. Available in medical libraries.

Clayman CB, ed. *The American Medical Association Encyclopedia of Medicine*. New York: Random House. 1989. Authoritative reference guide for patients with sections on irritable bowel syndrome and other disorders of the digestive system. Widely available in libraries and bookstores.

*Facts and Fallacies About Digestlve Diseases*. 1991. This fact sheet discusses commonly held beliefs about digestive diseases, including pancreatitis and gallbladder disease. Available from the National Digestive Diseases Information Clearinghouse, Box NDDIC, 9000 Rockville Pike, Bethesda, MD 20892. (301) 468-6344.

Frey CF, et al. Progress in acute pancreatitis. *Patient Care*, 1989; 23(5): 38–53. This review article for physicians is written in technical language. Available in medical libraries.

**National Digestive Diseases Information Clearinghouse**
Box NDDIC 9000
Rockville Pike
Bethesda, MD 20892
(301) 468-6344

The National Digestive Diseases Information Clearinghouse is a service of the National Institute of Diabetes and Digestive and Kidney Diseases, part of the National Institutes of Health, under the U.S. Public Health Service. The clearinghouse was begun by Congress to focus a national effort on providing information to the public, patients and their families, and doctors and other health care workers. The clearinghouse works with organizations to educate people about digestive health and disease. The clearinghouse answers inquiries; develops, reviews, and sends out publications; and coordinates informational resources about digestive diseases.

Publications produced by the clearinghouse are reviewed carefully for scientific accuracy, appropriateness of content, and readability. Publications produced by sources other than the clearinghouse also are reviewed for scientific accuracy and are used, along with clearinghouse publications, to answer requests.

# Chapter 45

# *Gallstones*

The gallbladder is a small pear-shaped organ located beneath the liver on the right side of the abdomen. The gallbladder's primary functions are to store concentrate bile, and secrete bile into the small intestine at the proper time to help digest food.

The gallbladder is connected to the liver and the small intestine by a series of ducts or tube-shaped structures, that carry bile. Collectively, the gallbladder and these ducts are called the biliary system.

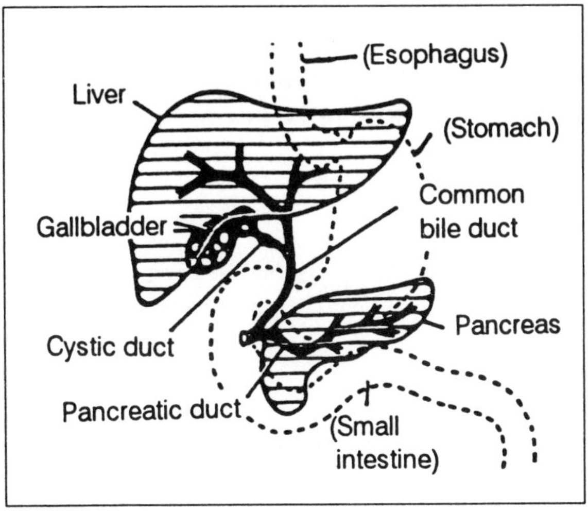


***Figure 45.1.***

---

NIH Pub. 93–2897.

Bile is a yellow-brown fluid produced by the liver. In addition to water, bile contains cholesterol, lipids (fats), bile salts (natural detergents that break up fat), and bilirubin (the bile pigment that gives bile and stools their color). The liver can produce as much as three cups of bile in one day, and at any one time, the gallbladder can store up to a cup of concentrated bile.

As food passes from the stomach into the small intestine, the gallbladder contracts and sends its stored bile into the small intestine through the common bile duct. Once in the small intestine, bile helps digest fats in foods. Under normal circumstances, most bile is recirculated in the digestive tract by being absorbed in the intestine and returning to the liver in the bloodstream.

## What Are Gallstones?

Gallstones are pieces of solid material that form in the gallbladder. Gallstones form when substances in the bile, primarily cholesterol and bile pigments, form hard, crystal-like particles. Cholesterol stones are usually white or yellow in color and account for 80 percent of gallstones. They are primarily made of cholesterol.

Pigment stones are small, dark stones made of bilirubin and calcium salts that are found in bile. They account for the other 20 percent of gallstones. Risk factors for pigment stones include cirrhosis, biliary tract infections, and hereditary blood cell disorders, such as sickle cell anemia.

Gallstones vary in size and may be as small as a grain of sand or as large as a golf ball. The gallbladder may develop a single, often large, stone or many smaller ones, even several thousand.

## What Causes Gallstones?

Progress has been made in understanding the process of gallstone formation. Researchers believe that gallstones may be caused by a combination of factors, including inherited body chemistry, body weight, gallbladder motility (movement), an perhaps diet.

Cholesterol gallstones develop when bile contains too much cholesterol and not enough bile salts. Besides a high concentration of cholesterol, two factors seem to be important in causing gallstones. The first is how often and how well the gallbladder contracts; incomplete and infrequent emptying of the gallbladder may cause the bile to become over concentrated and contribute to gallstone formation.

The second factor is the presence of proteins in the liver and bile that either promote or inhibit cholesterol crystallization into gallstones.

Other factors also seem to play a role in causing gallstones but how is not clear. Obesity has been shown to be a major risk factor for gallstones. A large clinical study showed that being even moderately overweight increases one's risk for developing gallstones. This is probably true because obesity tends to cause excess cholesterol in bile, low bile salts, and decreased gallbladder emptying. Very low calorie, rapid weight-loss diets, and prolonged fasting seem to also cause gallstone formation.

In addition, increased levels of the hormone estrogen as a result of pregnancy, hormone therapy, or the use of birth control pills, may increase cholesterol levels in bile and also decrease gallbladder movement, resulting in gallstone formation.

No clear relationship has been proven between diet and gallstone formation. However, low-fiber, high-cholesterol diets, and diets high in starchy foods have been suggested and contributing to gallstone formation.

## Who Is at Risk for Gallstones?

This year, more than 1 million people in the United States will learn they have gallstones. They will join the estimated 20 million Americans—roughly 10 percent of the population—who already have gallstones.

Those who are most likely to develop gallstones:

- Women between 20 and 60 years of age. They are twice as likely to develop gallstones than men.

- Men and women over the age of 60.

- Pregnant women or women who have used birth control pills or estrogen replacement therapy.

- Native Americans. They have the highest prevalence of gallstones in the United States. A majority of Native American men have gallstones by 60. Among the Pima Indians of Arizona, 70 percent of women have gallstones by age 30.

- Mexican-American men and women of all ages.

- Men and women who are overweight.
- People who go on "crash" diets or who lose a lot of weight quickly.

## What Are the Symptoms of Gallstones?

Most people with gallstones do not have symptoms. They have what are called silent stones. Studies show that most people with silent stones remain symptom free for years and require no treatment. Silent stones usually are detected during a routine medical checkup or examination for another illness.

## What Problems Can Occur?

A gallstone attack is usually marked by a steady, severe pain in the upper abdomen. Attacks may last only 20 or 30 minutes but more often they last for one to several hours. A gallstone attack may also cause pain in the back between the shoulder blades or in the right shoulder and may cause nausea and vomiting. Attacks may be separated by weeks, months, or even years. Once a true attack occurs, subsequent attacks are much more likely.

Sometimes gallstones may make their way out of the gallbladder and into the cystic duct, the channel through which bile travels from the gallbladder to the small intestine. If stones become lodged in the cystic duct and block the flow of bile, they can cause cholecystitis, and inflammation of the gallbladder. Blockage of the cystic duct is a common complication caused by gallstones.

A less common but more serious problem occurs if the gallstones become lodged in the bile ducts between the liver and the intestine. This condition can block bile flow from the gallbladder and liver, causing pain and jaundice. Gallstones may also interfere with the flow of digestive fluids secreted from the pancreas in to the small intestine, leading to pancreatitis, an inflammation of the pancreas.

Prolonged blockage of any of these ducts can cause severe damage to the gallbladder, liver, or pancreas, which can be fatal. Warning signs include fever, jaundice, and persistent pain.

## How Are Gallstones Diagnosed?

Many times gallstones are detected during an abdominal x-ray, computerized axial tomography (CT) scan, or abdominal ultrasound that has been taken for an unrelated problem or complaint.

When actually looking for gallstones, the most common diagnostic tool is ultrasound. An ultrasound examination, also known as ultrasonography, uses sound waves. Pulses of sound waves are sent into the abdomen to create an image of the gallbladder. If stones are present, the sound waves will bounce off the stones, revealing their location.

Ultrasound has several advantages. It is a noninvasive technique, which means nothing is injected into or penetrates the body. Ultrasound is painless, has no known side effects, and does not involve radiation.

## How Are Gallstones Treated?

### *Surgical Treatment*

Despite the development of nonsurgical techniques, gallbladder surgery, or cholecystectomy, is the most common method for treating gallstones. Each year, more than 500,000 Americans have gallbladder surgery. Surgery options include the standard procedure, called open cholecystectomy, and a less invasive procedure, called laparoscopic cholecystectomy.

The standard cholecystectomy is a major abdominal surgery in which the surgeon removes the gallbladder through a 5- to 8-inch incision. Patients may remain in the hospital about a week and may require several additional weeks to recover at home.

Laparoscopic cholecystectomy is an new alternative procedure for gallbladder removal. Some 15,000 surgeons have received training in the technique since its introduction in the United States in 1988. Currently about 80 percent of cholecystectomies are performed using laparoscopes.

Laparoscopic cholecystectomy requires several small incisions in the abdomen to allow the insertion of surgical instruments and a small video camera. The camera sends a magnified image from inside the body to a video monitor, giving the surgeon a close-up view of the organs and tissues. The surgeon watches the monitor and performs the operation by manipulating the surgical instruments through separate small incisions. The gallbladder is identified and carefully separated from the liver and other structures. Finally the cystic duct is cut and the gallbladder removed through one of the small incisions. This type of surgery requires meticulous surgical skill.

Laparoscopic cholecystectomy does not require the abdominal muscles to be cut, resulting in less pain, quicker healing, improved cosmetic results, and fewer complications such as infection. Recovery is usually only a night in the hospital and several days recuperation at home.

The most common complication with the new procedure is injury to the common bile duct, which connects the gallbladder and the liver. An injured bile duct can leak bile and cause a painful and potentially dangerous infection. Many cases of minor injury to the common bile duct can be managed nonsurgically. Major injury to the bile duct, however, is a very serious problem and may require corrective surgery. At this time it is unclear whether these complications are more common following laparoscopic cholecystectomy than following standard cholecystectomy.

Complications such as abdominal adhesions and other problems that obscure [the surgeon's view of the gallbladder] are discovered during about 5 percent of laparoscopic surgeries, forcing surgeon to switch the standard cholecystectomy for safe removal of the gallbladder.

Many surgeons believe that laparoscopic cholecystectomy soon will totally replace open cholecystectomy for routine gallbladder removals. Open cholecystectomy will probably remain the recommended approach for complicated cases.

A Consensus Development Conference panel, convened by the National Institutes of Health in September 1992, endorsed laparoscopic cholecystectomy as a safe and effective surgical treatment for gallbladder removal, equal in efficacy to the traditional open surgery. The panel noted, however, that laparoscopic cholecystectomy should only e performed by experienced surgeons and only on patients who have symptoms of gallstones.

In addition, the panel noted that the outcome of laparoscopic cholecystectomy is greatly influenced by the training, experience, skill, and judgment of the surgeon performing the procedure. Therefore, the panel recommended that strict guidelines be developed for training and granting credentials in laparoscopic surgery, determining competence, and monitoring quality. According to the panel, efforts should

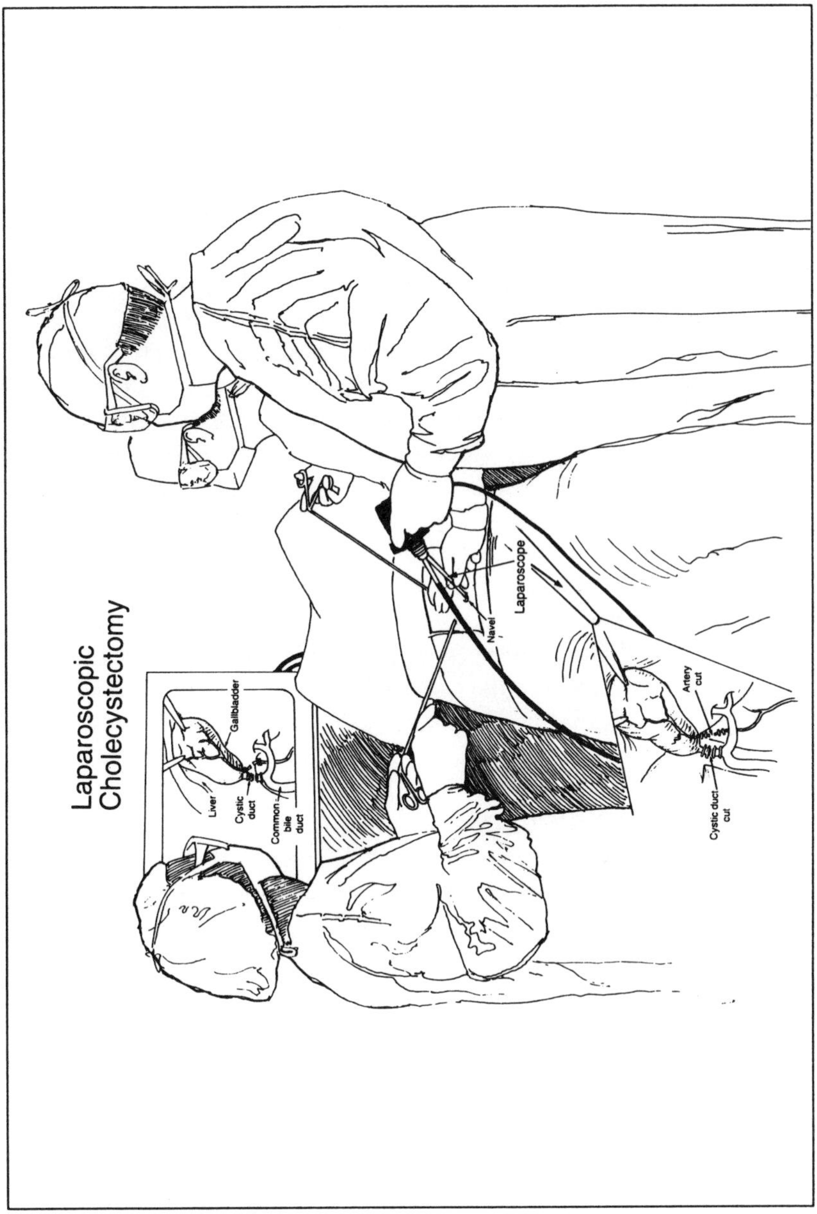
Laparoscopic
Cholecystectomy
Gallbladder
Liver
Cystic
duct
Common
bile
duct
Navel
Laparoscope
Artery
cut
Cystic duct
cut

*Figure 45.2.*

continue toward developing a noninvasive approach to gallstone treatment that will not only eliminate existing stones, but also prevent their formation or recurrence.

### *Non-Surgical Treatment*

In addition to surgery, nonsurgical approaches have been pursued but are only used in special situations and only for gallstones that are predominantly cholesterol.

Oral dissolution therapy with ursodiol (Actigall®) and chenodiol (Chenix®) works best for small, cholesterol gallstones. These medicines are made from the acid naturally found in bile. They most often are used in individuals who cannot tolerate surgery. Treatment may be required for months to years before gallstones are dissolved.

Mild diarrhea is a side effect of both drugs; chenodiol may also temporarily elevate the liver enzyme transaminase and mildly elevate blood cholesterol levels.

Two therapies, contact dissolution with methyl-tert butyl ether instillation through a catheter placed into the gallbladder and extracorporeal shock-wave lithotripsy (ESWL), are still experimental.

Each of these alternatives to gallbladder surgery leaves the gallbladder intact; so stone recurrence, which happens in about one-half the cases, is a major drawback.

## Additional Readings

Gupta, KL. Cholelithiasis: New Options for Diagnosis and Treatment of Its Complications. *Senior Patient* 1991; 3(1): 42, 44–46. Article for health professional explores new options for diagnosis of gallstones and treatment of complications.

Lewis, R. Gallbladder: An Organ You Can Live Without. *FDA Consumer* 1991; 25(4): 13–15. Article for a lay audience reviews current information about gallbladder function and disease.

Traverso, LW. Laparoscopic Cholecystectomy. *Practical Gastroenterology* 1991; 15(4): 15, 21, 25–27. Article for health professionals discusses surgical technique of laparoscopic cholecystectomy.

*Your Gallstones: Diagnosis and Treatment.* 1991. Digestive Disease National Coalition, 711 Second Street, NE, Suite 2, Washington, DC 20002; (202) 544-7497. Brochure outlines causes, diagnosis, and treatments of gallstones.

**National Digestive Diseases Information Clearinghouse**
Box NDDIC
9000 Rockville Pike
Bethesda, MD 20892
(301) 468-6344

The National Digestive Diseases Information Clearinghouse is a service of the National Institute of Diabetes and Digestive and Kidney Diseases, part of the National Institutes of Health, under the U.S. Public Health Service. The clearinghouse was authorized by Congress to focus a national effort on providing information to the public, patients and their families, and doctors and other health care professionals. The clearinghouse works to educate people about digestive health and disease. The clearinghouse answers inquiries; develops, reviews, and distributes publications; and coordinates informational resources about digestive diseases.

Publications produced by the clearinghouse are reviewed carefully for scientific accuracy, appropriateness of content, and readability. Publications produced by sources other than the clearinghouse are also reviewed for scientific accuracy and are used, along with clearinghouse publications, to answer requests.

# Chapter 46

# *Gallstones and Dieting*

## *What Are Gallstones?*

Gallstones are clumps of solid material that form the gallbladder. They may occur as a single, large stone or many small. Gallstones are a mixture of compounds, but typically they are mostly cholesterol.

One in ten Americans has gallstones. However, most people with gallstones don't know they have them and experience no symptoms. Painless gallstones are called *silent gallstones*. For an unfortunate minority, however, gallstones can produce can cause painful attacks. Painful gallstones are called *symptomatic gallstones*, because they cause symptoms. In rare cases gallstones can cause life-threatening complications. Symptomatic gallstones result in 600,000 hospitalizations and more than 500,000 operations each year in the United States.

## *What Causes Gallstones?*

Gallstones develop in the *gallbladder*, a pear-shaped organ beneath the liver on the right side of the abdomen. It's about 3 inches long and an inch wide at its thickest part. The gallbladder stores and releases *bile* into the intestine to aid digestion.

Bile is a fluid make by the liver that helps in digestion. Bile contains substances called *bile salts* that act like natural detergents to

---

NIH Pub. 94–3677. Originally published as *Dieting and Gallstones.*

break down fats in the food we eat. As food passes from the stomach into the small intestine, the gall bladder releases bile into the *bile ducts.* These ducts, or tubes, run from the liver to the intestine. Bile also helps eliminate excess cholesterol from the body. The liver secretes cholesterol into the bile, which is then eliminated from the body via the digestive system.

Most researchers believe three conditions are necessary to form gallstones. First, the bile becomes supersaturated with cholesterol, which means the bile contains more cholesterol than the bile salts can dissolve. Second, an imbalance of proteins or other substances in the bile causes the cholesterol to start crystallizing. Third, the gallbladder does not contract enough to empty its bile regularly.

## Are Obese People More Likely to Develop Gallstones?

Yes. Obesity is a strong risk factor for gallstones.

Scientists often use a mathematical formula called *body mass index (BMI)* to define obesity. (BMI=weight in kilograms divided by height in meters squared. The accompanying table shows BMI in pounds and inches.) For example, an obese woman who is 5 ft. 4 in. tall (64 in.) and weighs 174 pounds has a BMI of 30. The more obese a person is, the greater his or her risk of developing gallstones. Several studies have shown that women with a BMI of 30 or higher have at least double the risk of developing gallstones than women with a BMI of less than 25.

Why obesity is a risk factor for gallstones is unclear. But researchers believe that in obese people, the liver produces too much cholesterol. The excess cholesterol leads to supersaturation in the gallbladder.

## Are People on a Diet to Lose Weight More at Risk for Developing Gallstones?

Yes. People who lose a lot of weight rapidly are at greater risk for developing gallstones. *Gallstones are one of the most medically important complications of voluntary weight loss.* The relationship of dieting to gallstones has only recently received attention.

One major study found that women who lost 9 to 22 pounds (over a 2-year period) were 44 percent more likely to develop gallstones than women who did not lose weight. Women who lost more than 22 pounds were almost twice as likely to develop gallstones.

*Figure 46.1.*

**BODY WEIGHTS IN POUNDS ACCORDING TO HEIGHT AND BODY MASS INDEX***

| | Body Mass Index (kg/m²) | | | | | | | | | | | | | |
|---|---|---|---|---|---|---|---|---|---|---|---|---|---|---|
| | 19 | 20 | 21 | 22 | 23 | 24 | 25 | 26 | 27 | 28 | 29 | 30 | 35 | 40 |
| **Height (in.)** | **Body Weight (lb.)** | | | | | | | | | | | | | |
| 58 | 91 | 96 | 100 | 105 | 110 | 115 | 119 | 124 | 129 | 134 | 138 | 143 | 167 | 191 |
| 59 | 94 | 99 | 104 | 109 | 114 | 119 | 124 | 128 | 133 | 138 | 143 | 148 | 173 | 198 |
| 60 | 97 | 102 | 107 | 112 | 118 | 123 | 128 | 133 | 138 | 143 | 148 | 153 | 179 | 204 |
| 61 | 100 | 106 | 111 | 116 | 122 | 127 | 132 | 137 | 143 | 148 | 153 | 158 | 185 | 211 |
| 62 | 104 | 109 | 115 | 120 | 126 | 131 | 136 | 142 | 147 | 153 | 158 | 164 | 191 | 218 |
| 63 | 107 | 113 | 118 | 124 | 130 | 135 | 141 | 146 | 152 | 158 | 163 | 169 | 197 | 225 |
| 64 | 110 | 116 | 122 | 128 | 134 | 140 | 145 | 151 | 157 | 163 | 169 | 174 | 204 | 232 |
| 65 | 114 | 120 | 126 | 132 | 138 | 144 | 150 | 156 | 162 | 168 | 174 | 180 | 210 | 240 |
| 66 | 118 | 124 | 130 | 136 | 142 | 148 | 155 | 161 | 167 | 173 | 179 | 186 | 216 | 247 |
| 67 | 121 | 127 | 134 | 140 | 146 | 153 | 159 | 166 | 172 | 178 | 185 | 191 | 223 | 255 |
| 68 | 125 | 131 | 138 | 144 | 151 | 158 | 164 | 171 | 177 | 184 | 190 | 197 | 230 | 262 |
| 69 | 128 | 135 | 142 | 149 | 155 | 162 | 169 | 176 | 182 | 189 | 196 | 203 | 236 | 270 |
| 70 | 132 | 139 | 146 | 153 | 160 | 167 | 174 | 181 | 188 | 195 | 202 | 207 | 243 | 278 |
| 71 | 136 | 143 | 150 | 157 | 165 | 172 | 179 | 186 | 193 | 200 | 208 | 215 | 250 | 286 |
| 72 | 140 | 147 | 154 | 162 | 169 | 177 | 184 | 191 | 199 | 206 | 213 | 221 | 258 | 294 |
| 73 | 144 | 151 | 159 | 166 | 174 | 182 | 189 | 197 | 204 | 212 | 219 | 227 | 265 | 302 |
| 74 | 148 | 155 | 163 | 171 | 179 | 186 | 194 | 202 | 210 | 218 | 225 | 233 | 272 | 311 |
| 75 | 152 | 160 | 168 | 176 | 184 | 192 | 200 | 208 | 216 | 224 | 232 | 240 | 279 | 319 |
| 76 | 156 | 164 | 172 | 180 | 189 | 197 | 205 | 213 | 221 | 230 | 238 | 246 | 287 | 328 |

**Each entry gives the body weight in pounds (lb.) for a person of a given height and body mass index. Pounds have been rounded off. To use the table, find the appropriate height in the left-hand column. Move across the row to a given weight. The number at the top of the column is the body mass index for the height and weight.*

*Adapted with permission from Bray, G.A., Gray, D.S. Obesity. Part I. Pathogenesis. West J. Med. 1988; 149: 429-41.*

Other studies have shown that 10 to 25 percent of obese people develop gallstones while on a *very-low-calorie diet*. (Very-low-calorie diets are usually defined as diets containing 800 calories a day or less. The food is often in liquid form and taken for prolonged periods, typically 12 to 16 weeks.) The gallstones that developed in people on very-low-calorie diets were usually silent and did not produce symptoms. However, about a third of the dieters who developed gallstones did have symptoms, and a proportion of these required surgery.

*In short, the likelihood of a person developing symptomatic gallstones during or shortly after rapid weight loss is about four to six percent.* This estimate is based on reviewing just a few clinical studies, however and is not conclusive.

## Why Does Weight Loss Cause Gallstones?

Researchers believe dieting may cause a shift in the balance of bile salts and cholesterol in the gallbladder. The cholesterol level is increased and the amount of bile salts is decreased. Going for long periods without eating (skipping breakfast, for example), a common practice among dieters, also may decrease gallbladder contractions. If the gallbladder does not contract often enough to empty the bile, gallstones may form.

## Are Some Weight Loss Methods Better Than Others in Preventing Gallstones?

Possibly. If substantial or rapid weight loss increases the risk of developing gallstones, more gradual weight loss would seem to lessen the risk of getting gallstones. However, studies are needed to test this theory.

Some very-low-calorie diets may not contain enough fat to cause the gallbladder to contract enough to empty its bile. A meal or snack containing approximately 10 grams (one-third of an ounce) of fat is necessary for the gallbladder to contract normally. But again, no studies have directly linked a diet's nutrient composition to the risk of gallstones.

Also, no studies have been conducted on the effects of repeated dieting on gallstone formation.

## Are People Who Have Surgery to Lose Weight Also at Risk for Gallstones?

You bet. Gallstones are common among obese patients who loose weight rapidly after gastric bypass surgery. (In gastric bypass surgery, the size of the stomach is reduced, preventing the person from over-eating.)

One study found that more than a third (38 percent) of patients who had gastric bypass surgery developed gallstones afterward. Gallstones are most likely to occur within the first few months after surgery.

## Should People Who Already Have Gallstones Try to Lose Weight?

Scientists know that weight loss increases the risk of gallstone formation. However, they don't know whether weight loss increases the risk of *silent* gallstones becoming *symptomatic* gallstones or of other complications developing. In addition to painful gallstone attacks, complications include inflammation of the gallbladder, liver, or pancreas. These are usually caused by a gallstone getting lodged in a bile duct.

Although excluding people with pre-existing gallstones from a weight-loss program seems prudent, there is no evidence to support this action. If people have had their gallbladders removed, there is little risk of them having gallstones or bile problems while participating in a weight-loss program.

## What Is the Treatment for Gallstones?

Silent gallstones are usually left alone and occasionally disappear on their own. Usually only patients with symptomatic gallstones are treated.

The most common treatment for gallstones is surgery to remove the gallbladder. This operation is called a *cholecystectomy.* In rare cases, drugs are used to dissolve the gallstones. Other nonsurgical methods are still considered experimental.

The drug *ursodeoxycholic acid* prevented gallstones from forming in one clinical trial of patients on very-low-calorie diets. However, the drug is costly. Given the small proportion of patients who develop symptomatic gallstones on very-low-calorie diets, it is not known if ursodeoxycholic acid would be a cost-effective drug to recommend for all patients undergoing such diets, though people with pre-existing gallstones may benefit from this drug.

## Are the Benefits of Weight Loss Greater Than the Risk of Getting Gallstones?

There is no questions that obesity causes serious health risks. Obesity had been linked to heart disease, stroke, high blood pressure, high cholesterol levels, and diabetes. Obesity has also been associated with higher rates of certain types of cancer, such as gallbladder, colon, prostate, breast, cervical, and ovarian cancers.

Weight loss also reduces the risk of heart disease by lowering cholesterol levels. Even a modest weight loss of 10 to 20 pounds can bring positive changes. And the psychological boost from losing weight, such as improved self-image and greater social interaction, should not be ignored.

Patients who are thinking about beginning a commercial diet program to lose a significant amount of weight should talk with their doctors. A physician can evaluate a patient's medical history, individual circumstances, and the proposed weight-loss program. Doctor and patient can then discuss the potential benefits and risks of dieting, including the risks of developing gallstones.

## Additional Reading

Claymen CB, ed. *The American Medical Association Encyclopedia of Medicine.* New York: Random House. 1989. This authoritative reference guide for patients has entries on the gallbladder, gallstones, and the biliary system. It is widely available in libraries and bookstores.

Everhart, J.E. "Contributions of Obesity and Weight Loss to Gallstone Disease" *Annals of Internal Medicine.* 1993, Vol. 119, pp. 1029–35. This article, written for physicians, shows how obesity as well as weight loss and low calorie diets increase the risk of gallstones.

*Gallstones*. NIH Publication. No. 93–2897. This fact sheet provides basic information about gallstones and treatment options. It is published by the National Institute of Diabetes and Digestive and Kidney Diseases and is available through the National Digestive Diseases Information Clearinghouse, Box NDDIC, 9000 Rockville Pike, Bethesda, MD 20892, Tel: 301-654-3810.

Weinsier RL, et. al. "Gallstone Formation and Weight Loss." *Obesity Research.* 1993, Vol. 1, No. 1: pp. 51–56. This review article, written for physicians, examines gallstone formation rates in patients on very-low-calorie diets, including the role that fasting and diet composition may play.

Yang H., et. al. "Risk Factors for Gallstone Formation during Rapid Loss of Weight." *Digestive Diseases and Sciences,* Vol. 37, No. 6 (June 1992), pp. 912–18. This article, written for physicians, discusses gallstone formation in patients on very-low-calorie diets.

## Rapid Weight Loss and Gallstones

As most people know, there are significant health benefits to be gained from losing excess pounds. For example, many people can reduce high blood pressure and cholesterol levels through weight loss. Overweight people are at greater risk of developing gallstones than people of average weight. However, people who are considering a diet program requiring very low intake of calories each day should be aware that during rapid or substantial weight loss, a person's risk of developing gallstones is increased.

# Index

# Index

Note: Page numbers in *italics* refer to illustrations; page numbers followed by t indicate tables.

## B

## C

## D

## F

## G

## J



## K

## M

## O

## P

## T

## V



## W

## X



## Y



## Z